ARTHRITIS AT *YOUR* AGE?

Late teens to early 50s: a friendly handbook

for young and youngish adults with a rheumatic disorder

Jill Holroyd

Donations will be made to appropriate charities from any profits
made from the sale of this book.

GRINDLE PRESS

For the special people who have enriched my
life: the most special, of course,
being my family, and Andrew

Published by the GRINDLE PRESS,
P O Box 222, Ipswich, Suffolk, IP9 1HE

First published 1992
© Jill Holroyd 1992

ISBN 0 9518816 0 4

British Library Cataloguing-in-Publication Data.
A catalogue record is available from the British Library.

Cover photography by Glyn Barney
Cover design by Paul Chambers

Camera-ready copy by Daisywheel, 98 Bell Road, Wallasey, Merseyside, L44 8DP
Printed by C H Healey, 49—55 Fore Street, Ipswich, Suffolk IP4 1JL

CONTENTS
This is a book for dipping into
Mix and match to suit your interests

IMPORTANT NOTES

NOTHING IN THIS BOOK IS INTENDED AS A SUBSTITUTE FOR YOUR MOST IMPORTANT SOURCE OF MEDICAL INFORMATION, WHICH SHOULD *ALWAYS* BE YOUR DOCTOR.

Disclaimer

Some common abbreviations

ARC	Arthritis and Rheumatism Council	JCA	Juvenile chronic arthritis
AS	Ankylosing spondylitis	OT	Occupational Therapist
CAB	Citizens' Advice Bureau	RA	Rheumatoid arthritis
DLF	Disabled Living Foundation	SAE	Stamped addressed envelope
DRO	Disablement Resettlement Officer	SLE	Systemic lupus erythematosus/lupus
DSS	Department of Social Security	YPA	Younger person with arthritis

Some people whose comments are quoted have asked to remain anonymous. Pseudonyms are indicated by an asterisk *.

About the author

Jill Holroyd has had a fair (or unfair?!) quota of direct experience of rheumatic disorders herself, starting with juvenile chronic arthritis at the age of 10, followed by the later appearance in her mid-30s of systemic sclerosis, Raynaud's phenomenon and Sjøgren's syndrome, plus, along the way, four (sic) total hip replacements and an ankle arthrodesis.

She also has an honours degree in modern languages, works full-time for the British Council, and was at one time editor and chairperson of Young Arthritis Care's predecessor '130 Group', of people under 45 with arthritis.

ACKNOWLEDGEMENTS

I owe so much to so very many people who've helped with information and advice, and encouragement along the way. I can name only a few here, but thank you all, named or unnamed.

Thank you especially to Dr Frank Dudley Hart, for giving so generously of his time and invaluable wisdom in looking at the manuscript, and for his encouragement with the project.

Special thanks too to all the 'YPAs' (younger people with arthritis) who've shared with me their thoughts and advice and joys and tears, and allowed me to use these in the book: other people in turn will benefit from their generosity. Thank you to Pamela, Patsy, Peter, Jacqueline, Marilyn, Janet and Janet, Carol and Carol, Gail, Robin, Frances, Sue, Anne, Ken, Polly, Ron, and to very many others, named and unnamed in the text. Thank you to Babette for all your comments and encouragement, and thank you to Laura and Laura's mum. Thank you to Gwen, for your special inspiration, and to Phil Smith, to whom we YPAs owe so much for your years of inspired and dedicated work as Chairman of what was then called the '35 Group' for YPAs, now 'Young Arthritis Care'.

Thank you to the gallant YPAs on the cover: Barry Hayward, Mandy King, Jan Flower, Bernadette Sparks, and Glyn Barney, who also took the photos. Thank you to Darran and Becky Sparks, for appearing too. And thank you to Paul Chambers, for designing the cover.

For valued comments and for copyright permission, thank you to Kate Nash, Director of Young Arthritis Care; James Pollard, present Editor of *Arthritis News*; Lady Carol Holland, former Editor of *Arthritis News*; Cheryl Marcus, Founder, Editor and Trustee of the Lupus UK Group; Fergus J R S Rogers, Director, NASS (National Ankylosing Spondylitis Society); Dr L Gail Darlington MD FRCP, Consultant Physician; Dr George Lewith MA MRCP MRCGP, Co-Director of the Centre for the Study of Complementary Medicine, Southampton; and Marie Joseph.

Special thanks to my wonderful healthcare team at the Middlesex Hospital, and to my wonderful GP. Also to my family and to Andrew, for their understanding, encouragement and practical support while the book has slowly taken shape.

I would like to thank the following for permission to reproduce copyright material from the publications named:

Arthritis Care: *Arthritis News, Young Arthritis News, In Contact* and other publications. The Arthritis & Rheumatism Council for extracts from *ARC Magazine* and from other publications acknowledged in the text. Lupus UK Group: Dr G R V Hughes' *Lupus, a Guide for Patients*. NASS (National Ankylosing Spondylitis Society): *The NASS Guidebook for Patients*.

South Bank Publishing: *Practical Health* magazine 1987. Macdonald & Co (Publishers) Ltd: Dr F Dudley Hart's *Overcoming Arthritis*, Dr S Lipton's *Conquering Pain*, J Madders' *Stress and Relaxation*, L Hodgkinson's *Smile Therapy*, and *The Food Intolerance Diet Book* by E Workman, Dr V Alun Jones and Dr J Hunter.

Churchill Livingstone (Longman Group UK Ltd): Professor J M H Moll's *Manual of Rheumatology* and *Arthritis and Rheumatism*. Marie Joseph and Arrow Books (Random Century Group Ltd): Marie Joseph's *One Step at a Time. Living with Arthritis*. Tavistock Publications Ltd (Routledge): Professor D Locker's *Disability and Disadvantage*.

Peters Fraser & Dunlop Group Ltd: Professor P Parish's *Medicines: A Guide for Everybody*. Blackwell Scientific Publications Ltd: *Lecture Notes on Rheumatology* by Dr J Edmonds and Dr G Hughes. Sheldon Press: C Haddon's *Women and Tranquillisers* and Dr P M Shaw's *Meeting People is Fun*.

W & R Chambers Ltd: H Unsworth's *Coping with Rheumatoid Arthritis*. Elliot Right

Way Books: Mr D Wainwright's *Arthritis and Rheumatism*. Oxford University Press: Professor K Hardinge's *Hip Replacement: The Facts*, and Dr J T Scott's *Arthritis and Rheumatism: the Facts*.

Dr V Coleman for permission to quote from his *Natural Pain Control* (Century Arrow). HarperCollins Publishers Ltd: C Peck's *Controlling Chronic Pain* and G Stuart's *Private World of Pain* (George Allen & Unwin, now Unwin Hyman of HarperCollins). Methuen London: *Families and How to Survive Them* by J Cleese and R Skynner.

Pergamon Press plc: C L Wiener's article *The Burden of Rheumatoid Arthritis: Tolerating the Uncertainty*, published in Vol 9 of *Social Science and Medicine*, 1975. Souvenir (Educational & Academic Ltd) Press Ltd: Dr A Burnfield's *Multiple Sclerosis* and B Zilbergeld's *Men and Sex*. John Murray (Publishers) Ltd: L Mitchell's *Simple Relaxation*.

Methuen & Co: H Edwards' *Psychological Problems. Who Can Help?* and D Thomas' *The Experience of Handicap*. The Disability Alliance Educational & Research Association: *Disability Rights Handbook*. Martin Secker & Warburg Ltd: C Ward's *How to Complain*. The Disabled Living Foundation: P Jay's *Coping with Disability*. Dr Tony Smith and Consumers' Association Ltd: article by Dr Tony Smith in *Self Health* no 11, June 1986. Dr G Lewith for permission to quote from his *Alternative Therapies* (Heinemann).

Exley Publications Ltd: D Aslett's *Who Says It's a Woman's Job to Clean?* Skill (National Bureau for Students with Disabilities) for permission to quote from their 1986/87 Annual Report. The Open University: *005 — Occupational Information — A Supplement for Students with Disabilities*. Avery Publishing Group Inc, Garden City Park, New York, USA: Robert H Phillips' *Coping with Lupus*.

RADAR (Royal Association for Disability and Rehabilitation): *Employers' Guide to Disabilities* by M Kettle and B Massie (Woodhead-Faulkner in association with RADAR). HMSO: *Code of Good Practice on Employment of Disabled People*. Dial UK (National Association of Disablement Information and Advice Lines): *Dialogue* 1987.

J M Dent (Publishers): Dr W Greengross's *Entitled to Love*. Andre Deutsch Ltd: Ogden Nash's 'A Word to Husbands' from *I Wouldn't Have Missed It*. The Eurospan Group: *Towards Intimacy* by the Task Force on Concerns of Physically Disabled Women. SPOD (Association to Aid the Sexual and Personal Relationships of People with a Disability): extract on page 224.

The Volunteer Centre UK: P Stubbings' *New Resources for Old Tasks: Disabled People as Volunteers* (out of print). The Multiple Sclerosis Society of Great Britain and Northern Ireland: extract from *MS Bulletin*. J B Lippincott Company, Philadelphia, PA, USA: extract from 'Outcomes of Self-Help Education for Patients with Arthritis' by K Lorig and others, in *Arthritis and Rheumatism* vol 28, 1985.

William Heinemann Ltd: Corbet Woodall's *A Disjointed Life*. Lennard Associates: M Leitch's *Living with Arthritis*. Relate (National Marriage Guidance Council): S Litvinoff's *The RELATE Guide to Better Relationships*. The British Medical Association: extract from the *Annals of the Rheumatic Diseases* on page 294. Liz Gill and *The Times*: extract on page 223.

I have tried without success to trace the copyright holder of the extracts I quote from *Stigma — the Experience of Disability*, edited by P Hunt and published by Geoffrey Chapman, 1966. I am grateful for permission from Arthritis Care to quote from *In Contact*, from which the two poems on pages 194-195 are taken; I would also have liked to contact the unnamed authors, but have been unable to trace them.

Thank you to
Dr A J Burnfield for
permission to quote from
his *Multiple Sclerosis*
(Souvenir Press Ltd).

Chapter one

WHY THIS BOOK'S FOR YOU

Hello! We'd like you to know that you're not alone. There are quite a few of us out here, all with different tales to tell and ideas to share. Some of us are feeling pretty lousy at the moment; others feel surprisingly good. I'm sitting here with my ankle in plaster, after an operation which I hope will put paid to the pain in it. The rest of me feels fine (touch wood) so once the plaster's off I'll get back to the office.

I'll share with you here some of my own and other people's experiences in dealing with arthritis. There *are* 'ups' as well as 'downs', and there's a lot you can do to encourage the 'ups'. It isn't always easy to cope, but it *is* possible.

You may be lucky and have such a mild form of arthritis that a small dose of drugs or other medical treatment (or maybe nothing) is all that's needed to keep you leading a normal life. Or maybe you're not so lucky, and find that drugs and medical treatment alone won't solve all your problems. You might find it's affecting you socially, financially and emotionally as well, bringing problems for which solutions have to be found, or ways of adjusting to those problems which can't be solved or changed. If so:

"you need to find a new lifestyle, which takes account of your difficulties and how to deal with them. It's a whole new way of thinking...You have to accentuate the positive and take control of your life. It's a mistake to grit your teeth and carry on through pain and damage. Equally, it's a mistake to give up. It's your body. It's your arthritis. You can use your mind to outwit it!" (Heather Unsworth, senior occupational therapist at Odstock Hospital, Wiltshire, in *Practical Health* magazine, Aug/Sept 1987)

You'll need help from other people of course, professionals and non-professionals. You and your doctor come first. Then people such as occupational therapists, social workers, and voluntary organisations, like 'Young Arthritis Care', run by and for younger people with arthritis. Above all, of course, worth their weight in gold if you have them, are an understanding partner, family, and understanding friends.

Please don't underestimate your own capacity to help yourself, too. It may mean a struggle, and take time. But *fight*. It's worth it, as we 'old-handers' and experts like rheumatologist Dr Frank Dudley Hart would agree, *"It is a disease that you must fight mentally as well as (with the brakes on) physically."* (In his book *Overcoming Arthritis*, Macdonald Optima).

I hope this book will help you put together your own personal DIY kit, your own personal plan of campaign to outwit the arthritis. It's a book for dipping into, as and when needed. You'll find different bits relevant at different times, depending on what the arthritis has cooked up for you and what's going on around you. We're all different. So too will be each 'Outwit Arthritis Kit' (OAK − 'great OAKs from little acorns grow...').

If the going's difficult, please don't despair. Sometimes the arthritis may make things particularly miserable for you. If so, don't blame yourself for 'not coping'. Just hang on in there until the arthritis is a bit quieter again. Please don't be put off by the seemingly amazing things some people have got up to, despite the arthritis, and don't think that everyone except you must be an uncomplaining ever-smiling saint who *always* copes magnificently. We've each had our share of getting downhearted, or feeling thoroughly depressed:

"I don't know about you, but I often feel, when reading of other young arthritics...that they are wonderfully brave, courageous people − not a bit like me, in fact. Am I, I

wonder, the only arthritic in the world who, far from shouldering my burden lightly, occasionally, when the pain is bad, takes it out on the kids, and has been known to argue with the Almighty as to where exactly I fit into this divine plan of His? We all get discouraged from time to time. Personally I find it reassuring and encouraging to learn of others who have experienced such setbacks and overcome them." (Mary*, when 30, married, with RA and two young sons.)

On page 82, you'll find two more excerpts from Mary's diary which you might like to read. One written when she was feeling very low; the other when she was feeling totally different, bubbly and happy. Hard to believe they're both by the same person, but they are. Look too at the comments she made fourteen years later, on page 76.

What's special about this book ?

- *It's for and about a different age group* Most publications about arthritis concentrate on the *over* 60s. But nearly a million younger people have arthritis too, or what doctors prefer to call 'rheumatic disorders'. That million includes over 15,000 children. Older people with arthritis certainly have their problems. How I wish they didn't, but we younger people have many different, as well as similar, problems, and this book's 'younger' approach will, I hope, be helpful. (The Lady Hoare Trust and Joseph Rowntree Foundation Family Fund specialise in providing support and information to youngsters under 16, so I'm not including information specific to that age group.)

- *It focuses on the 'younger' types of arthritis* Most older people with 'arthritis' have the form called osteoarthritis, and in most (not all) it's limited to one, or only a few joints. In our age group, however, the chances are you've been diagnosed as having a form of chronic inflammatory arthritis, such as rheumatoid arthritis (RA), or anky-losing spondylitis (AS), or lupus (SLE) or perhaps, if the arthritis started before you were 16, juvenile chronic arthritis (JCA, often called Still's disease). In its possible impact on body and on lifestyle, chronic inflammatory arthritis can be very different from osteoarthritis. Much of what follows is about RA and other types of chronic inflammatory arthritis like JCA or AS, but some of the general non-medical points may be helpful even if your particular disorder is one of the many other 200 or so 'rheumatic disorders'.

- *A friendly book* I hope you'll find this a *friendlier* handbook than the usual helpful but often impersonal patient handbooks around. I know it's not always easy to get to meet people in the same boat. Yet meeting and sharing tips and friendly advice can be so helpful. That's why I've included lots of quotations from other people like you, who have direct experience of 'living with arthritis'.

- *Non-medical aspects* Though we may not feel 'disabled', and modern medicine can lessen the damage the arthritis can cause, there may still be physical, psychological, financial, and social difficulties: problems with jobs, personal relationships, marriage, children, leisure activities, over and above already well-documented practical problems of mobility, personal care, household adaptations, etc, as well as, of course, the physical illness itself. Your main source of medical advice and information should, of course, *always* be your doctor. This book concentrates mainly on the non-medical aspects of 'living with arthritis'.

- *A different sort of disability* Lots of useful information can be found in 'publications for disabled people'. But many of us, younger people with arthritis (YPAs for short), don't readily see ourselves as 'disabled'. We don't readily identify with publications that concentrate on people with severe and very visible disabilities often very different from our own. Sometimes the arthritis is visible; sometimes not. Some of us know only too well the problems that can, surprisingly, come from an *in*visible illness. If you're not in a wheelchair people may not believe you're ill or disabled, especially if you're young and *look* healthy.

● *What to call us?* I'll mainly use the term 'younger person with arthritis' (YPA for short). Not perfect, but I hope you'll accept it. Sometimes I'll call us 'disabled people', though not 'the disabled' – a term which encourages other people to forget we're all individual people first and foremost, and all very different at that. There are other words we may use too, of course, especially when lightening the tone talking to other people, for instance 'the hopalong people' or 'young dodderers' or 'young hippies' (if we've had a hip replacement), or 'spondies' (if we have AS). A useful device for some people is to see and talk about the arthritis as an obnoxious character called Arthur Itis. Blaming this scheming, unpredictable intruder in our lives helps remind ourselves and other people that the arthritis is no fault of ours and that the way my or your body behaves is quite different from the way I or you *want* it to behave. Arthur Itis is the one to blame if we drop something on the floor or are too tired to go to the cinema, or whatever.

● *Some assumptions* Though some of us use wheelchairs from time to time, most of us aren't full-time wheelchair users. I'm writing this book with that assumption in mind, but I'm assuming too that you may nevertheless have problems getting around, so will include plenty of information to help you get things by post or phone. I hope that much will also be relevant if you *are* a full-time wheelchair user, but please bear in mind that you'll need to look elsewhere too for practical information specific to your needs.

Tips on using the book

It's a BOOK FOR DIPPING INTO, so don't feel you have to plough laboriously through it page by page! After you've read this chapter, go on to pick out what's of special interest to you. Here are some suggestions for a first sample dip:

● The phone numbers on page 112. Do you know about the Wyeth Helpline, for instance? You can phone free, any weekday afternoon, and speak to friendly, trained counsellors at Arthritis Care. They have rheumatic disorders, too, so understand problems.
● Infokit suggestions on pages 112 - 114. All sorts of free or cheap information you can send away for, all full of signposts to yet more helpful discoveries.
● Sanity-savers and gadgets galore. Send off for all the commercial suppliers' leaflets listed on page 144. You'll be amazed at what delights you'll find in their pages.
● Some thoughts on why arthritis can create misunderstandings between us and other people – chapter 25, page 190 onwards.
● Armchair shopping goodies on page 177, and hordes of hobby ideas – page 280 onwards...

The book concentrates on non-medical, rather than medical information, but gives you signposts to guide you in finding out more about aspects which interest you. Addresses are listed in Appendix 2. The fact that something's included in the book does *not* imply recommendation: you must use your own judgement, and seek advice where appropriate.

As we go along I'll mention lots of books and publications which you might find useful. I've tried to keep to low-priced paperbacks and other publications, easily obtainable by post. Remember too you can keep costs down by borrowing many of them from your local public library. Chapter 15, page 114, goes into more detail about buying and borrowing books, and includes a note about a firm which supplies masses of different paperbacks by post.

Last but not least...

This book's written not just to help *you*, but so that you can, I hope, help the rest of us out here. We all need to do what we can to change public attitudes, which at 'best' mean we encounter strange looks in the street or hurtful remarks about 'being lazy' or 'putting it on'. At worst though such attitudes and ignorance can actually stop us getting the right medical treatment. It's horrific to think that even nowadays a teenage girl with continuing joint pains could be brushed off by her GP saying she's just got 'cold in her joints' or 'growing pains' when in fact she's got RA.

Listen to the report *Arthritis in the Eighties* by the Arthritis and Rheumatism Council (ARC), which urged us to demand improvements in rheumatological services:

> *"a steep price is being paid by many thousands of uncomplaining sufferers, experiencing pain and discomfort and the hazard of becoming needlessly more deformed and disabled. [Inequity in provision] is compounded by...people's ignorance. There is evidence that, in contrast to many other fields of medical endeavour, people have unreasonably low expectations of services for relief of their rheumatic suffering. As a result they do not always demand help that could be rendered, which eases the pressure on decision makers...We hope the silent army of sufferers will now assimilate this lesson, and demand services of similar quality for themselves."*

The Royal College of Physicians Committee on Rheumatology commissioned a report (1988) on District Rheumatology Services throughout Britain. It recommended that there should be at least one full-time consultant rheumatologist, plus supporting staff, in every health district, one for every 150,000 people. The report pointed out that arthritis is the biggest single cause of physical disability, accounting for about a third of the total of physically disabled people. The proportion rises to almost one half of people over retirement age.

The report said that much of this disability could be prevented, or at least considerably reduced in severity. Opportunities are lost because the level of rheumatological knowledge on the part of GPs remains unsatisfactory, and this is made worse by insufficient rheumatologists – the ratio of rheumatologist to population is nearer to one for every 220,000 people rather than the recommended 150,000. In Yorkshire there's only one rheumatologist for every 360,000 people. In 1990 the *British Journal of Rheumatology* said that the situation had changed little since the 1988 report.

Let's educate people into taking arthritis/rheumatic disorders seriously. Rheumatic disorders aren't 'just a part of growing old'. Attitudes need changing and far more resources should be devoted to these medical conditions which can strike at any age, and which can, if untreated, cause considerable pain, misery and other problems. Much can already be done in the way of treatment – far more could and should be done.

Grant me the serenity to accept the things I cannot change,
The courage to change the things I can,
And the wisdom to know the difference.

Chapter two

RHEUMATIC DISORDERS:
What are they? What's the immune system?

"Oh yes, dear, you've got rheumatism, have you? Fancy, and at your age, too. Well, I know *all* about it. I get twinges meself", says one Older Dear, with 'odd twinges', to one Younger Dear who has RA and knows only too well that the two experiences are poles apart. Symptoms and treatment differ enormously.

The words 'arthritis' and 'rheumatism' are used very loosely. People tend to use 'arthritis' for any joint trouble, and 'rheumatism' for vague aches and pains and muscle twinges. Correctly used, 'arthritis' literally means 'inflammation of the joint' ('arthron' = joint, '-itis' = inflammation, as in 'tonsillitis' for instance). 'Rheumatism' is too vague a term to be used medically.

Medical experts prefer the general term 'rheumatic diseases', or 'rheumatic disorders'. They also talk about 'disorders of the musculo-skeletal system' or 'locomotor system' (the body's 'movement' system), though other body systems and organs can be involved in rheumatic disorders too. The general medical term actually covers some *200* very different conditions.

Some people experience a rheumatic disorder as just a slight, temporary nuisance. For others it may mean a lifetime of misery. For just a few, *very* few people, some rare types of rheumatic disorder and complications can even be fatal. For most of us YPAs, though, it means a sort of 'switchback' existence of ups and downs – sometimes black periods of utter misery but good and better times too. More detail in chapter 3 about some individual rheumatic disorders. For now, here's a brief summary of the main groups.

- The commonest rheumatic disorder is OA, *osteoarthritis* (more correctly called osteoarthrosis since inflammation doesn't necessarily occur). In Britain, it affects something like five million people, and on the whole doesn't start before the 50s.

- *Inflammatory arthritis* tends to start earlier, inflicting on a younger age group such nasties as rheumatoid arthritis (RA – about half a million people altogether), ankylosing spondylitis (AS – between 50,000 and 100,000), juvenile chronic arthritis (JCA – some 15,000), psoriatic arthritis, Reiter's syndrome, reactive arthritis (arthritis associated with an infection, eg German measles), gout. (There is an inflammatory condition confined to people aged over 50, polymyalgia rheumatica: although it causes pain and stiffness in the muscles around the shoulders and hips it doesn't appear to be an arthritis, but an inflammatory condition of arteries affecting the muscles.)

- *Many back disorders* are classified as rheumatic disorders, eg ankylosing spondylitis (AS). Others include lumbago, sciatica, displacement of the intervertebral disc (more usually, but inaccurately, called 'slipped disc').

- *Soft tissue rheumatic disorders* are common, affecting muscles, tendons, ligaments, etc. They're usually comparatively mild and temporary, and include bursitis, Housemaid's knee, tennis elbow, frozen shoulder, sports injuries to muscles and ligaments, Dupuytren's contracture in the hand (which former Prime Minister Margaret Thatcher had).

- *Connective tissue disorders* are a group of rather complicated disorders with ponderous names, including systemic lupus erythematosus (SLE or 'lupus' for short), systemic sclerosis (scleroderma), polymyositis and dermatomyositis, polyarteritis nodosa. They can affect different types of connective tissue throughout the body.

- *Other types of rheumatic disorder* include osteoporosis.

Rheumatic disorders account for 23% of all attendances in family doctor practices and 65 million working days being lost annually. That's even before you start thinking about their physical, social and emotional consequences (which this book will do).

Rheumatic disorders can affect anyone, at any age, even babies. Some are more common in men than women (eg AS, gout, Reiter's syndrome), or vice versa (eg RA, lupus).

"*Approximately five per cent of persons between the ages of 16 and 44 years have a rheumatic disorder, compared with 23 per cent for persons between 45 and 64, and 41 per cent of those aged 65 years and older.*" (ARC's *Arthritis and Rheumatism in the Eighties*, 1986)

Numerically speaking, most people with arthritis are over 50 and have osteoarthritis (OA). Books and information about arthritis usually concentrate on this age group. Older OA usually affects one, or just a few joints. *Not* a true picture for younger people with arthritis. So in this book, and when *I* use the term 'arthritis' loosely, I'm referring to the forms more common to our age group, like RA, AS, JCA, psoriatic arthritis.

Causes and cures

As there are so many different conditions classified as rheumatic disorders, there can be no one cause of or no one cure for 'arthritis', as such. The cause of rheumatic fever, which used to be one of the commonest serious diseases of childhood, *is* now known. Not so for disorders like RA and AS, yet, so for those there's no instant cure either, not yet, anyway. However there *is* plenty of research going on, and while we wait for a cure treatments are constantly improving. Chronic gout, for instance, is now fully controllable with a drug called allopurinol. (Look too at page 32, for more on the topic of no-cure-yet.)

Better understanding of our disorders means they can be better treated or 'managed'. Keep up-to-date with research by getting ARC's *Arthritis Today* magazine (page 113). It's thought that the cause or causes of something like RA, AS, lupus or Reiter's may be a particular 'jackpot' combination of factors. We may perhaps have a 'genetic predisposition' which alone does nothing unless and until it's combined with one or more 'trigger factors' – perhaps infection by a bacteria or virus (though the disorders themselves aren't infectious or contagious), perhaps something environmental, perhaps something hormonal. It's even possible the same condition may have different causes in different people.

Whatever the cause, in inflammatory arthritis the body develops an 'auto-immune' reaction, a sort of allergic reaction to bits of itself. Instead of your immune system defending your body against foreign invaders it mistakenly (and painfully) turns on itself. More about the immune system on page 14.

A short anatomy lesson
(Miss this out if you prefer!)

As rheumatic disorders are mainly disorders of the musculo-skeletal system, learning a little about the system's bits and pieces will help you understand not only what's gone wrong, but also why and how different treatments work. For instance:

- *why* you should rest an inflamed joint,
- *why* you should balance rest with exercise, 'prescribed', careful exercise that is, to

stop the muscles wasting leading to deformity and disability
- *why*, in AS, exercise is *the* most important treatment, to stop the particular bone development which can fuse together bones in the spine.
- *why* and how some drugs work – painkillers for instance, which damp down messages from a painful joint to the brain, or anti-inflammatories, which work to reduce pain-causing and damaging inflammation in a joint. And so on...

Any of the bones and joints of the musculo-skeletal system and/or the body tissues in and around them, like muscles, tendons, bursae, blood vessels, skin, can be affected. It just depends which particular disorder has chosen you as its victim.

But even then, no two experiences of the *same* rheumatic disorder are exactly the same. Even the same disorder in the same individual can change mysteriously from hour to hour or day to day or month to month. Remember that *does* mean things can and do get unexpectedly better as well as unexpectedly worse.

Bones (some 206 of them!) form the body's framework. Bones connect with each other at *joints*. Not all joints move, but those that do are called *synovial joints*. Joints are connected, stabilised, and moved by *soft tissue* (muscles, tendons, ligaments). Next time you cook a chicken, look first at the joints and how they move and fit together. Joints in the back have a different structure from synovial joints.

A *synovial joint* is enclosed in a joint capsule, lined with a fine skin-like *synovial membrane* (or synovium). This contains *synovial fluid*, which lubricates the joint, like oil (though it's much more complex). Fluid increases in an inflamed joint, causing swelling.

The surface of each adjoining bone in the joint capsule is covered by a white shiny rubbery substance called *articular cartilage* (not the same as cartilages removed from knee joints). Synovial fluid pumps in and out of its fine sponge-like surface as the joint moves or rests. The cartilage contains no nerves to act as pain-transmitters. That's why symptoms of early OA, which starts in the cartilage, tend to be stiffness, rather than pain. But when a rheumatic disorder starts elsewhere, eg in the bone, or synovial membrane (as in RA), pain is a much earlier symptom, because these bits have a rich nerve (and blood) supply.

Muscles which move bones and joints are called skeletal muscles. Some are attached directly to the bone, while others are attached by extra strong fibrous bands or cords called *tendons*. When muscles contract, joints move. Some tendons run through sliding tunnels which are lined by a sheath of the same type of synovial membrane as the joint capsule, and can similarly become inflamed (tenosynovitis) and possibly damaged.

Tendons can be displaced sideways, pulling bones (eg finger joints) in the wrong direction. Sometimes in RA a tendon can become so weak that it breaks, and the attached muscle and joint no longer work properly, leading to a 'dropped finger' appearance. Special splints may be used to encourage the tendon to heal. (Though my fingers have 'dropped' so I can't straighten them, after several years in remission they *have* regained remarkable strength.)

Muscles can be very strong, those in your thighs, for instance – the quadriceps muscles or 'quads' physios are so fond of, and rightly so. Weak quads make life really difficult, but simple exercises can keep them strong. Each muscle fibre receives 'relax' and 'contract' signals via the nervous system, is fed with oxygen and other energy-producing substances (eg glycogen) through the blood, and produces waste products (eg lactic acid).

Doctors and physios sometimes talk about muscles *going into spasm*. The muscles tighten, to try to prevent a painful joint moving. In an arthritic knee for instance this means you tend to walk with the knee slightly bent. Unfortunately the muscles are then in danger of weakening and wasting, leading to greatly increased pressure within the knee as it bears weight, and increasing the danger of joint damage and deformity.

The first step in counteracting this is treatment with painkillers and/or heat or cold to relieve the pain so you then, coached by your physio, can work on strengthening the weakened muscles. Stronger muscles help prevent possible damage and deformity. In the prolapsed disc ('slipped' disc) of backache, bedrest aims to relax the back muscles which are in painful spasm, and aims to protect the displaced disc tissues.

Ligaments are another part of the musculo-skeletal system. They hold together bones, cartilage, and other parts of the body. A *bursa* is a sort of protective cushion of body tissue, which lies between a tendon and and a bone, or between other moving parts. It's lined with a membrane like the synovial membrane, and can become inflamed and painful (bursitis) in disorders like housemaid's knee.

That's a brief picture of the main musculo-skeletal bits and pieces. Different disorders affect different bits in different ways. Gout, for instance, is an inflammatory arthritis in which 'urate' crystals are deposited in and around the joints, resulting in excruciatingly painful inflammation, if left untreated. In OA it's the joint cartilage (insensitive to pain) which is first affected, and pain follows later, as pain-sensitive bits like the bone become involved.

RA on the other hand starts in the very pain-sensitive synovial membrane, which becomes inflamed and swollen, and can lead to thinning and destruction of the smooth cartilage and bone. Synovial fluid increases and swells the joint, stretching the stabilising ligaments and tendons, leading to weakness and possible deformity, if untreated. AS usually starts in the bones of the lower back, with inflammation of the 'enthesis', the place where muscle is attached to the bone. 'Soft tissue' disorders affect body tissues around the joint rather than the joint itself. For more about:

- pain and the system of nerves which transmits pain, see chapter 11;
- joint care, see chapter 6;
- anatomical detail about other bits of the body which can sometimes be affected, eg the circulatory system (blood vessels, heart), eyes, lungs, skin, etc, dip into the general books on rheumatic disorders, listed on page 16, or read a good up-to-date school biology textbook.

The immune system

This is the body's internal self-defence system. Abnormalities with the way it works are closely linked with many rheumatic disorders. Normally it works well. The body's natural reaction is to fight anything it identifies as foreign. For instance it responds to a first attack of measles or other invader infection by producing *antibodies*, to fight and conquer the infection, the *antigen*. Some of these antibodies remain in the body ready to leap into action again at the first sign of any repeat infection and quash it at once. Vaccines are a way of artificially stimulating antibody production, to protect the body against infections, and 'confer immunity'.

Many rheumatic disorders, for instance RA and lupus, are described as *auto-immune disorders* ('autos' = self, in Greek). Instead of beneficially fighting a foreign invader, the body for some unknown reason mistakenly fights its own tissue, causing damage. (You might have noticed that the full name for the illness 'AIDS' is 'auto-immune deficiency syndrome'. AIDS *isn't* a rheumatic disorder but an entirely different type of   immune disorder where the immune system weakens and ultimately gives up fighting completely.)

Blood tests tell the experts something about past or present fighting inside the body by its immune system. All sorts of different antibodies (or 'immune complexes') may be identified. One of these is the *rheumatoid factor* (discovered in 1940), found in *some* but by no means all, people with RA. Having the factor doesn't automatically mean you'll get RA. Masses of people *with* rheumatoid factor never develop RA.

So by itself the rheumatoid factor doesn't tell us much about why someone does or doesn't develop RA. It may be only one of a particular 'fruit-machine' combination of environmental, physical, infectious or possible genetic factors which trigger release of the unwanted 'jackpot'. It's even possible that the same disorder may have different causes in different people. Researchers are working hard to unravel these mysteries.

Similarly, the *LE cell* test used for people with lupus (SLE) isn't positive in *everyone* with lupus though another more recently developed test, for *anti-DNA antibodies*, does give a positive response for practically everyone with lupus. In lupus various auto-antibodies circulate in the blood, and can cause problems wherever they end up, eg rashes in the skin, damage to blood vessels, or trouble in the kidney, lungs, joints, and occasionally the brain.

HLAs are another bit of the immune system. An HLA (*Human Leucocyte Antigen*) is a sort of biological trademark in our genes, which helps an individual immune system to distinguish between what is or isn't part of the body for which it is responsible. We each have only eight out of a vast range of possible HLAs. Someone needing a kidney transplant needs to find a kidney with a perfect or almost perfect match of HLAs, to avoid it being rejected by the immune system. Identical combinations are hard to find. HLA incompatibility is similar to blood group incompatibility, where a bodyful of, say, blood group A will reject an infusion of blood group B.

Someone with AS may read that over 90% of people with AS have HLA number B27 (though it's present in only about 7% of the normal population). People with Reiter's syndrome also usually have HLA B27. Many other disorders are associated with a particular HLA. HLA DR4, for instance, is found in 70% of people with RA, but in only 25% of the general population.

Immunosuppressives are sometimes used to treat severe problems in rheumatic disorders. They suppress activity in the immune system, and hopefully any harmful auto-immune activity. Unfortunately they also suppress beneficial immune activity, putting the body at risk of attack by outside infections. That's why they're only used with the utmost care and caution by doctors.

Professor John Dwyer, Professor of Medicine at the University of New South Wales, has written a layperson's guide to the immune system *The Body at War* (Unwin, 1989).

Chapter three

MORE ABOUT SOME INDIVIDUAL
RHEUMATIC DISORDERS

As I'm not a doctor, I won't go into a lot of medical detail here, though I do believe it's well worth finding out about your own particular rheumatic disorder so you can understand what's happening to your body and what you and your doctor can do about it. I'll concentrate on the main disorders affecting our age group. You'll find more information on these and others through the books and organisations mentioned here and in other chapters.

A word of warning! *Don't* imagine everything you read about will happen to you. *Do* choose your reading with care. There's a lot of misleading information around about arthritis, written by out-of-date, non-experts. Even medical textbooks are quickly out-of-date, the language isn't easy to understand, and they can sometimes be horribly frightening (especially the pictures). If anything that you read worries you, *do* please ask your doctor about it. I once spent weeks in misery having completely misinterpreted one very worrying thing I read!

The best reading matter tends to be that written for patients by doctors and other reputably qualified professionals with a specialist and up-to-date knowledge of rheumatology. Especially good are the publications produced by the Arthritis and Rheumatism Council (ARC).

General books on rheumatic disorders (see also Appendix 1)
Here's a list of general books, written by healthcare professionals. I'll mention others dealing with specific disorders as we go along.
- ARC publications (mostly free, but send an SAE) include *Introducing Arthritis*; handbooks on *Rheumatoid Arthritis, Osteoarthritis explained, Gout, Ankylosing Spondylitis, Lupus, Backache, Pain in the Neck*. Others deal with shoes, chairs, new hip and knee joints, etc. Send an SAE to ARC for an up-to-date list.
- Arthritis Care's *Information for People with Arthritis* (free, but send A5 SAE)
- Dr Frank Dudley Hart's illustrated and very readable *Overcoming Arthritis* (Dunitz/Macdonald Optima)
- Professor J M H Moll's *Arthritis and Rheumatism* (Churchill Livingstone)
- Professor Malcolm Jayson and Professor Allan Dixon's *Rheumatism & Arthritis. The Commonsense Guide to the Problems and the Latest Treatment* (Pan)
- Dr J T Scott's *Arthritis & Rheumatism. The Facts* (Oxford University Press)
- Consultant orthopaedic surgeon Mr Denys Wainwright's *Arthritis & Rheumatism. What They Are – What You Can Do to Help Yourself* (Elliot Right Way)
- Dr Vernon Coleman's *Arthritis* (Severn House)
- Senior occupational therapist Heather Unsworth's *Coping with Rheumatoid Arthritis* (Chambers)
- Kate Lorig and James F Fries' *The Arthritis Helpbook* (Souvenir Press)
- Dr A Clarke, L Allard, B Braybrooks' *Rehabilitation in Rheumatology* (Martin Dunitz) (see page 293)
- Dr John Shenkman's *Living with Arthritis* (Franklin Watts). Designed for youngsters, so particularly clear and well-illustrated.

Self-help/patient support groups

Great source of information. Most produce helpful regular newsletters. The main groups for people with arthritis (of whatever type) are the Arthritis and Rheumatism Council (ARC), which concentrates on research plus education of patients and professionals, and Arthritis Care, which concentrates on social and welfare aspects. Young Arthritis Care is run specially by and for under 45s with arthritis. Read more about these groups on pages 113, 118 and 123. There are other groups, which concentrate on specific rheumatic disorders, and I'll mention those in this chapter, under the relevant disorder.

Ankylosing spondylitis (AS)

What is it and who gets it?

'Ankylos' is Greek for stiffness, 'spondylos' the word for spinal vertebra, 'itis' indicates inflammation. In the old days people with AS were, unfortunately, immobilised in plaster for weeks (quite the wrong treatment), and developed a characteristic posture of rounded shoulders, flat chest, back bent in a stiff curve with the head and neck held forwards.

In the spine of someone with AS the 'enthesis' becomes inflamed (the place where a muscle is attached to the bone). The bone responds by growing out from both sides of the back vertebra. Unless you keep mobile there's a danger of one vertebra becoming fused to the next, to form a stiff 'ankylosed' joint, leading to the old pokerback posture. Exercises aim to prevent that happening.

AS is the third commonest rheumatic disorder after OA and RA. Estimates of people with AS in Britain vary between 50,000 and 100,000. It's 2½ times commoner in men than in women, with an average age of onset of 24 years old. Most people with AS (over 90%) have a particular cell group called HLA B27 (see page 15), which may be significant, though there are far more people (four out of five) with HLA B27 who *never* get AS than do. So screening for HLA B27 in healthy individuals would prove nothing about their chances of getting AS.

What symptoms might you get?

No two people experience AS in exactly the same way. Only some of this may apply to *you*.

- Usually starts with pain, aching, stiffness in the lower back or buttocks. Rest tends not to relieve the pain and stiffness.
- Stiffness may be worse in the early morning, but improves with exercise.
- Problem may (or may not) spread higher up the spine, and to the neck.
- Other joints may (or may not) become involved, eg hip, shoulder, knee, ankles.
- You may feel generally unwell too, very tired, and perhaps lose weight.
- Understandably you may experience anxiety and frustration, especially early on, before the AS settles down and before you've learnt how best to cope.
- Some people develop iritis, inflammation of the iris, which surrounds the pupil of the eye. If you suddenly develop a slight blurring of vision, or a red eye, action must be taken quickly to prevent eye damage. Take yourself to the casualty department of an eye hospital, or if there isn't one near you, then go to any hospital accident and emergency department, and insist on seeing the ophthalmologist on call, who will understand the relationship between the AS and the eye condition uveitis.
- Some specially tender areas may develop, eg under the heel bone, or your 'seat' bone.
- There may be chest problems, related to inflammation in the sternum joint and ribs where they articulate with the vertebrae.

Management of AS

Blood tests and X-rays and particular symptoms can help identify AS, though correct diagnosis may take a while. Once it's confirmed you *must* 'leap into action' (*almost* literally), to keep your spine mobile, and to prevent deformity. This really is an illness where the person who can most help you is *you*, yourself.

- Exercise is *the* essential treatment. You'll be taught progressive spinal exercises and chest expansion, which you must practice daily, preferably twice a day. Make the exercises as much a habit as cleaning your teeth. (NASS cassettes may help – see below)
- Rethink your posture, environment, and, if necessary, your job with advice from the physio and OT, to avoid spinal strain. Invest in a good upright chair, and, crucial, a good firm mattress. Avoid slouching. Keep your head erect.
- Keep as fit as possible generally. Many sports are good for you, especially swimming. Check which ones with your doctor and physio.
- No drugs actually alter the course of the disease itself, but they may be prescribed to relieve pain and stiffness so that you're better able to exercise and to get around. NSAIDs (eg indomethacin or naproxen) may be used. Unlike RA, aspirin isn't usually used, nor gold or penicillamine, and steroids seldom. Phenylbutazone is occasionally used, but only under hospital supervision so you can be closely monitored for any problems.

ARC's booklet on AS is reassuring:

> *"In its early stages AS causes considerable pain but effective treatment is available to relieve this, even though the discomfort is not always abolished. Later the disease becomes much less active, or even inactive. You will most probably be able to carry on with your work and lead a normal life..."*

Read: NASS's *Guidebook for Patients*

Group: National Ankylosing Spondylitis Society (NASS). Regular newsletter, also audio and videocassettes of a home physiotherapy programme, and booklets *Stretch, Relax and a Little Bit More* and *Living with Ankylosing Spondylitis*. More than 60 NASS branches provide physiotherapy after working hours, one evening a week.

Back pain

It's been estimated that some 2% of the population go to their doctor every year because of backache, and some 19 million working days a year are lost (ARC estimate 1988). Although it's so common, severity and causes vary considerably. You should seek medical advice if you have persistent back pain. It could be a symptom of AS or a prolapsed disc ('slipped disc') or something else. For AS exercise will be prescribed; for a prolapsed disc, it's likely to be just the opposite, complete bed-rest. So correct diagnosis is essential. Other back pain may be due to wear and tear, small fractures, over-stretched muscles, accidents, awkward lifting and carrying, ageing, sporting injury, or other stresses and strains.

Read: ARC's *Backache*, and Chapters 1 and 2 of Jayson and Dixon's *Rheumatism and Arthritis*, mentioned earlier

Group: National Back Pain Association. Membership includes quarterly magazine *Talkback*

Gout

What is it and who gets it?
Gout *isn't* caused by over-eating or over-drinking, as such, but *is* caused by the way your body deals with what you eat. It's an 'error of metabolism', with a tendency to run in families. Metabolism is the process by which the body changes the food we eat and the

oxygen we breathe into usable substances like protein, fats and carbohydrates. Waste products are produced at the same time, among them 'purines', which break down into 'uric acid'. Normally the body easily gets rid of this uric acid, but someone with gout either can't get rid of it adequately through the kidneys or produces too much. The excess is deposited in the form of crystals in the affected joint.

Gout's most common in men and women over 40, though there's also a very rare type which affects children and younger adults. It's commoner in men than in women. Some people only ever have one or two attacks of acute gout. Others may have repeated attacks. The great thing is that gout can be effectively controlled, for life, if necessary, by medication.

What symptoms might you get?
An acute attack usually (70% – 90%) starts in the big toe, with very intense pain, swelling and redness. Other joints which may suffer include the ankle, knee, fingers, elbows, wrists. The pain can be so severe that you can't bear *anything* to touch the joint, not even a light sheet. But remember, gout *can* be treated effectively.

Management
Quick diagnosis and early treatment are important. Untreated, continuing gout can lead to permanent joint damage and deformity. Treatment for a one-off, acute attack, differs from long-term treatment for repeated attacks.

Read: ARC's handbook *Gout*

Juvenile chronic arthritis (JCA)
(often called Still's disease)

What is it and who gets it?
JCA is inflammatory arthritis lasting at least three months, which starts in a baby or child aged under 16. Many of you may, like me, have started out with JCA. There are several different types or subgroups of JCA, estimated to affect between 1 in 1,000 and 1 in 1,500 children (some 15,000 in Britain). Overall it affects more girls than boys, though the ratio varies in each subgroup. The good news is that more often than not, JCA ultimately burns itself out, and the aim of treatment is to ensure that when that happens, the child has as few physical, educational and social limitations as possible. ARC's report *Children and Arthritis* comments:

> *"It has been shown that, with good management, which can now be provided, 70% of the children who get arthritis early in life make a good recovery. Specialists are now able to overcome most of the complications resulting from the disease. And even for the remaining 30% of the children who do not make a full recovery, and whose arthritis persists in adulthood, many are able to lead reasonably normal lives."*

What symptoms might you have?
Symptoms differ according to the subgroup. The main subgroups are:
- *Systemic arthritis* Usually begins in very young children. Thought to affect boys and girls in equal numbers. Marked by persistent fever and illness as well as joint pain, and may lead to joint damage. There's a characteristic swinging temperature, often higher in the afternoon or evening, and a characteristic patchy measles-like rash.
- *Polyarthritis* Means inflammation of *many* joints (five or more), and can occur at any age, more usually in girls than boys. May start with joint trouble alone, or the child may also feel generally unwell.
- *Pauci-articular arthritis* Means only a *few* joints involved (four or less). May start in

just one joint, eg knee. Though general health's usually little affected, there's risk of eye disease (chronic iridocyclitis), with a danger of serious eye problems, even blindness. So it's essential to have regular eye checks, as problems can otherwise go unnoticed (there's no redness or pain warning sign).

- *Juvenile ankylosing spondylitis* Affects mainly boys, aged 10 and over. Usually starts in one or two leg joints (eg hips, knees, ankles), and may move to the lower back. There's a risk of eye problems (acute iridocyclitis), so consult an ophthalmologist at the first sign of a painful red eye (see the note on page 17 about adult AS.)
- *Adult-type rheumatoid arthritis* Affects mainly girls, aged 11 and older. Usually starts in the small joints of the hand and feet, sometimes the knees, and there may sometimes be elbow nodules. Early diagnosis is essential so treatment can be started to avoid possibly serious joint damage.
- *Psoriatic arthritis* Occurs especially in children aged about nine or ten. Scaling skin disease, with usually mild arthritis in only one or two joints.

Management of JCA

Some JCA clears up quickly. In other children longer term treatment is essential and includes:

- Careful management by doctor, physio, OT, and other people, plus cooperation of parents and child in what may be a long and difficult course.
- A rest and exercise programme specially tailored to the individual child, including the use of 'rest' and 'work' splints, aims to avoid muscle wasting, joint damage, and deformity, and aims to maintain good function. It's essential to keep this programme going regularly at *home* and not just under the eagle eye of the physio. Hopefully hard work now will be rewarded by future benefits.
- Constant attention to joint care and good posture, ensuring the right sitting and lying positions, as well as walking, standing and action movements, with the same aims as the rest and exercise programme.
- Prescribed drugs, chosen from those used for adults.
- Sometimes surgery may be necessary.
- Remember the child's a 'whole person', not 'an illness' or 'an invalid'. It's essential not to let his or her educational, social, and personal development suffer. 'Brainpower' rather than 'brawnpower' becomes even more important for someone with a frail body. Integration to 'normal' life should be encouraged, and over-protection avoided, as it can add social handicaps to any physical handicaps. Adolescence is a trying time for anyone, even more so for a YPA. Skills and talents and strength of character need to be gently encouraged to develop, plus as much independence and self-reliance as possible too. Accentuate the positive and minimise the negative.

Read: ARC's *When Your Child Has Arthritis* (for parents) and
            When a Young Person Has Arthritis (for teachers)
Groups: Lady Hoare Trust. Young Arthritis Care

Osteoarthritis (OA)

What is it, who gets it, and what are the possible symptoms?

Osteoarthritis is the most widespread rheumatic disorder. About five million people have some form of OA. Most are over 50, though it does sometimes start earlier. It probably affects slightly more women than men. OA's not primarily an inflammatory disorder like RA or AS (though inflammatory episodes do occur). In most people it's limited to one, or only a few joints, rather than affecting the whole or a large part of the body as in inflammatory arthritis.

OA in a joint doesn't necessarily cause symptoms or get worse: it may stay the same, get easier for a time then bad again, or, sometimes, it may become easier and stay that way. *"Most people with OA don't become crippled or severely disabled and maintain a normal life"* (ARC). Severe OA in a knee or hip may cause pain, misery, frustration and disability, but joint replacement operations can bring relief.

The most commonly affected joints are one (sometimes more) of the following: knees, hips, hands, big toe ('hallux valgus'). A characteristic type of OA in non weight-bearing joints appears mainly in the joints at the end of the fingers and the joint at the base of the thumb. Small knobs form called 'Heberden's nodes' after the doctor who first described them. Though they may be painful to start with, usually they are or become painless.

Exactly what happens in OA and why isn't yet fully understood. Sometimes there's an obvious predisposing factor, where 'secondary OA' develops following repeated small injuries or a single minor injury (eg in footballers or long-distance runners, or women after years of wearing badly fitting shoes), or perhaps as a result of an inherited or congenital joint abnormality.

It's called 'primary OA' where there's no obvious pre-disposing factor, though age or 'wear and tear' processes may have something to do with it. Various theories suggest there may be a failure in the joint's lubricating mechanism, or an abrasive process set up by tiny crystals deposited in the joint, or the bones may not be 'elastic' enough to cope with repeated 'impact shock', due to jogging, being overweight, etc.

The articular cartilage (forming the slippery, protective end of bone) in an OA joint gets thinner and rougher, so the bones end up rubbing against one another. Synovial fluid increases and thickens, and spurs of new bone tissue (osteophytes) form at the edge of the joint. Cartilage stops growing after childhood, so if it's damaged has only a limited ability to heal itself. The joint swells, becoming distorted and stiff, leading to aches and pains, tenderness, muscle wasting, and limited movement.

Stiffness rather than pain may be the earliest symptom, as there are no pain-sensitive nerves in the cartilage where OA starts. Pain comes after using the joint, and in later OA, at rest and the end of the day. There may be a creaking, grating, cracking sensation with movement, and limitation in range. There are usually ups and downs in discomfort, with bad spells and better spells.

Management of OA
- Reduce stress on the joint and avoid activities which cause pain.
- Use a stick. Due to a leverage effect, up to as much as 75% of your weight can be taken off the hip joint if you use a stick correctly (see page 181).
- Keep your weight down. Being overweight stresses joints. Apparently at least four times the body weight is borne by your hip and knee joints when you walk. To understand this, the less scientifically minded of us may be helped by observing how an object dropped on to a hand feels heavier than the same object simply resting on that hand.
- Consult a physio for advice on balancing exercise and rest, usually based on 'little and often' and 'take it gently', plus advice on regularly taking the joint through its full range of movement.
- Consult an OT for help in overcoming practical problems and advice on joint care (eg a small raise on a shoe or rubber heels may help a hip problem).
- Keep warm and avoid damp. OA in some people seems to respond to changes in the weather, though it's not *caused* by the weather. Cold and damp may make you more aware of joint pain. Muscles may tense and small blood vessels feeding the joints may become constricted.
- Pain control: physios use methods like infra-red, short-wave diathermy, wax baths, to ease pain. Ask about home-made ways of achieving the same effect − eg hot-water bottle, flannel-wrapped bag of frozen peas, warm underwear/overwear.

- Keeping mentally occupied is a good form of natural pain-control.
- Drugs may be prescribed to control pain, but the other pain control methods described above should be tried first.

Read: ARC's *Osteoarthritis explained*
Group: Arthritis Care

Osteoporosis

In osteoporosis bones become fragile and break more easily than usual, due to a deficiency in the bone structure. Most at risk are women around the menopause, especially those who've had an early menopause, or who have had both ovaries removed in an operation.

Read: ARC's *Thin Bones*
Group: National Osteoporosis Society

Psoriasis and arthritis

What is it and who gets it?
Psoriasis (Greek word for itch) is an itchy and distressing skin condition which appears as raised red patches of skin covered with silvery scales. It usually affects knees, elbows and scalp and there may be 'pitting' of the nails. It isn't infectious or contagious nor is it caused by poor standards of hygiene.

Psoriasis is a vast acceleration of what happens in everyone's skin, where skin cells slowly mature as they work their way to the surface, before being shed, usually unnoticed, as dead cells. The process normally takes some 21 to 40 days, but psoriatic cells are thought to do the same in only two to seven days, and so rapidly and chaotically that even live cells reach the surface and accumulate visibly with the dead ones.

About 1% of the population suffers from psoriasis, but only about 5% of people with psoriasis also develop arthritis. Psoriatic arthritis usually starts between the ages of 30 and 50, though can occur earlier, even in children. Psoriasis may be linked with arthritis in several different ways:
–   as psoriatic arthropathy, superficially similar to RA, but with differences. Fewer joints may be affected, and unlike in RA, joints near the *tip* of the finger may become painfully swollen
–   as psoriatic spondylitis, which resembles AS
–   appearing, by sheer coincidence before, after, or at the same time as RA
–   as psoriatic arthritis mutilans, where both skin and joint disease may be so severe that intensive medical and nursing care is needed.
Both psoriasis and arthritis are conditions that wax and wane, sometimes better, sometimes worse, sometimes disappearing altogether.

Read: *Psoriasis*, by Dr Ronald Marks (Macdonald Optima)
              Learning to Live with Skin Disorders, by Christine Orton (Souvenir)
              Psoriasis – A Practical Guide to Coping, by Dr C Wilson (Crowood)
              Overcoming Disfigurement, by Doreen Trust (Thorsons)
Groups: Psoriasis Association. Young Arthritis Care. The British Red Cross runs a helpful Beauty Camouflage Care Service.

Raynaud's phenomenon (named after a 19th century French doctor)

Raynaud's may occur by itself (primary Raynaud's), or in tandem with another illness, for instance RA, lupus, systemic sclerosis (secondary Raynaud's). The blood supply to the extremities (usually fingers and toes) is interrupted. Affected parts become white and numb, later turning purple, and then red with a burning sensation, pain, or numbness. An attack may be triggered by temperature changes, emotion, or stress.

Anyone, at any age, may get Raynaud's, though women are affected nine times more than men. It can be mild, or so severe that ulcerations form. If these are left untreated they may become gangrenous and amputation may be necessary. Cause and cure are unknown. Keeping the extremities, and the body itself warm may help, plus avoidance of situations likely to cause an attack. Special heated socks and mittens, and tiny portable 'heat packs' are available from the Association. Drugs help some people (eg nifedipine).

Read: *Raynaud's – A Handbook for Patients* by Anne H Mawdsley
        Raynaud's – A Better Understanding by Mr K Lafferty, FRCS
        (Both available from the support group, below)
Group: The Raynaud's and Scleroderma Association

Reiter's Syndrome (RS)
and other arthritis associated with infection

There are three main ways in which arthritis can be associated with an infection:
- *Infective, septic, or suppurative arthritis* If bacteria get into a joint (eg through the blood) it can become red and very hot, with acute pain and tenderness, and there may be high fever. This can happen in a joint damaged by RA/OA, or, rarely, around a joint prosthesis. Treatment is with antibiotics and sometimes joint drainage.
- *Arthritis associated with viral infections* Sometimes occurs in people who get infections such as infective hepatitis B, mumps, smallpox, glandular fever, rubella (German measles). The arthritis usually goes quickly. Treatment is with aspirin and anti-inflammatory drugs.
- *Reactive arthritis* Arthritis which occurs as a *reaction* to infection. There are three main groups: (1) rheumatic fever, (2) arthritis following a bowel infection, (3) arthritis following a sexually acquired infection:

    Rheumatic fever used to be one of the commonest serious diseases of childhood, and it's still prevalent in developing countries. In 1928 25% of the patients at Great Ormond Street Hospital had it. Unlike other rheumatic disorders the cause *is* known – it follows infection with a microbe called (something of a mouthful) Group A beta-haemolytic streptococcus. Main symptoms are fever, joint swelling and pain, and, more seriously, heart inflammation and damage.

    Reiter's syndrome (RS) can be type (2) *or* type (3) reactive arthritis. It's commoner in men than women, and usually starts in young adults, though can also occur in children. RS is a combination of urinary and eye (conjunctivitis) problems, and the joint problems of arthritis. Treatment is with antibiotics, pain-killers and anti-inflammatory drugs (NSAIDs), occasionally steroids, physiotherapy, joint and muscle care, rest, and help and advice on coping with any practical and personal problems. Like many rheumatic disorders it's hard to predict how it'll affect any one person; but there are usually periods of remission, sometimes lasting years, between flare-ups.

    Reiter was a German military doctor who identified the syndrome in soldiers fighting in the trenches in the First World War Battle of the Somme, where bowel infection was common.

Rheumatoid arthritis (RA)

What is it and who gets it?
The body develops an auto-immune reaction (see page 14), a sort of allergic reaction to

bits of itself. Instead of your immune system defending your body against 'foreign invaders' it mistakenly and painfully turns on itself, inflaming and swelling the thin synovial membrane which lines the joint.

Most of you reading this probably know only too well all about RA from your own personal experience, and know how it can at times affect the whole body, not just the joints. Though it can affect anyone, at any age, it usually starts before the age of 45, more usually in women than in men. It affects about 0.8% of the adult population in Great Britain (about half a million), though many people are only mildly affected.

RA may start overnight or very gradually, usually in the smaller joints, particularly hands and wrists, and/or in the feet, with pain, joint swelling and stiffness (particularly in the early morning), and a general feeling of being unwell, a sort of 'fluey' feeling. But it varies tremendously, and no two people experience RA in exactly the same way. Some people are more or less back to normal fairly quickly. Others continue to have greater or lesser joint pain and swelling, with perhaps a flare-up from time to time.

RA's a fluctuating, variable disorder, with bad times and flare-ups, but also, thank goodness, good and better times too. It's misleading to call it progressive. The good or better times are wonderful, though joints and body still need to be treated with respect. The bad or worse times we could well do without, but as with so many things, most of us, with support and encouragement, work out ways of adapting. Listen to Phil (a mum, and former Chairman of the 35 Group for YPAs) who knows the ups and downs only too well:

> "If anyone had told me 15 years ago, when I was first diagnosed, that I would cope, manage to bring up not one, but two children, remain married, have a demanding, fulfilling, enjoyable job, work full-time and drive thousands of miles each year, that I would dance (occasionally), swim, go on holiday and enjoy life, I don't think I would have believed them."

What symptoms might you get?

Remember, no two people with RA experience it in exactly the same way. The number and types of joint affected vary considerably, even at different times in the same person. Only some of these may apply to you:

- Morning stiffness, which might last for 20 to 30 minutes or even several hours, and stiffness at other times too, for instance after inactivity.
- Pain, inflammation, tenderness, swelling, of joints and surrounding areas.
- Limitation of joint movement, eg loss of grip strength, muscular power, mobility, what writer Grace Stuart so aptly called 'the strange powerlessness of the arthritic joint'.
- You might feel generally unwell and get tired easily. Some people may be anaemic and/or lose weight. You might feel depressed. Not surprising, especially in the early days, before you've really fathomed out what's happening, and learnt how best to cope.
- Some people develop rheumatoid 'nodules' around the elbow, others don't. Other parts of the body may (or may *not*) be affected too, even eyes, lungs, blood vessels, heart.

When the RA's particularly active, we talk about having a 'flare-up'. The joint linings and other body tissues become inflamed. The body's defences are activated, as they are if you have a cut that goes septic, and heat, swelling and pain result. But the inflammation doesn't clear up quickly like a septic cut. It may persist, as chronic inflammation.

> "The inflammation in rheumatoid arthritis has been likened to a forest fire. If it is raging furiously, then bed rest and and full drug treatment are required, if grumbling and almost out, simple analgesics and/or anti-rheumatic drugs as required. Like a forest fire, certain areas (joints) may flare up for a time and require attention and then settle." (ARC magazine, spring 1988)

Management of RA

- Medical help from GP, rheumatologist, and other healthcare specialists. Help with inflammation control and pain relief (using periods of rest, splintage, supports, and heat, as well as drugs), and help with understanding the disorder and working out ways of coping. Advice on what should be done and what should be avoided, so you know how best to help yourself.

- Advice from physios and OTs on joint care, energy conservation, and the right exercise/rest programme for your individual needs. It'll probably take a while to work out the right balance for you, and how best to 'pace' yourself in your daily life. Various simple joint care guidelines can help prevent your joints taking too much strain and help limit joint damage. Wear rest and work splints if prescribed for you. OTs and physios can also advise you how best to manage at home and work, how to 'keep going'. Do ask for *early* referral to physio and OT; don't wait till the damage is done.

- More about rest. It's one of the best treatments for inflammation and joint damage, though it *must* be balanced with prescribed exercise to keep joints from stiffening up too much and to stop the muscles becoming weak. The joint or joints become *very* vulnerable and must be treated with great care and respect, to minimise possible damage to the joint cartilage, joint capsule, ligaments, and tendons.

   In a bad flare-up your doctor may prescribe complete bed-rest, at home or in hospital for a few days. Professor J M H Moll, Head of the Centre for Rheumatic Diseases, Sheffield, writes: *"Rest..is a particularly useful form of treatment, although patients may not be impressed by the idea of being admitted to hospital 'only for rest'. (Perhaps if it were termed 'horizontal hypokinesia' it would be more respected by patients!)"* (*Manual of Rheumatology*, Churchill Livingstone, 1987)

- More about exercise. Important for keeping your muscles strong and functioning as well as possible. The joints should be moved fully each day and muscles exercised as prescribed by your physio. *Don't* chicken out of doing them every day at home just because you haven't got a fierce physio standing over you!

- Drugs. Though there's no miracle cure (yet), drugs, used as part of a total management programme, can help keep the disorder bearable. More about drugs in chapter 5.

- Surgery may sometimes be necessary, 'minor' (eg release of trapped nerves) or 'major' (eg hip replacement). More in chapter 8.

- 'Natural' pain control – more about this in chapter 11.

- Support and adjustments, as necessary, to cope with any personal, psychological, social, domestic, money, or job problems. Help can come from a variety of sources: hopefully this book will help you identify them.

ARC's booklet on RA summarises everything helpfully:

   "Although rheumatoid arthritis is a common, persistent joint disorder, which sometimes causes serious problems, most sufferers have only modest problems. There is no cure yet and the disease is not fully understood. But there is a wide variety of treatments, and knowledge is increasing rapidly. It takes time and common sense to get used to having arthritis and to learn how best to adapt to it, but help is available...

   "Much can be worked out with common sense. The principle is to keep doing everything you want to but, if necessary, to adapt things to protect joints and to have a little respect for the condition. Don't be too proud to accept help and advice when it makes sense. Learn to accept and live with rheumatoid arthritis, while leading as normal a life as possible."

Read: ARC's *Rheumatoid Arthritis Explained*
            Heather Unsworth's *Coping with Rheumatoid Arthritis* (Chambers)
Groups: The Arthritis and Rheumatism Council. Young Arthritis Care and its parent body Arthritis Care.

Sjøgren's syndrome
(pronounced Showgren's)

Another auto-immune disorder where dry eyes (kerato-conjunctivitis sicca) and dry mouth (xerostomia) sometimes accompany other rheumatic disorders (RA, lupus, systemic sclerosis). Dry eyes occur in about 15% of people with RA. Eyes may feel persistently 'gritty', tired, and sensitive to light. Mouth and throat may feel dry, and possibly ulcerate. Dry skin may be itchy. Other parts of the body may be affected. Cause and cure aren't known yet. Eye drops may ease eye discomfort, and frequent sips of fluid may help the dry mouth. Replens may help a dry vagina. Aqueous cream may ease dry skin. Preventive dental care is important.

Groups: British Sjøgren's Syndrome Association.
             Raynaud's and Scleroderma Association

Systemic lupus erythematosus
(SLE or 'lupus' for short)

What is it and who gets it?
'Systemic' means it affects various parts of the body; 'lupus' is a word used medically to describe some skin rashes (Latin word for wolf – people used to think the rash looked like a wolf bite); 'erythema' is used medically to describe the red colour of inflamed skin. Lupus usually starts in the teens or twenties, or, rarely, in children. More women than men are affected (nine women to every man).

Lupus is a connective tissue disorder. Since connective tissue occurs throughout the body, binding or connecting cells and tissues together, lupus can rear its ugly head almost anywhere, not just in the skin and joints. Like RA it varies tremendously and unpredictably from person to person. It may disappear as mysteriously as it came. Usually though it waxes and wanes, with quieter periods alternating with flare-ups.

Nowadays the outlook is far better than in even the recent past, so *do* beware of reading even slightly out-of-date books, as ARC's handbook for patients warns:
"If you happened to look it up in a medical book in the public library, you might become worried; it is often described as very serious and sometimes fatal. You need not worry. This idea is out of date because, at the time when such books were written, only severe cases were ever diagnosed by doctors."
Dr Graham Hughes is reassuringly up-to-date
"..it is not uncommon for the disease to appear acutely in the late teens or twenties, and, following treatment, to subside. The majority of patients, given careful management, can possibly ultimately succeed in stopping treatment – a fact which until recently was not widely appreciated." (In *Lupus, a Guide for Patients*)

What symptoms might you get?
Remember, everyone has a different version of lupus, and only *some* of these symptoms may apply to you:
- Skin rashes, for instance a pink rash on the cheeks which might ironically be mistaken for the ruddy glow of good health, or a 'butterfly' shaped rash over cheeks and nose. Skin may be 'photosensitive', reacting to sunlight with a severe rash.
- Joint, muscle and tendon inflammation and pains. Someone with lupus may first think they have RA, but the joints are rarely damaged as they can be in RA.
- Flu-like symptoms – fever, tiredness, headaches, in addition to aches and pains and weakness.
- Hair. There may be some temporary hair loss during a flare-up.
- Raynaud's phenomenon, which I described on page 22. Circulatory problems in the

fingers so they go cold and numb, turning white then purple.
- Other areas where lupus inflammation may occur include the blood vessels, digestive system, heart, lungs, kidneys, brain. Blood pressure may be raised.
- Depression can occur, especially during a flare-up.
- Rarely fits (like epilepsy) may occur.

Management of lupus

Lupus can be difficult to diagnose, because symptoms may be confused with another illness, RA for instance. Blood tests help confirm the diagnosis, and someone with lupus symptoms should be referred to hospital for a DNA blood test. Treatment aims to relieve pain and other symptoms, to damp down inflammation, and help you lead as normal a life as possible. It may take a period of trial and error to work out the best individual treatment for you, but hang on in there.
- Drugs. People with lupus may be sensitive to some drugs (eg antibiotics) and develop rashes after taking them. In mild lupus drugs are kept to a minimum, with occasional use of pain-relievers (eg aspirin) and anti-inflammatories (NSAIDs). In more active lupus drugs such as anti-malarials, steroids, or immunosuppressives may be used. Drugs may also be used to treat raised blood pressure if appropriate.
- Rest when you need to, and watch your general health. Avoid possible trigger factors, eg sunlight or ultra-violet light, if you're one of the 50% or so people whose lupus reacts badly to sunlight. Where possible, avoid highly stressful situations, and try to avoid becoming over-tired or over-doing things.
- Keep extremities and body warm to avoid Raynaud's problems. Sometimes drugs may help with the Raynaud's.
- Seek help from doctor, OT, social worker, etc, to help you lead as normal a life as possible. You might find joining the Lupus Group helpful. Try to keep up with interests and hobbies and keep mentally active.
- Pregnancy requires special care. Discuss with your doctor well before becoming pregnant (see page 229). It's rare for children of people with lupus to develop lupus themselves.

Read: ARC's *Lupus*, and both from Lupus UK:
            Lupus, a Guide for Patients by Dr Graham R V Hughes
            Coping with Lupus (Avery Publishing) by Robert H Phillips, PhD
Groups: Lupus UK Group (research and welfare).

Systemic sclerosis (scleroderma)

'Scleroderma' comes from the Greek, 'sclero' meaning hard, and 'derma' meaning skin, ie hard skin, but the hardness (too much collagen) isn't limited to the skin, and can affect any connective tissue in the body. The internal organs (lungs, heart, kidneys and gut) and their blood supply may become damaged. Raynaud's (page 22) and Sjøgren's (page 26) may occur too. Scleroderma's quite rare, affecting only three in a million people (one of them being me, and another being Anne Mawdsley, founder of the Raynaud's and Scleroderma Association). It's commoner in women than men, and most common between the ages of 30 and 50. Alas it's not possible to predict the course of the disease in any individual – it may be mild or severe, and the cause is still unknown.

Read: *Scleroderma – A Handbook for Patients* by Anne H Mawdsley (from the Association)
            ARC's *Scleroderma – A Booklet for Patients*
Group: Raynaud's and Scleroderma Association.

Chapter four

YOU AND YOUR DOCTOR

A different sort of illness

Until arthritis rears its ugly head, for most of us visits to the doctor have probably been for a 'common' illness, like chickenpox or flu, or for something like a twisted ankle or broken bone. These problems usually have a fairly clearcut beginning, middle and end, plus clearcut symptoms and treatment. The doctor can easily tell you just what to do for the best, and roughly how long it'll take before you're back on form.

Arthritis, needless to say, just has to be different. Like you, we other YPAs have been through fears and frustrations and anger too, because of its peculiarities. We've been puzzled by the wait for a definite diagnosis. Alarmed to learn there's no cure − yet. Discovered there's often a 'trial-and-error' approach to treatment; what works for you with your RA might be totally wrong for me and my body and *my* RA, though what I try next might be ideal, or possibly the fifth-next treatment... Baffled that the doctor wouldn't (because s/he simply couldn't) predict what was going to happen. Discovered that 'time and patience' form part of the prescription, just when you're impatient for results. And oh, the frustration at being told 'you'll just have to learn to live with it' − and asking why? how? Feeling alone and helpless. Yes, things can seem dismal, especially in the early days.

However there *is* a bright side. Gloom does clear with time and experience, with information, and with help and support from other people. More, much more about all that later. I hope it might help if we look here at why the early days of the arthritis-doctor-you triangle can seem so frustrating. Otherwise it's easy to lose faith in your doctor and treatment.

Some of the problems are because of the peculiarities of the arthritis, some because of our reactions and difficulties in understanding what's going on, and because we haven't yet learnt the skills of being an 'expert patient' (see page 33 onwards); other problems may be because of the doctor's inadequate knowledge of rheumatology, his or her inexperience at dealing with a chronic rather than acute illness, or simply personality problems.

Ideally you and your doctor need to establish a good working relationship, based on mutual respect, where each listens to the other and fully appreciates the special contribution *each* of you can make, as allies, to the fight against the arthritis. It's a partnership that might have to last a long time.

Some of us have been lucky enough to find a correct diagnosis and wonderfully supportive doctor right away. Others haven't. I've seen both extremes and some in between! The first doctor I saw with my aches and pains, when I was ten, diagnosed and treated me for flat feet. When that didn't help, he said the arches were too high. It wasn't until an agonising year later that I found another doctor who made a correct diagnosis, and then backed it up with effective treatment and support.

A few years later another doctor alienated me by saying 'Stop worrying about it. Go out and enjoy yourself' − instead of trying to understand and help me work through the physical and emotional agony I was suffering. Happily I now have a wonderful medical team in my GP, rheumatologist and orthopaedic surgeon. They can't give me a magic cure, but they do give me continuing support and understanding, and help me tackle specific problems as they crop up.

What we most certainly don't want, but sometimes get, alas, is a doctor like Liz W's*:

"He wanted to put me into a home as I was very dependent physically, but I'm blessed with fantastic parents. They wouldn't hear of it...He'd told me there was no future for me as a person in 'the outside world', well I couldn't accept that either so after a few days at home I contacted my local Disablement Resettlement Officer, he got me the interview for my job and the rest is past history. Two weeks before I started work I had to return to the doctor – when I told him of my plans he said 'you won't last a week'. – I've been there for 12 years – needless to say I didn't go to see him any more!"

Why can diagnosis sometimes be such a problem?

The trouble is that inflammatory arthritis takes so many different forms and even the same condition can start in many different ways. Maybe you were gradually aware of recurring aches and pains, and stiffness, in hands or feet or other joints. Or perhaps it started dramatically, taking you completely by surprise, so that several joints were suddenly acutely swollen and painful, and you could hardly move. Or it could have started with something completely different, like skin trouble, or a rash, as in psoriatic arthritis or lupus. With around 200 different rheumatic disorders, to say nothing of thousands of other conditions, the doctor's got plenty to choose from. Horribly frustrating for you, wondering what on earth's happening and just wanting to have it over and done with.

Marie Joseph, the writer, was 24 years old, with a small baby and a husband just back from the air force, when she found she had RA:

"My wrist grew steadily more painful, and I developed twinges in my knees, but refused to acknowledge them, working on the theory that the human body can only cope with one pain at a time. I found a way of fastening a nappy with my left hand and my teeth, and discovered that opening doors, turning on taps, holding a pencil, became virtually impossible..." (*One Step at a Time*, Arrow Books)

Corbet Woodall, former BBC TV newsreader, was 38, and on his second honeymoon when he noticed a *"permanent nagging pain in my hands and feet"*. Soon his hands looked a trifle swollen. Luckily he mentioned it to a doctor friend, who quickly worked out it was RA.

As a young man, Norman Cousins developed ankylosing spondylitis. It started with a slight fever, then rapidly worsening general feeling of achiness. Soon he found it difficult to move his neck, arms, hands, fingers, and legs, and at one point, his jaws were almost locked. The bones in his spine and almost every other part of his body felt *"as though I had been run over by a truck."* (*Anatomy of an Illness*, Bantam 1987)

Phil Smith, former Chairman of the '35 Group' for YPAs, had her first attack of RA when she was expecting her first baby:

"It started with aches and pains in one arm right at the end of the pregnancy. I came out of hospital two weeks after Christopher was born and a few days later I felt a bit fluey. I went to bed but when I tried to get up for his night feed I literally couldn't move." In spite of her swollen joints, her doctor wasn't sure at first what was wrong with her. *"Then I went back and mentioned that my mother had arthritis, could I have it too? That was it. I was diagnosed at once. In a way I was lucky. Being diagnosed quickly meant I could start taking drugs to ease the inflammation and prevent the joints being permanently damaged."* (In *Woman* magazine, 5 May 1984)

Diagnosis is based on masses of questions about your symptoms and medical history, a physical examination, plus special tests (eg blood tests to look at the Erythrocyte Sedimentation Rate (ESR), tests for the 'rheumatoid factor' (see page 14), a urine test, maybe X-rays and goodness knows what else. Maddeningly, tests aren't always conclusive – for instance the rheumatoid factor isn't always present in the blood of someone with RA, and even if it is – it's also found in perfectly healthy individuals who never develop it. A strongly positive test, however, usually means active RA or lupus. Early AS pain down the legs may be misinterpreted by an inexperienced doctor as sciatica (a disc in the back pressing down on a nerve). So all in all, making a correct diagnosis isn't always straightforward, and may take time.

Why do some doctors seem unhelpful?

Alas, some doctors (not all by any means) don't always seem as helpful as we'd like. Let's look at some of the reasons why there may be problems. These help to explain why we need to work at being as fully informed as possible about the disorder itself and ways of dealing with it. My feeling is that it helps everyone if we try to understand these problems rather than pretend they don't exist. Once we've got them out of the way we can look at our doctors' many undoubted talents!

One major problem is slowly disappearing, thanks to work by rheumatologists and ARC on improving the education and training of GPs. At medical school too many GPs were taught too little about rheumatology, despite the fact that *"in aggregate approximately 23 per cent of patients seen by GPs have some sort of rheumatic condition"* (ARC's report *Arthritis and Rheumatism in the Eighties*). It's depressing to read a report as recent as 1986 identifying a major problem as *"deficiencies in the rheumatological training of many earlier generations of general practitioners, so that inappropriate use is often made of rheumatological services and many patients who could be helped at primary level are deprived of such help."* Rheumatology's a rapidly changing and highly complex area, and it's crucial for doctors to keep up to date.

I've mentioned this problem not to depress you, but so that, firstly, you're not surprised at finding it's sometimes up to *you* to put ideas into your doctor's head (but *tactfully* – s/he *has* spent years acquiring considerably more medical knowledge than most of us). Secondly, so that you might be inspired to add your voice to patient-pressure to get such problems sorted out. National provision of rheumatologists is still woefully poor. They're needed not just to treat patients, or carry out research, but to educate GPs and other healthcare professionals too.

Fortunately the picture's slowly changing, and many doctors do make special efforts to increase their knowledge, through in-service courses and publications from ARC and other organisations. Recently, GPs particularly interested in the rheumatic diseases have formed a 'Primary Care Society', which meets several times a year.

GPs need more training, too, in how best to help a patient deal generally with an unpredictable chronic illness. Some GPs already have these skills, others don't. When curing isn't yet possible, they need to expand their caring skills, and be fully aware of other sources of help (not just medical) to guide us to.

Other 'doctor problems' may simply be due to personality. There's the 'aloof and distant approach', where s/he identifies the illness, hands you a prescription, and more or less says go away and get on with learning to live with it. Or there's the doctor who knows his curable illnesses back-to-front but is flummoxed at having to deal with an 'incurable' illness. S/he may be very caring, but upset at not knowing how to help, or may not want to admit to uncertainty in case you lose confidence in him/her. S/he ends up telling you little or nothing at all, and you may feel angry and upset as a result.

Not nearly as helpful as the doctor who's honest about problems and what s/he doesn't know, but who reassures you there *are* ways of 'managing' the arthritis, and reassures you of unfailing support as you learn to outwit it. Different approaches work for different people at different times, and your doctor-patient partnership will need to keep working on this, together.

Good communication's essential, with each of you respecting and listening to the other. Fortunately it's now being realised that much more time should be spent on teaching medical students 'communicating skills'. Cambridge University even has a full-time teacher of doctor-patient communication skills. Kathleen McGrath's book (page 39) includes tips on improving the doctor/patient communication process.

Referral to a specialist
Some people are treated entirely by their GP; others will be referred to a hospital rheumatologist, nearby if you're lucky, or you might have to travel quite a way. GPs build up expertise in many areas, but it's the rheumatologist who has the most thorough and up-to-date knowledge of the more complicated rheumatic disorders.

These usually require a team approach. You and your GP start the ball rolling, drawing upon other experts as required, eg rheumatologist, physio, OT, nurse, social worker, chiropodist (see pages 37 - 39). The team spreads outside the medical profession to include family and friends, and perhaps a self-help group.

Referral to a specialist has to be through your GP (even if you want private treatment from that specialist). If your GP doesn't refer you, ask what s/he thinks of the idea. Try something like 'I'd be interested in having a specialist opinion...' If you know where the nearest rheumatology clinic is, you could add 'I believe there's a rheumatology clinic at... Could you please refer me there?' Find out where from reference books in your library, or from your local Community Health Council (CHC – see page 119) or Arthritis Care. Check how easy or difficult it might be for you to get there, but don't let difficulties put you off: many can be overcome.

If your GP won't agree to refer you, then ask (politely) why not. You could discuss his view with, perhaps, your Young Arthritis Care Contact or local CHC. With the more complicated disorders you really should seek specialist advice as early as possible. So much can be done, especially if they're caught early and treated with up-to-date expertise. I'd rather be referred to a specialist who says there's little or nothing after all to worry about, than endure the possibly long-term serious effects of delayed or refused referral.

Referral might mean just a one-off visit with advice from the specialist to your GP on how best to continue treating you. Or specialist and GP might decide to work together, each keeping the other informed about progress. A common misunderstanding is that the specialist is superior to the GP. In fact the GP doesn't hand over responsibility for you to the specialist. S/he's just asking for supplementary support and know-how. Specialists have great expertise, but in a comparatively narrow area. It's still your GP who oversees your care, and holds full details of your medical history. Your GP can act as an interpreter, explaining to you what the specialist has recommended, and discussing in more detail the advantages and disadvantages of proposed forms of treatment in the context of your particular circumstances, which s/he may know more about than the specialist. Referral for other services, eg physiotherapy, occupational therapy, is also best done through your GP/rheumatologist, though referral isn't always compulsory (page 38).

What can you and your healthcare team do? – 'Managing' the arthritis

What you probably want first is relief from pain and stiffness, and help to get going again. And information – what exactly have you got, will it get worse, how long will it last, what's the cure, what can your doctor do for you, what *shouldn't* you do, and what *should* you do for the best?

Treatment for inflammatory arthritis means much more than a prescription for drugs, and 'management' is a better way of describing what happens. The best approach for each person varies according to diagnosis, severity of symptoms, previous treatment, drug history, age, particular personal circumstances, and how things progress. A trial-and-error approach may be necessary, especially with drugs – you and your healthcare team may need to try out several different ones before finding out what's best for you.

At the centre of your management team is *you*, and you need to find out (with help where necessary) how best *to help yourself*, eg how and when your drugs should be taken and what they're expected to do, how best to balance rest and exercise, how to avoid joint-straining habits and activity, how to adjust your lifestyle to cope, etc.

Yes, arthritis *is* manageable. But what about that bleak word 'incurable', thrown at you? True, the cause and cure of most rheumatic disorders like RA and AS aren't yet known, so there's no 'instant cure' yet, *but*:

- you may have RA or another inflammatory arthritis in a mild form – lots of people do – and it may remain mild and even disappear altogether, possibly very quickly.
- many inflammatory arthritic conditions are 'fluctuating' disorders. There are ups as well as downs, better periods as well as worse periods.
- your disorder may become less active, even inactive. A 'remission' may last a few days, weeks, months, years, or even for ever. This can happen in children, for instance, as they leave their teenage years, or during the menopause. There is *always* this hope of a remission at the back of our minds.
- there's plenty going on in research. While we wait for a cure, better understanding of auto-immune disorders like RA and lupus means treatments are constantly improving, and chronic gout, for instance, is now fully controllable.
- there's so much you can do to help yourself, and to help others help you. Outwitting the arthritis means learning new skills. Like learning to drive a car or a new language, it takes time and dedication, but *is* possible.
- last but not least – out here there are plenty of us who would like you to know that it most definitely is possible to live with RA or AS or whatever and enjoy life, even if you and we'd most definitely prefer to be *without* it. People with arthritis *do* keep jobs, *do* marry and have children, *do* do their fair share of enhancing the lives of other people, *do* give as well as 'take'. People *do* learn how to cope with a variable disorder, how to get through the bad or worse times and how to make the most of the good or better times when they appear.

Generally speaking, managing the arthritis will involve one or more of the following (plus other more specific bits and pieces where necessary):

Medical and practical management:
- Explanations and information from the doctor (not all at once!) to help you understand your disorder and what you and your team can do about it.
- Drugs. Prescription of drugs, information about them, and a continuing review of how they and your body are getting on together. More about drugs in chapter 5.
- Physiotherapy. Guidance on rest and exercise, joint care, posture, use of splints, walking devices, use of heat, cold, hydrotherapy, manipulation. Some physiotherapy overlaps with OT help (see chapter 6).
- Occupational therapy (OT). Guidance and help with adjusting your lifestyle, and with learning to be as independent as possible. Help with learning to make the most of reduced time, energy and strength, and help with sorting out difficulties in personal care, domestic activities, mobility at home and outside, leisure activities, work.
- Referral to other specialists and sources of information and help as necessary.

Non-medical, emotional and psychological aspects:
- Effective medical and practical management will help you cope psychologically, too. Pain control, advice on joint care, helpful gadgets are all 'sanity-savers', each doing their bit to cut down on frustrations and anger and misery.
- Sometimes help from a social worker may be appropriate, eg advice on social and financial problems, on children, family difficulties.
- Other people can do so much to help you keep going. Our nearest and dearest, just 'being there', can give love and courage and moral support. Sometimes, though, the whole 'You plus Nearest-and-Dearest plus Arthur Itis' triangle can create its own problems to be worked through. More about arthritis and close relationships in later

chapters. Sometimes you may need to turn to outsiders who can give support with less emotional involvement. Good friends or neighbours, maybe, or a patient support group, or a good social worker, or welfare officer at work, even the Samaritans. Some of us live on our own, far from family, and may need even more help from outsiders.

● Your healthcare team can help with non-medical problems too. Your doctor, especially, will certainly want to know about anything worrying you, and just might have a solution. Good doctors know too how helpful simply the right attitude of caring and taking an interest can be. Often it's not specially important what s/he says, just the simple act of them taking an interest is helpful. JCA has been my companion for many years. My medical treatment doesn't change much from consultation to consultation, but my rheumatologist's understanding and interest continues. That's just as important as drugs or physiotherapy, though not always rated as highly as it should be. If your doctor doesn't have the right personality or sufficient time you might find other healthcare team members more supportive, eg the physio, or OT, or home help.

Professor David Locker, of St Thomas' Medical School, did some detailed research into the experiences of 24 people with RA, and he recognised clearly that:

"Medicine has other important functions which go beyond mere therapeutic intervention. It is a source of knowledge... It is also a source of hope... [Patients] also looked to medicine and its practitioners for social and psychological support and, arguably, this was its most significant contribution...It appeared that much was to be gained when doctors maintained an interest in their clinical condition and their personal and social affairs, if only because they felt valued as a result." (*Disability and Disadvantage*, Routledge/Tavistock, 1983)

● Though your healthcare team can help you find out about sources of non-medical help, they simply can't know everything. So the more you can find out for yourself too, the better. I hope this book will give you plenty of information and ideas to help you help yourself. Given time and persistence and information and experience so much that seems insoluble can be sorted out. Helping yourself can make you feel good too, can make you feel more independent and 'in control' again.

● Experience and tips of other people with your type of arthritis can help. Many have become experts at 'living with arthritis'. Better *not* to seek their advice on medical aspects, though. Leave that to the medical experts.

● If you're tempted to try some form of 'alternative/complementary medicine', read chapter 10, and check first with your doctor that it won't do any harm. Some people do find help that way, but you do need to be sure it won't harm you or cost a fortune.

Some tips on being an expert patient

Remember you're in partnership with your doctor. S/he's the medical expert, but you, the patient, can do a lot to help make the most of that expertise.

Getting organised

Get two foolscap cardboard wallets from a stationer's, or use a couple of large envelopes or cardboard boxes or plastic carrier bags. The first is for your personal 'Medikit', the second is for your 'Infokit' (see page 112). Keep in your Medikit things like:

● addresses, phone numbers, working hours, of your healthcare team
● your personal 'medical notebook' for your own notes on treatment, drugs, etc (a pocket-sized one could go with you to the doctor's)
● appointment cards (in a perspex season ticket holder, with the next appointment visible on top
● your NHS card, your national insurance number, address of local DSS office, details of

your firm's sick leave regulations, your 'Green Card' (if registered disabled), pharmacist treatment card (if yours issues them)

- information from physio/OT (exercises, rest plan, joint care tips, etc)
- your 'Personal Needs list' (if applicable), quick self-reminder, eg when visiting a new doctor, writing for a college place, phoning a hotel to see if it's accessible. (My Personal Needs List includes high chair (over 24" from ground) and bed (over 28" from ground), non-slip mat in bath, shoes with 1¼" heel, no buckles, etc.)
- name and address of local Young Arthritis Care Contact plus address and your membership number, plus details for any other relevant groups
- your 'Personal Abilities List' (your 'PAL'!) as a reminder and a morale-booster in times of doubt!
- plus anything else you can think of...

Homework: preparing for visits to the doctor

Worries are understandable. Will you get there on time and in reasonable shape? Will you remember the questions you want to ask? Do some seem too stupid to ask? What questions will the doctor ask you? Will there be time for everything? Will it all be too rushed and feel a let-down afterwards? A little homework beforehand will help cut down on nervousness and forgetfulness. It'll help increase mutual respect, too.

Don't forget appointments! After each visit note the next right away in a diary and on a wall calendar, hanging up where you can check it regularly (by the telephone?). If you can't keep an appointment phone well in advance to explain. If you have problems getting to appointments, find they're too frequent, or whatever, talk to the doctor or nurse and see if between you you can't solve the problem. Write a polite letter if that's easier.

Keep your personal medical notebook always handy to jot things down between visits. For instance, questions about your drugs, about something you've read and don't understand, about things you find you can't do, or are specially worrying you. Sort them into some sort of order just before the appointment. Don't produce a vast encyclopaedia! But a few careful, concise questions/thoughts/worries/ideas can help both you and your doctor.

If you're going to have lots to talk about you could try asking well beforehand if it's possible to have a 'double appointment'; or, a trick I occasionally find helpful, write a letter to the doctor at least a week beforehand, putting some of the more important points (keep a copy to take with you as a reminder). For instance I needed my doctor's considered opinion on my mobility allowance application, and on an ankle op, so I wrote a letter first. It helped me get my thoughts in order and gave the doctor time to prepare a helpful response.

Prepare beforehand for doctor's questions that crop up regularly. For instance, s/he will ask: 'How are you?' You: 'Well, I've been feeling reasonably OK most of the time, except for two particular problems – my left wrist and right ankle.' Prepare for pain/stiffness questions. For instance, where do you feel the pain? When? Early morning? After exercise? After rest? How long does it last? What sort of pain – stabbing? dull ache? Does it radiate/spread out? What seems to make it better or worse? Some doctors and patients develop their own pain measurement system, eg using a scale of 1 to 10, where 10 is utterly unbearable and 1 is minor discomfort. I think and talk about pain in 'noise' terms, so a minor pain is a 'whisper' or 'quiet', getting 'louder' until it screams.

Jot down any seemingly insoluble non-medical worries too, even if you've no idea whether or how the doctor might help, eg 'I'd really like to have a baby, doctor, but my husband just doesn't see how we could cope' or 'My wife keeps nagging me to help around the house; – she doesn't seem to understand how stiff I am and what an effort everything is.' Step number one in finding a solution is to talk about it. If the doctor doesn't have an answer, s/he might know someone else who can help.

Bear in mind that contact with a GP or specialist doesn't have to be limited to face-to-face appointments only. For people like us with mobility problems and a possibly long-term disorder, sensible use of letters and telephone is a useful occasional alternative. By telephoning, I don't mean ringing up and demanding to speak to the doctor there and then, but a phone call to say something like "I'm worried about 'x' (eg side-effect with a drug) – could the doctor possibly phone me back when s/he's got a moment?" Some surgeries have special times for dealing with non-urgent problems over the phone.

Actual visits

Early visits concentrate on diagnosis, explanations, and advice on treatment. At follow-up visits your doctor will check how you're getting on, and probably continue to look at specific joints, may measure particular movements, grip strength, ask what you can/can't do, ask about morning stiffness, stiffness at other times, swelling, tenderness, pain, fatigue, your weight, how you're getting on with drugs/other treatment/aids/splints, arrange tests (blood, urine, etc). Don't forget early referral to a physio and OT is a good idea.

Getting there   Plan beforehand how best to get there, and allow plenty of time. Wear easy-to-manage clothes in case the doctor needs to examine you or wants a sleeve rolled up for a blood-test. Take any gadgets you might need. There's usually someone around to help but I always like to take my own stocking puller-on and folding 'easy-reach' gadget, for instance. Don't forget your medical notebook and questions. You might want to take a friend/relative along for practical or moral support; your partner, maybe, to help him/her better understand what's happening. It might help oil any squeaky wheels in your relationship.

How you feel during the visit   If you feel nervous, why not tell the doctor, so s/he understands? Your homework will help too. Don't feel embarrassed about checking your notes in front of the doctor, or jotting down what s/he says. Your doctor makes notes; why not you too? Do you feel inhibited if students are present? You can ask beforehand to see the doctor alone, if you prefer, or, during the consultation, ask 'could I talk to you privately for a couple of minutes?'

Do you get bolshy and exasperated, rather than nervous? Try to keep things polite and friendly and avoid grumbling accusingly at the doctor. Explain how you feel and ask for support. You can express misery without blaming the doctor for it! Doctors are human too, and more likely to respond to encouragement than criticism. Remind yourself you're in partnership together, against the arthritis. Use the word 'we' as a simple reminder to both of you – for instance, 'is there something else we could try, doctor?', instead of confronting the doctor with a 'what are *you* going to do about things, doc?' approach.

If you've an unhelpful doctor, count to ten under your breath and vow to give him/her a fair chance while you (subtly) re-educate him/her. Re-read my earlier notes explaining some reasons for apparent 'unhelpfulness'. In the last resort you could change your GP (see page 37). If your specialist is unhelpful, discuss the difficulties with your GP.

Questions and answers   Be honest in your answers to the doctor's questions! So often we YPAs 'put on a brave face' to avoid boring other people with our problems, or whatever. This can become such a habit that we forget to drop the mask at the doctor's. Don't feel too proud or too brave or whatever to say how you really feel behind the mask.

Remember, doctors aren't mind-readers. And they're unlikely to know your notes and case history back to front. So, for instance, if you've developed a slight rash, and think 'oh, it's not worth mentioning unless the doctor says something' you're wrong! – It's up to *you* to mention it. There are 1001 reasons why s/he might not ask the right question or notice anything, but it could still be important. When you see a different doctor from normal, it's *especially* important not to assume s/he's read your case history and knows all your allergies/peculiarities/drugs you're on/whether you're pregnant/whatever.

Keep time limits in mind, but don't let that stop you bringing up important points. Bring up the most important ones first, using your notebook as a reminder if necessary. For instance, when s/he says 'How are you?', you might reply 'Not too good, doctor. There are three main things I'd like to mention to you...'

Get worries into the open – is it infectious? hereditary? what about having children? could you end up in a wheelchair? what can *you* do to help yourself? etc.

Bear in mind that since there's still a lot to be discovered about rheumatic disorders there may not always be an answer, or the explanation might be horribly complex (some of the finer points of the immune system, for instance, are thoroughly mind-boggling), or you might need to look elsewhere for the answer. But, I repeat, don't hesitate to ask. Apart from anything else, it helps the doctor understand more about you. You won't necessarily get many answers at any one time, not just because time's limited, but also because the amount of information anyone can comfortably absorb at any one time is limited too. ARC publications will answer some questions, and help you prepare others for the doctor.

If you're puzzled by something the doctor says, do ask, and ask again if necessary. Ways I use to help myself listen and understand are repeating it back to the doctor slightly differently, asking a question, or jotting a note down, especially on medication. The doctor can check you've noted the drug name and dosage correctly, or could even write it for you.

If you don't agree or have doubts about something, say so, tactfully. For instance, 'What you suggested worries me a bit, doctor...' Apparently much treatment is misused or simply *not* used, because patients either don't understand or disagree, silently, with it. Talking about your doubts or difficulties might mean your partnership decides to try something else instead, or perhaps postpone the treatment for a while, like Phil:

> *"[My consultant] has been really great, understanding why I have refused to go in for treatment, and even gave me tea with sympathy when I needed it just recently. Anyway, we've come to a compromise and I've agreed to go in at the end of the week."*

Doubts or queries about drugs are common, so do talk them through. Be sure to understand what they've been prescribed for – stiffness? pain? inflammation control? what dosage, how often to take them, before or after meals, whether there are any special side-effects you should look out for, effect on daily routine, etc (see chapter 5).

Before you leave summarise out loud what plans you've made together about drugs, treatment, etc, and what to do if a problem comes back, or gets worse.

After a visit

Make a note of your next appointment in your diary and on your appointments calendar. Think about what happened and get the important things clear in your mind. Work out how to fit advised changes into your life – eg fitting in a midday rest period, cutting down on particular physical activities. Work out how best to remember to take your drugs and how best to fit in regular prescribed exercises. You might think of questions about the treatment prescribed and wish you'd asked the doctor in the surgery. If so, leave a phone message for him/her or write.

Give any treatment a fair trial. Remember, a lot of arthritis treatment involves a sort of trial-and-error approach. Maybe one drug and your stomach don't get on together. Well, OK, the doctor can then suggest another drug, or maybe the same drug in a different form.

Factfile

The health services are going through many changes at present. For up-to-date information contact your local Community Health Council (CHC). CHCs provide information and advice on local health services and the NHS (see also page 119).

Two other bodies offering help and advice to patients are the Patients' Association (see page 122) and the College of Health (see page 119). Together with the Consumers' Association the PA has published *A Patient's Guide to the National Health Service* (cheapish), which covers all aspects from the consumer's point of view.

Finding a GP
GPs are listed in the Family Health Services Authority (FHSA, formerly FPC) list, available in most major libraries and post offices, Citizen's Advice Bureaux (CABs) and CHCs. The FHSA list includes information on partners in a practice and surgery hours. The *Medical Directory* (in most libraries) gives doctors' qualifications. Ask friends and neighbours for personal views, too, but allow for any possible bias!

Changing a GP
Look at the instructions on your NHS medical card. You can register with another GP without any special formalities, but check first that the new doctor will accept you as a patient. Take your NHS card along to the surgery of the new doctor and the administration staff there should be able to sort out any formalities for you. Bear in mind that it may take a while for your medical records to be transferred. Though it's not obligatory to ask or inform your old GP, it's polite and helpful, if you can let him/her know.

GP help away from home
You can obtain 'immediately necessary treatment' from any GP for up to 14 days, if you are away from home or have no permanent doctor.

Complaints
Procedures are complicated. Consult your local Community Health Council for advice. There are time limits, so don't delay seeking advice if you feel you do need to complain.

You and your rights
The National Consumer Council has published a free leaflet, and a low cost book *Patients' Rights: A Guide for NHS Patients and Doctors* (available from HMSO). The Patients' Association (page 122) publishes *Rights of the Patient: A Guide to the Patient's Legal Rights*.

One right we sometimes forget – You can choose *not* to have a particular treatment or examination (with a few exceptions like infectious illnesses). You're quite entitled to think for a while about what's recommended before deciding, or might want to discuss it futher with your GP. Remember too you can ask your doctor whether s/he can speed things up if you've been waiting ages for a hospital appointment: s/he may or may not be successful.

Going private
If you want private medical care from a specialist, you still need to be referred by a GP (NHS GP *or* private GP – it doesn't matter which). Some GPs may charge for making a private referral. (See also page 63, on going private.)

Who else might be in your healthcare team and what do they do?

Here are the names of some specialists, and what they specialise in: orthopaedic surgeon (bones and joints), dermatologist (skin problems including psoriasis, scleroderma, lupus rashes), ophthalmologist (eyes), gastroenterologist (digestive system and intestines), cardiologist (heart conditions), urologist (bladder, kidneys, urinary system), haematologist (blood problems), chest specialist, radiologist (supervises taking of X-rays (by a radiographer) and reports on results).

Nurses   All qualified nurses have the basic qualification SRN (State Registered Nurse) or SEN (State Enrolled Nurse). Studies for SRNs are more academically demanding than for SENs. SRNs may also have further specialist qualifications. Some nurses work in hospitals (see page 57), others are community nurses.

Dietitians   They usually work in hospitals, advising catering staff, doctors and patients on appropriate diets, eg for overweight patients, diabetic patients. In some areas GPs can refer patients directly to a local hospital dietitian.

Referral to paramedical services
It isn't always essential to be referred to other paramedical services via your GP or hospital specialist, though it's wise to try that route first, so that important details of your medical history can be passed on. Unfortunately, even with self-referral, there may still be a waiting list for appointments or treatment. RADAR's Health and Social Services Factsheet 1 gives more information about access to paramedical services, and what initials to look out for to ensure a particular paramedic is professionally qualified. Some paramedics can make home visits, and some are in private practice.

Physiotherapists   Physios work in hospitals and the community, usually receiving patients by referral, though you can refer yourself directly too. Only state-registered chartered physiotherapists (MCSP or SRP after their name) are allowed to work in the NHS.

Physios assess, treat, and rehabilitate patients by 'non-invasive methods' ie not using surgery or drugs. They're trained in manipulation, massage, movement, exercise, heat and cold treatments (eg wax and ice), electrotherapy, infra-red and ultra-sound, hydrotherapy, massage and traction, etc. (More about physios in chapter 6.)

Occupational therapists (OTs)   OTs are employed by hospitals and social services departments. You can refer yourself to the social services OT or be referred by GP or consultant. Make sure they have the initials DipCOT and/or SROT after their names.

OTs are trained to assess and help patients sort out functional and practical problems at home, at work, in personal care, mobility, leisure activities. They can advise on joint care and self-management, aids and adaptations, and can also liaise with other departments, eg about meals-on-wheels, home helps, if necessary. The OTs' three year full-time training includes medical, psychiatric, psychological and social subjects. (More about OTs in chapter 6.)

Chiropodists   They deal with foot problems. Treatment of painful corns, advice on shoe choice, etc, can make a real difference to some pain and mobility problems. Chiropodists can be seen with or without referral from your doctor, but be sure you see only a state-registered chiropodist, with the initials SRCh (the Society of Chiropodists can help you find one). SRCH means the chiropodist has completed a three year full-time course of training and is professionally approved by the NHS. Home visits can be arranged if you're housebound.

Only some people are eligible for free NHS chiropody treatment, including people under 18, people with diabetes, pregnant women and registered disabled people. In some areas, other people with a long-term illness may also qualify.

Subjects covered in chiropodists' training include theoretical and practical chiropody, anatomy, dermatology, life sciences, medicine, microbiology, pathology, pharmacology, surgery, local analgesia and skin surgery, appliance construction and shoe fitting. (See also page 55)

Orthotists They assess, fit and supply people with surgical splints, shoes and other appliances. You need to be referred by your GP and consultant.

Social workers Those working in local social services departments deal with community care services, providing help with financial or domestic problems, and liaison with other services and organisations. You can refer yourself for this help.

Pharmacists Make use of their drugs/medication expertise, as well as the doctor's, on questions like when best to take medicine, use ointment, possible side-effects, drug interactions with other medication, advice on drug storage, interactions with drinking and driving. If you need a prescription in an emergency, and a doctor isn't available, a pharmacist is allowed to supply it, but only if it's a medicine previously prescribed for you. Even then s/he may only provide a limited amount until the doctor can be contacted. (More about pharmacists on page 42)

Publications

CHCs, the Patients' Association, and the College of Health are the best sources of up-to-date information (see page 37), but some information in these two books may be relevant, too:

– *You and Your GP. A Handbook for Patients* by Kathleen McGrath (Bedford Square Press, 1990, available by post from Harper & Row Distributors). Packed with practical information to help you understand and make the most of GPs, specialists, and some aspects of the NHS. Kathleen McGrath trained and tutored in paediatric intensive care at the Great Ormond Street and Middlesex Hospitals, and is now Director of the Medical Advisory Service. MAS provides a central source of information and advice on healthcare treatments – from official organisations to the latest information on medical matters, and there's a MAS helpline, staffed by nurses, which provides medical advice of a non-diagnostic nature. (Send SAE for free leaflet about MAS; there's also a free leaflet with suggestions on how to improve the doctor/patient communication process.)

– *The Patients' Companion* by Dr Vernon Coleman (Corgi, 1986) is an 'all-in-one-guide to health care', full of information about the health services in Britain. Some of the 1986 edition will now be out-of-date, though some will still be helpful. A nice personal tone runs through it, so it's very readable, and Dr Coleman makes clear when he's expressing a personal view which might not be shared by others.

Chapter five

DRUG THERAPY

As yet, alas, the magic cure hasn't been found, but while we wait impatiently there are many different drugs the doctor can choose from to help us control pain, inflammation and stiffness, and make life more bearable. Different treatments work for different people at different times, so the first drug you try won't necessarily prove to be the most effective one for you and your unique body make-up. Don't despair. Persevere at working with your doctor to produce a tailor-made treatment. Try to be (dare I say it?) patient.

More about specific drugs later. First, some general points. A 'drug' is basically any substance that can alter the structure or change the way the body normally functions. Changes can be beneficial or harmful, or a mixture of the two. 'Drugs' used in medicine are intended to be beneficial. Some people place too much faith in drugs, others go to the other extreme and reject their help completely. However, used with care and respect, the right drug can keep you going and make life liveable again. Why make life more difficult than it need be?

Maximising benefits and minimising risks

Drugs alone won't solve all your problems. It's important to remember that drug therapy's only one item in a much larger 'Outwit Arthritis Kit'. The Kit should include *non*-drug pain control too, eg the right balance of rest and exercise, joint protection, control of body weight, pacing and planning of activities, keeping yourself occupied. 'Simple' traditional remedies such as warm-water bathing, or using a walking-stick to relieve pressure on a tender hip are examples of Kit items which may be just as effective, and sometimes more effective than a drug. Even if you have to take *some* drugs, these non-drug measures can help you keep drug dosage down with maximum benefits. (See also chapter 11.)

Stories about serious unwanted drug side-effects ('adverse drug reactions' – jargonised as 'ADRs') can be worrying, but need to be kept in perspective. As Dr Dudley Hart points out: *"Remember that any medicine, whatever its virtues, also has the power to do you harm"* (In *Overcoming Arthritis*). For every patient with arthritis who develops a problem with a drug there are many others who've benefited.

It surprises many people to learn that even 'alternative remedies', bought in health food shops, can cause unwanted side-effects, sometimes serious (see page 75). You can even overdose harmfully on the usually very healthy carrot! Drugs bought over-the-counter or that we've been using for centuries have their risks too. The familiar aspirin, originally derived from the willow tree, is very powerful, potentially even harmful, but used as prescribed, with care, can be beneficial too.

Even a cup of tea or coffee is a drug. Both contain caffeine, one of whose side-effects is to make you want to pass urine more frequently. Caffeine's also a stimulant – keeps you awake and alert – so don't complain about insomnia if you've been drinking coffee before going to bed! Not all side-effects are unwanted. Many of us actually like the side-effects of a drop or two of alcohol. Some side-effects turn out to be unexpectedly beneficial. Anti-malarial drugs unexpectedly turned out to be effective for some rheumatic disorders, for instance, so did gold, originally used for treating TB.

Since the thalidomide tragedy of the early 1960s, testing and regulation of new drugs has been tightened up though inevitably not all side-effects come to light before a drug is approved for public use. My personal preference is always where possible to go for a drug that's been in use for some time, where the risks are more likely to be known, and I try to find out all I can about it from a reliable source.

As with so many things in life (crossing the road, driving a car, etc) taking drugs for a rheumatic disorder is a calculated risk. Do the benefits outweigh any risks? Many side-effects are minor, and you and your doctor may decide they're worth living with for the sake of the benefits. It's also a question of ensuring everyone concerned (manufacturer, doctor and patient) is each doing their bit to minimise risks. I've included some notes and a booklist in this chapter to help you.

Choosing drugs

You, the patient, your GP and/or specialist each has a part to play in working out what's best for you and your unique body. It's essential that your past medical history, any allergies, any previous adverse drug reactions, your general health and habits are all taken into account. The doctor will also look at any other drugs you're already taking, to avoid harmful interactions, since many drugs don't mix well together.

It's your responsibility as well as the doctor's to make sure that everything important is taken into account, *especially* if you're seeing a different doctor from normal, as often happens. Don't take it for granted s/he's read your medical history thoroughly. Don't be too scared or over-awed to say anything. Much better to *say* you've got this or that allergy, or past liver disease, or are taking the contraceptive pill, or whatever, than to assume the doctor's done all the homework and thinking for you.

Mention any over-the-counter or alternative medicines you take too, for instance for colds, headaches, travel sickness, anti-malaria (on holiday), etc. Just because drugs are easy to buy *doesn't* mean they're free of possible side-effects, especially if mixed with other drugs. Someone with psoriasis, for instance, bought a non-prescription over-the-counter drug to prevent malaria when on holiday: it made him very ill.

Above all, if you're pregnant, or thinking of becoming pregnant, mention that too. You should *not* take any drugs (including alternative remedies) without your doctor's agreement, if you're pregnant, or planning a pregnancy.

Be sure you understand certain basic facts about the drugs prescribed for you. Use the checklist below to make notes in your own Medikit notebook about each drug, and get the doctor to check what you've written is accurate. Include too the dates you started each drug, changed dosage, discontinued, or whatever; and any particular benefits or other reactions you noticed. Your record will help you, and will help your doctor and pharmacist, and any new doctor, help you too. Here's what you ought to know: −

Drugs Checklist

1 *The drug's name.* The 'generic' name is the most important name, the name applied worldwide to a particular combination of drug chemicals, and the name the doctor writes on the prescription, eg 'indomethacin'. There's also a brand name, for example 'Indocid' is the brand name used by Thomas Morson Pharmaceuticals for the indomethacin they manufacture. Unbranded (BP − British Pharmacopaeia) products are usually cheaper than branded products.

2 *Its purpose.* To control pain? inflammation? To fight infection (antibiotic)? Or?

3 *Its strength* (normally expressed in milligrams). If the doctor prescribes 'three capsules a day' what strength is each capsule? Indomethacin, for instance, comes in capsules of 25 mg and 50 mg, or a 'sustained release' capsule of 75mg. It's also available as an elixir (liquid) containing 25 mg per 5 ml, and as a suppository

(100mg). A drug described as 'retard' or 'slow release' means it's released into your system in a steadily controlled way over a period of time, rather than all at once.

4   *Frequency.*   How many times a day should you take it, and when? Before meals? With or after meals? Before you go to bed? Would a glass of milk or cup of tea plus biscuit do if you're not due for a meal?

5   *Benefits.*   How soon are you likely to see any? Some drugs show quick results, others take days or weeks and you'll be disappointed if you expect instant improvement.

6   *Adverse side-effects and their symptoms.*   What are they? What should you do if you suspect side-effects? Many side-effects are mild and hopefully the doctor will have warned you about them. But if you don't know what to do, contact your doctor and ask. Remember your hospital specialist writes to your GP after any changes in treatment, so you could contact either if problems arise. Some side-effects can be dealt with easily, for instance you might avoid gastric side-effects by changing to aspirin in a soluble or specially coated form, or by taking an anti-inflammatory in the form of a suppository instead of by mouth. (See the note on RAD-AR on page 49.)

7   *Interactions.*   Might the drug react badly with any other drugs or foods? Should you avoid alcohol? Alcohol in your body can be dangerous mixed with other drugs. I always take the precaution of leaving a very wide gap between any drugs and alcohol. A few years ago I waited some five hours after taking one commonly prescribed painkiller before having a drink but still had the most horrific reaction. No one had warned me at all. That drug does now carry a warning.

8   *What about reducing or stopping the drugs?*   You should check with your doctor first, as some drugs, steroids for instance, can be dangerous if stopped suddenly. But s/he might say you can reduce a painkiller when you are feeling less pain.

9   *No-nos.*   Is there anything you *shouldn't do* while taking the drug, such as driving a car or operating machinery? Some drugs impair judgement and concentration, with potentially dangerous results.

10   *If you miss a dose.*   What should you do?

At the pharmacist's/chemist's

Remember, you can check drug queries with the pharmacist as well as the doctor, even on the phone if need be. S/he has had at least four or five years' university education and training and is an expert on drugs; make the most of that expertise. Pharmacies are gradually changing to encourage the public to make more use of them, and some have counselling areas where patients can be seen in private.

Some have a system of Patient Medication Records (PMRs) which list each patient's name, address, age, chronic illness, drug allergies and previous drug reactions, and medicines prescribed. Before a new prescription's dispensed the card is checked to avoid errors or potentially harmful interactions.

If, like me, you can't manage 'child-proof' medicine bottle tops, say so as you hand the prescription over. Screw tops, or the sort you can lever off with your teeth can be substituted. If there *are* children around though do make sure your medicines are kept locked away out of sight and reach. Draw a sad face on the label, so if they do get hold of a bottle by mistake the face reminds them how they'd feel if they take a taste.

Read the instructions carefully on the bottle or package. If you don't understand, ask the pharmacist to explain. For instance if it says 'one to be taken every six hours' does that mean 'every six hours, day *and* night'? Some drugs should be taken only with food and some only on an empty stomach. If you're not sure, ask. It's important, and one way of avoiding some side-effects.

If you run out of your regular drugs (eg on holiday in Britain) and can't immediately obtain a prescription, you can ask a pharmacist for an emergency three days' supply (five days if a public holiday's included), provided the drug's not on a controlled list. S/he will need convincing your need's genuine and you may have to pay the full price.

Reducing prescription costs

If you qualify for exemption, prescriptions are free. Even if you don't qualify, buying a 'season ticket', officially called a 'prepayment certificate', can reduce costs if you need prescribed drugs regularly. Once purchased, it covers the cost of all your prescriptions for a set period, eg four months or 12 months. You apply using form FP95 (or EC95 in Scotland), available through a post office or from the DSS Leaflets Unit.

People who qualify for exemption include children under the age of 16, anyone over retirement age, pregnant mothers and those who have had a baby during the past 12 months, people on a low income, or with certain medical conditions. Arthritis/rheumatic disorders *aren't* included, and would only qualify you if deemed 'a continuing physical disability which prevents [you] leaving [your] residence without help...'.

Ways of remembering to take your drugs and avoid mistakes

Choose the best system for you:

- Keep a simple chart listing the drug name and strength, and actual times of day it should be taken. Tick it off each time you take the drug.
- Each day sort out the tablets for that day into a container (eg pillbox, egg cup). Be sure you know which tablet is which. Remember to keep them out of reach of children. You can buy purpose-built pill containers in which to sort out daily or weekly doses, but you'll need to check you can manage to open and close them. One sort 'bleeps' as a reminder! (A watch with an alarm, or a kitchen timer would do too.) Some of the firms listed on page 144 supply special containers.
- If the medicine's only to be taken with food and you're not due for a full meal at the time, do at least line your stomach first with a large glass of milk plus a biscuit or two. Avoid taking tablets while lying down – they'll reach your stomach and work quicker if you're upright.
- Never give your drugs to anyone else, and never try anyone else's, even if they have some form of arthritis. Even the same form of arthritis differs considerably from person to person and treatment must be tailor-made for each individual. What suits someone else could be dangerous for you.

Warning cards and MedicAlert

If you're on certain types of drugs (eg steroids, anti-diabetic drugs, anti-depressants, sedatives, tranquillisers) or if you have a particular drug allergy you should carry a warning card with you. Some drugs can cause serious problems if combined with other drugs, or if you have dental treatment, or need any sort of emergency treatment. The card's a safeguard in case you have an accident, fall unconscious and can't explain which drugs you're on.

Some people wear specially engraved bracelets or necklaces giving details of their condition. Ask your pharmacist for details. You could consider registering with the Medic-Alert Foundation. Members wear a special bracelet or necklet on which their particular medical problem and membership number is engraved together with the

Foundation's 24-hour emergency hotline number. Medical professionals can make a reverse charge call from anywhere in the world and receive information supplied by the wearer's doctor instantly.

Injections

> *"You know, we do take some prodding and 'messing around with', don't we? I sometimes feel like a pin cushion after the blood tests and gold injections!"*

So says Marilyn S, with feeling. She developed psoriatic arthritis in her 20s. However much you hate the thought of injections, try to avoid tensing the area being injected. Train yourself instead to relax it. Don't watch the needle going in. Shut your mind off from that area. Imagine a barrier sealing it off from the rest of you. Switch your mind to something pleasant instead. Plan beforehand what you'll think about.

Suppositories

Less likely to irritate the stomach than preparations taken by mouth, as they're inserted in the anus (though they may irritate existing ulcers via the blood stream). Make sure they're retained and don't pop out again (if they're put in back to front they may be retained better!). Inserting them may be difficult for some arthriticky hands. Some drug companies have produced special inserters, so ask your doctor about these if you have problems.

Some specific drugs

Do read all the general notes above. They apply to any medication you take. Drugs come in a variety of forms: as tablets, slow-release ('retard') preparations, capsules, powders, granules, syrups, inhalants; or as externally applied creams, ointments or gels; or given as injections or suppositories. Whatever form they come in, *all* have to be treated with the greatest care and respect, to maximise benefits and minimise possible problems. Always read, understand, and follow instructions carefully.

Drugs used to treat inflammatory arthritis like RA are usually divided into those tried first – 'first line drugs', and 'second line drugs', used for patients who don't respond well to first line drugs. Approaches differ according to the specific rheumatic disorder and individual patient. Be guided by your doctor.

The anatomy notes in chapter 2 and those on pain and pain control in chapter 11 may help you understand how the drugs work in your body, and the BMA's and Professor Parish's books mentioned on page 49 give reasonably dejargonised descriptions of individual drugs, possible adverse reactions, special precautions, and dosages.

NO INFORMATION IN THIS BOOK IS INTENDED TO BE A SUBSTITUTE FOR YOUR PRIMARY SOURCE OF EXPERT INFORMATION, WHICH IS YOUR DOCTOR.

First line drugs

These can be divided into 'analgesics' (non-narcotic and narcotic painkillers) and 'analgesic/anti-inflammatories'.

Analgesics (painkillers)

These help relieve pain but don't actually tackle inflammation or affect the progress of the the underlying disorder itself. Some (eg paracetamol) also relieve any feverish symptoms. You should normally take them with food (or glass of milk) to avoid stomach problems, but check with the doctor. Never take more than the dosage prescribed. If you think you need an increased dosage consult your doctor first. Ask if you can reduce the dosage on good days.

Analgesics basically work in two different ways. The first group (non-narcotic analgesics) work at the site of the pain, blocking chemicals (prostaglandins) which carry pain messages to the brain. The second group (narcotic analgesics) work in the brain, making it ignore any pain messages it receives. Non-drug pain control methods are thought to work in these two different ways, as well – see chapter 11.

1 Non-narcotic analgesics Low-dose aspirin is one. In low dosage aspirin is a simple analgesic: in higher dosage it becomes an analgesic/anti-inflammatory. (More details in that section, below.) Another non-narcotic analgesic is paracetamol, a mild pain-reliever, useful for patients who can't tolerate aspirin. No effect on inflammation. Side effects are usually mild but paracetamol should not be used by patients with liver or kidney disease. Overdosage causes severe liver damage.

2 Narcotic analgesics Many (eg morphine) are very powerful and can produce drug dependence. They're not used routinely for people with long-term rheumatic disorders. However there are some that relieve moderate to severe pain, and these may sometimes be helpful for patients like us. Prolonged use at high dosage should be avoided. As Professor Parish explains, they must be treated with great respect:

"(They) differ markedly in structure and yet have similar actions and effects. Their adverse effects include nausea, vomiting, drowsiness, dizziness, constipation and respiratory depression. They differ in their onset and duration of action, in whether they are effective by mouth and in the way that individuals respond to them. They may all cause tolerance and physical dependence, and are potential drugs of abuse. They increase the effects of alcohol and other depressant drugs and they should not be taken by patients who drive motor vehicles and/or who operate machinery." (In *Medicines: A Guide for Everybody*, Penguin)

Other narcotic analgesics include:
- Codeine: Present in many drug combinations (including cough medicines and diarrhoea mixtures, available without prescription). Can cause constipation.
- Co-proxamol: Combination of dextropropoxyphene and paracetamol (eg Distalgesic, Paxalgesic)
- Co-dydramol: Combination of dihydrocodeine tartrate and paracetamol (eg DF118, Paramol)

Analgesic/Anti-inflammatories

Also known as NSAIDs (non-steroidal anti-inflammatory drugs). They work by blocking prostaglandins. Besides relieving pain they also reduce inflammation and swelling in the joints. There are many different NSAIDs, the best-known being, to many people's surprise, aspirin (high-dose, strictly as prescribed by the doctor). Examples of other NSAIDs are diclofenac sodium (eg Voltarol), ibuprofen (eg Brufen, Nurofen, Lidifen, Motrin), indomethacin (eg Indocid, Indomod, Imbrilon), naproxen (eg Naprosyn), piroxicam (eg Feldene), tiaprofenic acid (eg Surgam).

NSAIDs come in many different forms, too – eg tablets, capsules, syrups, powder, suppositories. Some need only be taken once or twice a day, others more often. Possible side-effects include indigestion and stomach problems, so you should always take them with food (except the suppositories of course, which are a good way of avoiding the problems as they bypass the stomach, so to speak!) Rub-in gels (eg Voltarol Emulgel, Feldene gel) or skin creams (eg Difflam) are another way of avoiding stomach problems.

Since there are so many different NSAIDs, in so many different forms, identifying what suits you best may take a while. You should take your prescribed NSAID regularly, and strictly in accord with the doctor's instructions. Don't vary the dosage or omit them unless s/he has first agreed. Ask about possible side-effects to watch out for, and what to do about them. Besides stomach problems some of the others may be nausea, skin rashes, dizziness, headaches, lightheadedness.

By the way, if aspirin's prescribed for you, don't spurn it just because it's so familiar. It's used for RA, though not appropriate to gout or AS. In *Arthritis Research: The Way Ahead* (1977) The British League Against Rheumatism wrote:

> "*It is not generally realised that aspirin has an anti-inflammatory effect in addition to its pain-killing properties, but this is why this drug is so widely used as an anti-rheumatic − it does more than just relieve pain.*"

Used correctly, aspirin can be effective, and it's reassuring to know it's been around such a long time. Gardeners and Latin enthusiasts may notice the similarity between aspirin's chemical name 'salicylate' and the Latin name of the willow-tree, 'salix', from which aspirin was originally derived.

Buzzing in the ears, indigestion or stomach bleeding may indicate side-effects with aspirin, and you should consult your doctor. A switch to another form, eg soluble aspirin, or a specially coated form, or something like benorylate (aspirin/paracetamol compound) may help avoid stomach irritation.

Phenylbutazone is an anti-inflammatory now restricted to patients with ankylosing spondylitis under hospital control.

Second line drugs

Your doctor might advise trying one of these if the first line drugs are insufficient. They're not appropriate though for OA or AS. Second line drugs may modify, halt or slow down the underlying disease process, but they're not first choice treatment because they have potentially serious side-effects and because the disease may stop spontaneously.

As they're powerful drugs, your treatment will need to be closely supervised and monitored. Don't let that put you off if your doctor is strongly in favour. Not everyone gets side-effects. With gold I was lucky, and didn't. Not everyone benefits but more people do than don't, and the effects can be dramatic. Be warned though that with second line drugs it takes a long time to see benefits (maybe four weeks to six months of closely supervised treatment) so don't expect immediate miracles, and they may have to be continued for many months or years if effective.

- *Gold-based drugs*   Gold has been used to treat RA since the 1920s. It's not used for OA, AS, or lupus/SLE, and should *not* be prescribed if you're pregnant. Gold may be given in the form of injections, eg sodium aurothiomalate (Myocrisin), or daily by mouth, eg Auranofin (Ridaura). The injected form is usually given weekly, starting with a small test dose. If there's no adverse reaction the dose is increased.

    Symptoms of adverse effects include skin rashes, mouth ulcers, bruising or bleeding, blood changes, skin sensitivity to sunlight, sore throat, fever, diarrhoea. You should have your blood and urine tested regularly, and should always carry a warning card showing that you're on gold.

    You *must* report any side-effects *at once*, however disappointing the discovery. You'll have to stop the treatment, though might be able to start again at a later date, depending on what your doctor says.

- *Penicillamine* (eg Distamine)   Related to penicillin though nothing like it in its effects. It should not be prescribed if you're allergic to penicillin. Given in tablet form, usually once a day, and is best taken on an *empty* stomach. As with gold, you must have regular blood and urine tests to monitor for adverse effects, and *must* report any side-effects at once (eg rash, sore throat, stomach problems). May cause a disturbance to taste but this is only temporary. Should not be prescribed at the same time as phenylbutazone, gold, antimalarials, immunosuppressives. Not usually prescribed if you're pregnant.

● *Antimalarials*   Used for RA, lupus/SLE, JCA. Usually given in tablet form, eg chloroquine (Avloclor) or hydroxychloroquine (Plaquenil). Like gold and penicillamine benefits are slow to appear. Again you'll need to be closely watched for side-effects, especially possible eye problems. Should not be prescribed if you've got eye abnormalities anyway, nor if you're pregnant, or have psoriasis. Should not be prescribed at the same time as phenylbutazone, gold, penicillamine, or immunosuppressives.

● *Sulphasalazine*   Given daily as coated tablets (eg Salazopyrin). On the whole gives fewer side-effects than other second line drugs, though may cause nausea, headache, rashes, fever and loss of appetite. Occasional blood counts necessary. You need to take plenty of fluids if you're on sulphasalazine, and eat plenty of green vegetables.

● *Corticosteroids*   When these were first introduced they were hailed as wonder-drugs. Symptoms of RA seemed to disappear almost overnight. But alas, used long-term, particularly at high dosage, they can produce serious side-effects and have to be used with extreme caution. (Corticosteroids are *not* the same thing as anabolic steroids, taken by some athletes.) Listen to experts Edmonds and Hughes:

> *"Steroids stand in a category of their own as the most potent anti-inflammatory agents available. There is, however, little evidence that they have beneficial long-term effects on the course of [RA]. Their suppressive effect on rheumatoid disease is dramatic but they are dificult to withdraw without disease exacerbation. Since rheumatoid arthritis is a chronic illness, introduction of steroids may commit the patient to long-term therapy, which, even in modest doses, may cause many side-effects. "*(In *Lecture Notes on Rheumatology*, Blackwell Scientific, 1985)

Used properly however, under the expert supervision of a rheumatologist, steroids (eg Prednisolone) can sometimes be beneficial, for instance in an active flare-up of lupus, or for saving vision in giant cell arteritis. Possible side-effects include stomach troubles, disorders of blood pressure, bones, skin, and delayed wound healing, mood changes, and a characteristic swelling of the face ('moon face') and body. Steroids may aggravate diabetes mellitus. Long-term use in children may retard growth.

A major problem is that a form of dependency develops. Steroids are a stronger version of corticosteroids produced naturally by the body. During periods of stress, anxiety or injury, the body needs and produces more natural corticosteroids. But the body of someone on artificial steroids can't respond like this, with potentially dangerous consequences, unless extra steroids are administered (for instance in an accident, acute infection, surgery, or even some dental procedures). The following rules must be followed if you're on steroids:

● *Always* carry a warning card with you and before any treatment (surgical, dental, treatment of an infection, prescription of any other drugs) explain you're on steroids. You might want to wear a MedicAlert bracelet or necklet (see page 43)

● Follow your doctor's instructions exactly and never take more than prescribed.

● Watch your weight carefully. You may put on weight.

● *Never* stop taking steroids suddenly. You could become seriously ill as this would leave your body without steroids before it could start making its own again. If your doctor decides to stop or reduce the drug s/he will help you do it over a long period, so that your body can gradually readjust itself.

● If ever you're sick and unable to take your tablets, contact your doctor, for urgent advice. S/he may need to give you an injection of cortisone.

● The effects of steroids last a long time, so you should carry your warning card with
you for two years after any course of steroids, however brief.

Locally-acting corticosteroid injections

If a joint is particularly inflamed and painful, steroids may be injected directly into that
joint. Since their effect is localised the problems of steroids taken by mouth are avoided.

Other drugs

Some drugs are limited to use in a specific rheumatic disorder, eg allopurinol, probenecid,
colchicine, for gout. Other drugs may be prescribed to treat any other disorders you may
have, eg for anaemia, psoriasis, infections. Your doctor will need to be careful to avoid
adverse interactions between one drug and another. Immunosuppressive drugs (eg azathio-
prine, cyclophosphamide), may be used in very severe rheumatic disorders which can't be
controlled in any other way, and methotrexate, a folic acid antagonist, is also used, given
once a week by mouth or by injection.

Minor tranquillisers and sleeping pills (benzodiazepines)

Benzodiazepines used as tranquillisers/sedatives include chlordiazepoxide (Librium),
diazepam (Valium), lorazepam, alprazolam (Xanax); those used as sleeping pills include
nitrazepam (Mogadon), temazepam (Normison). Taking these continuously to help cope
with something like RA isn't a good idea. They may sometimes be useful in the short term
(more about that later), but long-term use will only add to your problems.

Common side effects include drowsiness, blurred vision, unsteadiness, and lack of
coordination. You lose your ability to be alert and concentrate, so should not drive or
operate machinery, and looking after children could be a problem. Accidents could
happen. These side effects could lead to problems in family relationships, social life, work,
housework, etc. The effects last long after you've taken the drugs. The greatest problem is
the danger of physical and psychological dependency (addiction). You could come to rely
on them so much that you and your body couldn't function without them. If they're
withdrawn abruptly, sleeplessness, anxiety, fits, and hallucinations may occur.

At times of crisis it's only natural for people to feel anxious and stressed. Especially so
if the crisis is something you at first don't understand and fear you can't do anything
about, like RA or lupus. As I've said before, many of us out here have felt that way too. But
we can tell you too the picture *isn't* as bleak as it may seem at first.

With something like RA you need to *sharpen* your ability to cope, not blunt it with
tranquillisers. Read chapters 13 and 14, which aim (as does this whole book) to get you
started on other ways of 'de-stressing' the situation in an effective long-term way, so
you've got a real alternative to tranquillisers and sleeping pills (and likewise other
potentially harmful drugs like alcohol and tobacco.)

To find out more about the potential risks of tranquillisers and sleeping pills, with
guidelines to help you use them as safely as possible if there really seems no alternative,
read Celia Haddon's *Women and Tranquillisers* (Sheldon Press). Men: don't be put off by
the title, it's for you too! (She concentrates on the benzodiazepine family of drugs, and
doesn't write about major tranquillisers (antipsychotics) used in major psychiatric illness
or antidepressants used to treat depression.)

Sometimes, used sparingly and correctly, tranquillisers/sleeping tablets may be
temporarily helpful. Celia Haddon gives a tranquilliser safety plan and important rules for
anyone thinking of taking them:

 *1 Do not take them unless you need them. There are many alternatives to tranquillisers
    and sleeping pills, try them first.*
 2 *Take as small a dose as possible.*

3 *Take the pills for as short a time as possible.*
  It is much more sensible – if you must take sleeping pills – to take them intermittently, never more than three nights continuously. Use them to break a pattern of insomnia, then leave them aside for as long as possible.

Benzodiazepines do, in any case, soon lose their effectiveness as sleeping pills or tranquillisers. The British Committee on the Safety of Medicines reported on benzodiazepines in 1980, and agreed with American studies which *"show that most hypnotics (sleeping pills) tend to lose their sleep-promoting properties within three to fourteen days of continuous use "*. Tranquillisers too are usually effective for only a few weeks at most.

I have a very small supply of prescribed sleeping tablets, kept strictly for a real emergency where I'm locked into a vicious circle of pain and insomnia, which I haven't been able to break with non-drug measures. Just one or two nights with a sleeping tablet breaks the vicious circle and renews the strength to keep going.

Sleeping pills are handed out too freely to hospital inpatients. Refuse them unless you're really desperate, and instead try simple things like an eye mask (to block out the light, eg from Chester-Care or home-made), ear plugs (from any chemist, to block out the noise, eg Boots 'muffles'), meditation, or listen to tapes or read to pass the time. At home you could add a comforting warm drink of milk and honey, and cosy hot-water bottle.

If you're already a long-term user of tranquillisers/sleeping tablets, don't stop suddenly, or you could suffer severe withdrawal problems. Ask your doctor to help you with a withdrawal plan. If s/he's unhelpful read Celia Haddon's book, or SRN Shirley Trickett's *Coming off Tranquillisers and Sleeping Pills* (Thorsons) and seek help from a self-help group like Tranx. Self-help groups can offer plenty of help and encouragement as you learn to live without the drugs.

Booklist

Some of the books listed on page 16 include sections on drugs. Other sources of information:
– Ask your doctor or pharmacist for a patient information sheet, or write to the manufacturer.
– The British Medical Association's excellent *Guide to Medicines and Drugs* (Guild Publishing/Dorling Kindersley) explains how drugs work, how to use them sensibly, special precautions, possible adverse effects, and drug interactions. (By post from RA-DAR, an organisation set up to improve the collection of data on adverse drug reactions, and which aims to make information more accessible to patients.)
– Professor Peter Parish's *Medicines: A Guide for Everybody* (Penguin paperback) includes arthritis-related drugs, how drugs work and a comprehensive list of drugs, with possible adverse effects. It's detailed, and regularly updated.
– You could also look in a library at books produced for the medical profession, but do beware of (a) baffling and scary medical jargon and (b) immediately imagining you've got all the symptoms described! General drugs books include Martindale's *The Extra Pharmacopoeia* (Pharmaceutical Press), *British National Formulary* (BMA/Pharmaceutical Press) and *MIMS* (Haymarket Publishing). There's also *A Manual of Adverse Drug Interactions*, edited by J P Griffin, P F D'Arcy, C J Speirs (Wright, 1988). Books dealing more specifically with anti-rheumatic drugs include H A Bird and V Wright's *Applied Drug Therapy of the Rheumatic Diseases* (Wright, Bristol, 1982), J M H Moll, H A Bird, A Rushton's *Therapeutics in Rheumatology* (Chapman and Hall Medical, 1986), and *Drug Treatment of the Rheumatic Diseases* (Adis Press), edited by F Dudley Hart.
– *The Drug and Therapeutics Bulletin* (Consumers Association), aims to provide information independent of the pharmaceutical industry and commercial pressures.

Chapter six

PHYSICAL CARE, REST
AND EXERCISE PROGRAMME (PREP)

"Exercise is another must *in getting joints going. Even if it is only possible to do two or three of one exercise each day, gradually build it up and keep a chart of your progress. After about three weeks you should see some improvement."*

So says Anne Ryman, who's lived with RA for several years. Jacqueline S is now in her 50s, but has lived with it since her 20s. Careful balancing of rest and exercise has paid off:

"If your doctor says rest and don't worry please try and do just that. Rest is vitally important as is exercise but try to strike a happy medium. Don't too do much of either.

"I have always been very lucky in that I am not deformed in any obvious way. My hands and wrists give me a lot of trouble and I have limited movement in my wrists but I've worked hard to keep my fingers straight. My legs are also straight for the same reason, hard work and exercise...It's only when I move that it becomes obvious I have anything wrong with me but if I move slowly and keep myself straight people don't notice. It's difficult getting up after a meal in a restaurant or getting out of the car. After even a short journey it takes me a while to loosen up. My very worst time of day is getting up in the morning. What a blessing a hot shower can be."

A good 'physical care, rest and exercise programme' ('PREP') is a highly essential item in your Outwit Arthritis Kit. It won't cure your arthritis, but it can make a vast difference to your muscles and joints, and to your ability to cope. Don't think of it as 'just' a half-hour exercise programme in the physiotherapy department. Prescribed exercises should be done regularly at home too, as an important part of your PREP.

PREP principles really apply to almost everything you do. Think of 'exercise' as moving your body or any part of it; *not* using your body or part of it as 'rest'. Relieving strain on a joint in some way (for instance by using splints or changing the way you use it) is also a form of 'rest' for that joint. You'll need to learn (with helpful advice, and time) how to rest and exercise correctly, and how best to balance the two.

Good joint care is important, too. Be constantly aware of how you use (and how not to *ab*use) your joints in everything you do, all day long. Even if all you're doing is sitting still, how you sit matters and affects the bones and joints and muscles where the arthritis is lurking. So too does something like the way you get up from a chair, walk, stand, open a jar, hold a saucepan, carry a bag, use a pen, deal with bending, reaching, gripping, and so on and on. Like learning to read or write, with time it'll become second nature, so persevere.

Get advice from the experts

Your GP or rheumatologist may help with some PREP advice, but the specialists are the physiotherapist and the occupational therapist (OT). Ask for a referral as soon as possible after diagnosis, and *before* problems set in. Therapists (especially those attached to rheumatological units) can do a lot to help prevent damage and deformity developing. Listen to a physio and an OT quoted in *Practical Health* magazine (Aug/Sept 1987):

Ron Harrison, superintendant physiotherapist at the Royal National Hospital for Rheumatic Diseases, Bath, says: *"Twenty years ago, people who came to us for treatment were quite passive. These days, we work with patients, tell them what to expect and devise a self-care regime they can do at home. Regular exercise is very important – especially with rheumatoid arthritis and ankylosing spondylitis. It helps prevent the joints from stiffening up. You need to build an exercise routine into your daily lifestyle – just as you clean your teeth. If you move every joint properly, every 24 hours, they will stay mobile. We can advise you what to do.*

You also need exercise to maintain muscle strength. If a joint flares up painfully, you will tend to stop using that part of the body. What you don't use you might lose. So we devise exercises that keep muscles strong until the flare-up goes away.

We also advise you how to rest. If you rest a joint in a bad position, permanent stiffness or deformity can set in quickly. You need to adopt the right habits from the start. Sometimes we devise splints to ease pain or hold the joint in the correct position."

Heather Unsworth, senior OT at Odstock Hospital, Salisbury, Wiltshire, says: *"People tend to think occupational therapists just teach you to weave baskets, but we do much more. We help you find ways to cope with ordinary everyday tasks. We look at you as a whole person with an individual lifestyle, and we devise ways for you to do what you want, without straining or damaging your joints. Our main aims are to prevent pain and maintain function.*

It's important to learn to recognise your own personal body signals – the pains that tell you you're doing something harmful. We analyse the tasks you want to perform and find solutions to the problems. We teach you to do the same for yourself, too.

We are also the experts on aids and equipment, from small gadgets to structural adaptations in the home. Through us, you can apply for help with the costs. Here again, we are trained to look at you as a whole person, with a mind as well as a body. Our job is to design ways around, so you can do things that matter to you."

Do seek 'personalised' advice and only from the experts. It's wrong to generalise (as some books do) about 'exercises for arthritis'. Each type of arthritis/rheumatic disorder requires a different approach, and each person needs a different sort of PREP to fit in with their body and their lifestyle.

The basic rules differ in each condition. Take OA, RA and AS, for instance. In OA general rest isn't usually necessary since it normally affects only individual joints, and by the time a joint's become painful and worn-down it's usually better to keep it (and the muscles) going than to try to rest it too much.

For someone with RA, however, rest is very important, especially during a flare-up, though the joints should also be put through a full range of movement (ROM exercises) at least once a day (more, once the flare-up has eased). 'Pacing' and 'planning' of activity is important too, with periods of rest and avoidance of unnecessary stresses and strains.

In AS the emphasis is on keeping going. Exercise and mobility are crucial. It's important to keep joints moving, because if they're allowed to rest too much they can seize up completely. Someone with AS will be taught an extensive range of exercises and must keep at them each and every day (look back at AS on pages 17 and 18).

However, we don't all have easy access to good physios and OTs, and even when we do it's not always easy to remember all the dos and don'ts. You'll find information to help listed at the end of this chapter.

Prescribed exercises or 'what you don't use you lose'

With these you aim, gently, to put all your joints through their full range of movement (ROM) at least once a day. Though physiotherapy can't cure, it can strengthen weakened muscles, increase your range of movement and ability to do things and become more independent. By working to keep joints mobile you'll also help avoid putting too much strain on other joints which might later be affected by the arthritis. The feeling of doing something to help yourself is good too, and in itself a form of 'natural pain control'.

Muscles tend to 'go into spasm' (see page 13) to try to prevent a painful joint moving, but unfortunately are then in danger of weakening and wasting, which increases stresses and strains in the joint. Physiotherapy aims first to relieve muscle spasm (eg by easing or numbing the pain, with heat or cold) and then gradually to restore painfree movement. Strong muscles will help joints 'take the strain'.

Some exercises are 'passive', where someone else moves the joint for you and you don't use your own muscles. Some are 'isometric' where you work on the muscles only, without moving painful inflamed joints at all. Others are 'active', where you do move your joints, using your own muscle-power, or have some assistance – 'assisted active'. Your physio will prescribe a programme appropriate for you to follow regularly at home.

Exercising at home

- You can't exercise easily if you're in pain. Time an exercise session for when your painkillers are working and when you're not too stiff or tired. Get the physio's advice on home-made pain-control methods, eg heat: using hot-water bottle, warm water, a towel wrung out in hot water used as a soothing compress, wax 'baths' for hands (using a special sort of paraffin wax); cold: using a packet of frozen peas (wrapped in a flannel), ice cubes in a hot-water bottle.

- Regularity's important and, eventually, produces benefits. Besides, making something a habit makes it much less of an effort to do. Don't be discouraged if progress is slow. Keep at it!

- Make the session a pleasure rather than an effort. Play your favourite music. Keep a chart to tick off with glee each time you've finished. Reward yourself afterwards with a nice cup of tea or whatever.

- Don't be too ambitious to start with. If you're too energetic you'll only end up making the joints more painful and swollen. Stop if this happens and take it more gently next time. Learn to understand your body's signals, so you know just how much to do and when to rest.

- 'Little and regular' is better than a marathon only now and again. Increase the amount you do very slowly, coaxing the movement a little bit further each time. Don't keep at it until you make any pain worse; that'll only put you off trying again. If the exercise causes pain, time how long the pain lasts afterwards so you can tell the physio and ask for advice on what to do.

Fitting muscle and joint exercise into everyday activity

Prescribed exercises can also be fitted into ordinary activity. For instance standing at the bus-stop or sitting on an office chair you can work (unnoticed) on strengthening your buttock muscles and 'quads'. While watching TV gently exercise your fingers by squeezing and releasing a spongy ball. Ask your physio for other tips.

Watch your posture; slouching strains the joints and can lead to deformity. Ask for advice on the best standing, sitting, lying and working positions. Stand as if the top of your head were linked to a star!

Get advice from your doctor or physio about any sports. Generally speaking, swimming, in warm water, is excellent exercise (see page 289). The buoyancy of the water takes strain off joints and lets muscles move easily and as fully as possible. Hydrotherapy is prescribed exercise in very warm water, supervised by a hydrotherapist/physio, and very good it is too. Ask your physio if there are any gentle exercises you can do while having a bath. Swimming instructor Judy Jetter and OT Nancy Kadlec have produced an illustrated book *Arthritis and Back Pain: Exercises for the Bath* (Bantam, 1987), intended for use with doctor/physio advice. Your physio might also give the OK to some cycling, or gentle dancing. But avoid anything that jogs or twists joints, or subjects one or more to repeated pressure or strain (eg jumping or weightlifting!). It's important not to over-do things, but often difficult to judge when to stop, especially if you're enjoying yourself. One rheumatologist advises:

"In general, if exertions and exercises make joints more painful or swollen for an hour or so afterwards, this is permissible, but if the pain or swelling is still present two or more hours afterwards, the activity has been too much, and if things are still worse next morning, far too much!

"...Feet and knees affected by rheumatoid arthritis can be improved by walking on even ground for suitable periods but worsened by standing for hours on hard surfaces or walking for long distances over rough, hard or uneven surfaces.

"What is 'too much' in rheumatoid or any other inflammatory arthritis differs for every patient, and it is best to keep to the one to two hour rule mentioned above. If symptoms are worse for hours or days after any particular activity that activity has probably been too much, but a temporary mild aggravation of an hour or two often followed by an improvement in the general state, is not only permissible, but may well prove to be beneficial." (In *ARC magazine*, summer 1988)

Rest and relaxation

"Rest can vary from reducing an activity which over-uses a joint, to complete bed *rest. There are several stages in between.*

It may be helpful to change to lighter work or spend one to two hours *resting on the bed* each *day.*

Try different ways, to help you *decide what is best for* you. *Resting on a bed is generally more beneficial than sitting in a chair.*

Resting is not giving-in.

Your body will need *more rest when you have a flare-up. Relaxation requires skill and practice."* (Heather Unsworth, in *Coping with Rheumatoid Arthritis*, Chambers)

After taking physio and OT advice, in the end it's up to you to find the correct balance of rest and exercise for you and your body. On page 232 two mums with small babies say how they fit rest periods into the day.

Learn how to relax mentally, as well as physically. Both forms of rest are skills that, once learnt, can help you cope with the physical and emotional strains of arthritis. (See too chapter 11 on pain, and chapter 14 on simple self-help anti-stress techniques.)

Splinting is another way of resting and supporting one or more joints. ('Working' splints are used too, to help prevent deformity while a joint's in use.) Heather goes into a lot of persuasive detail in her chapter 'Why Splint?' and quotes someone who's 32 and had RA for nine years:

"I wish I had known earlier just how important splints were in helping to prevent deformity and as a resting aid. I feel that if better, neater, more comfortable splints had been given to me earlier, I would not be so bad now as I might actually have worn them..."

Lightweight plastic can be used for splints. They're moulded to the right shape after being heated or immersed in hot water, and are lighter than plaster of Paris. Neck collars or callipers also help 'rest' joints, relieving them of strain. It's important that any of these devices should fit comfortably. If you're not happy, don't just banish them to the back of a cupboard, but get back to the physio or OT and explain, and see if they can be improved or replaced.

Other 'resting devices' are those which help relieve weight on a joint. Simply using a walking stick can relieve considerable pain and pressure on an arthritic hip, for instance. Worth trying, even if it takes some getting used to (see page 181).

There's another form of 'rest' you might be prescribed. You might be asked to go into hospital for a 'rest' if you've been having a particularly bad time. In actual fact it won't be 'just rest', but a programme of carefully planned rest and relaxation combined with drug treatment and physiotherapy.

Joint protection

Re-think the way you use your joints, and body generally. *How* you do things is important. Both physio and OT can advise you. Young Arthritis Care's Personal Developmemt courses (see page 123) include joint care. The books I mention at the end of this chapter will help too, and the 'short anatomy lesson' on page 12 might help with understanding why joint care's important. Advice will differ according to your particular type of arthritis and difficulties, but here are some general ones for someone with RA:

- Keep pressure off small joints, especially in your hand. For instance take weight on your forearms not knuckles when getting out of a chair, close a drawer with your behind or foot, and carry a shopping bag over your shoulder, rather than in your hand.
- Avoid gripping tightly or for too long. 'Little and often' is better than non-stop. Enlarge the diameter of handles. Use levers and other gadgets to help.
- Spread the load or get help. Avoid handling heavy things. Avoid too much strain on individual joints: use two hands rather than one, for instance.
- Don't stay in one position too long.
- Avoid very vigorous movements, or jogging, or twisting movements.
- Rest your joints *before* they become painful.
- Use every gadget and labour-saving device you can afford.
- Think before you start. Is an activity really necessary? If yes, think through the most sensible way to do it *before* you start.
- Redesign your work areas to avoid unnecessary bending, stretching, or walking.
- Accept some help but try not to become inactive. Ration what you do to what's most essential or most pleasurable.
- Try not to be a perfectionist!

Rethink your environment, with assessment and advice from the OT. Get the right sort of chair (firm, correct height) and bed (firm, good height, light bedclothes). Get OT advice before spending lots of money – the right solution *isn't* necessarily the most expensive. Far from it! There are plenty of ways to make life easier, eg gadgets and tricks to help with washing and grooming, using the loo, eating and drinking, sexual activities, baby and child care, aids for the kitchen, cleaning, washing, shopping, writing, reading, phoning, gardening, working, studying, driving, travelling. Look at chapters 20 – 24 for a start.

Rethink, with your OT's help if necessary, how you use your time and limited 'energy rations'. Page 158 may help, too. 'Pacing and planning' at work and at home saves wear and tear on nerves and joints, and helps conserve energy and avoid unnecessary fatigue. Think before you act. Work out what can be 'eliminated' (eg ironing, drying dishes, car cleaning), what can be 'facilitated' (eg with labour-saving devices), and what can be 'delegated' (eg by getting other people to do things).

Divide essential activity into periods of 'work' and 'rest', and *make* yourself take the planned rest ((eg half an hour's housework, then 15 minutes rest). Re-think how you look at tasks – for instance instead of thinking 'there's a pile of ironing to be done', think 'I can afford to spend half-an-hour ironing, then I must stop'. Work out what's *really* essential and save your energy rations for that. Try to avoid the great temptation of *over-*

doing things on your 'better' days. (Heather Unsworth puts it beautifully: *"Today's over-enthusiasm is tomorrow's 'OUCH'!"*)

Physio and OT can also give you advice on foot care. So too can a State Registered Chiropodist: regular attention can benefit mobility and pain relief, eg through removal of corns and callouses, relief of painful pressure ulcers, work on weakened muscles to relieve strain and deformity in toe joints and advice on footwear (see page 156).

Further information

– Much the best patient handbook for someone with RA is Heather Unsworth's *Coping with Rheumatoid Arthritis* (Chambers, 1986), full of PREP tips and helpful diagrams. As an OT she's an expert, and she explains and illustrates clearly just how to fit joint care, rest and exercise into everyday activity. Chapters include 'Posture: Resting, Working and Driving Positions', 'Resting, Planning and Energy Conservation', 'Exercise', 'Why Joint Care is Important', 'Guidelines for Joint Care', 'Foot Care', 'Why Splint?'.

– For someone with AS, NASS (the National Ankylosing Spondylitis Society) has an exercise booklet and excellent physiotherapy audio and video cassettes (recorded by physiotherapists of the Royal National Hospital for Rheumatic Diseases, Bath) – just the thing to keep you at it, each and every day! Local branches have regular group physiotherapy sessions. (See page 18)

– Some ARC publications will help with your PREP, for instance the information sheets on *Exercise, Choosing a Chair*, and *Your Home and Your Rheumatism*, a booklet with diagrams and photos showing how you can spare your affected joint or joints, or your back.

– *The Arthritis Helpbook* by Kate Lorig and James F Fries (Souvenir, 1983) is based on a successful arthritis self-management programme at the Stanford Arthritis Centre in California. Diagrams and photos show exercises, how to protect your joints, 'self-helpers: 100 hints and aids', relaxation techniques, etc.

– Young Arthritis Care (page 123) arranges Personal Development Courses from time to time, in different parts of the country

– The general publications on arthritis listed on page 16 include information on physiotherapy treatments. There's quite a bit in Wainwright, for instance.

Chapter seven

HOSPITALS

General information

As out-patients or in-patients, we YPAs are likely to have a fair amount to do with hospitals. You might like to know where to find out more about them:

-   Two reference books – expensive, but look for them in your library: *The Hospital and Health Services Yearbook* (Institute of Health Services Management, London) which lists all hospitals, health centres, NHS administrative offices, etc, in the UK, and *The Directory of Hospitals* (Longman), which is an annual listing of all UK hospitals (NHS and independent), plus names of consultants at each hospital.

Contact your local Community Health Council for the most up-to-date information specifically on local hospitals.

-   The College of Health's *Guide to Going into Hospital* (College of Health, London) is cheap, and worth getting if you're going to be an in-patient. You'll feel more confident knowing beforehand what to expect, how best to prepare, admission procedures, what to take with you, what happens at each stage after arrival, who to ask about what, going home, etc.

Hospital waiting lists

The College of Health (see page 119) runs a helpline (081 983 1133, Monday to Friday 10 am till 4 pm, for doctors and patients to help them find the shortest waiting lists for operations. For information about specific operations see chapter 8. The College also publishes:

-   The *Guide to Hospital Waiting Lists*, (cheapish), which gives you an idea of how long or short the waiting lists for admission to hospital are in every health district in the country for eight specialities: trauma and orthopaedics, general surgery, ear, nose and throat, ophthalmology, plastic surgery, gynaecology, oral surgery and urology.

You could ask for referral to another hospital or surgeon, though you don't have a specific right as an NHS patient to have your request granted. Bear in mind that you'd need to be able to attend for an out-patient consultation first, and probably follow-up visits too.

Who's who in the team looking after you?

The *Consultant* heads the team. S/he has spent many years specialising in a particular area of medicine. You could be referred to a Consultant in rheumatology or orthopaedics, for instance. Besides treating some patients directly a Consultant may also teach and carry out research. As an NHS patient you don't have an automatic right to direct treatment by the Consultant in person.

You may instead see and be treated by the *Senior Registrar* or *Registrar*, who come next in the hierarchy, and are responsible to the Consultant. They're aiming to be Consultants, and already have several years' general and specialist training and experience behind them.

Below the Registrar comes the *Senior House Officer (SHO)* and the *House Officer* (or *Houseman*). The Houseman is a newly qualified doctor working on a six-month contract. Every doctor must work as a Houseman before becoming fully registered and being allowed to work outside the hospital service. The SHO has completed this requirement and is beginning specialisation.

The Houseman is the doctor you'll see most of as an in-patient. When you first arrive, s/he will take your detailed medical history, examine you thoroughly, prescribe any drugs you'll need in hospital, and arrange various tests. This is the time to mention any allergies, the drugs you're already taking (don't forget to include any drugs for depression, anxiety, steroids, the contraceptive pill), even if it seems strange to have to go over everything already in your notes. It's also a good time to ask questions about what's going to happen. If the Houseman doesn't know the answer, ask if s/he could find out for you. Many people mistakenly save all their questions until the Consultant's *ward round* when time and privacy are very limited. Try to get at least some of them answered beforehand. Remember however that it's the Consultant who's ultimately responsible for any decisions made about you. S/he might not always agree with what other members of the team have told you.

Other people you may see are the physiotherapist and occupational therapist, radiographers and other paramedicals or medical technicians. (See also pages 37 – 39.) If you have any personal, domestic, social or financial worries, ask Sister if you can see the hospital social worker for help. S/he's also the person, together with the occupational therapist, to help arrange any necessary support services for when you're discharged.

Who's who in the nursing team?
You can tell who's who by the uniform they wear (eg belt, cap, colour of dress/tunic). The *Ward Sister* heads the team (call her 'Sister', not 'Nurse'!). If a male nurse is in charge, he's called the *Charge Nurse*. Then come the *Staff Nurses* who are *SRNs* (State Registered Nurses) who have completed a three-year training course (call them 'Staff Nurse'). Next come the *State Enrolled Nurses* (SENs) who have completed a two year training course. There may also be student nurses and nursing auxiliaries, who don't have nursing qualifications.

Do put questions and worries to the nursing team as well as the medical team. They work closely together, and the more experienced nursing team members often have specialised knowledge of medical and surgical procedures. They can help explain some of what the doctors have told you, and make sure other questions and worries get through to the doctors.

Ask the nursing team to explain some of the ward routine to you. It helps, for instance, to know when the Consultant and/or Senior Registrar are going to make their ward round. Ask, too, when the nurses' shifts start and end, as they usually spend time round about then in conference or 'hand-over', a good time to avoid asking for bed-pans, etc, if possible! Find out about mealtimes and visiting times too.

Financial aspects
See DSS leaflet NI9 *Going into Hospital: What Happens to Your Social Security Benefit or Pension?* Some benefits may be reduced or stopped. See DSS leaflet H11 *Your Hospital Fares* if you're on benefits or a low income: you may qualify for help with hospital fares. *The Disability Rights Handbook* (see page 127), has chapters on 'Going into hospital' and 'Hospital – one year on'; and the Disability Alliance has also produced *The Hospital Patients' Handbook*, a guide about how going into hospital affects benefits.

Suggestions and complaints
If you have ideas for improving services in your hospital, or are unhappy with something, you could try having a word with the Sister or Charge Nurse at the clinic you attend, or write to the General Manager of the hospital.

Chapter eight

SURGERY

Hip replacements are the best-known form of surgery for people with arthritis. Successful total hip replacement has been one of the most exciting developments of recent years. In November 1962, at Wrightington Hospital in Lancashire, Professor John Charnley performed the first successful operations. Improvements have continued since then. More than 250,000 people in Europe and North America undergo the operation each year, and over 90% function successfully.

Other joints can now be replaced (the general technical term is 'replacement arthroplasty'). The second most frequently replaced joint is the knee. Work's also been done on replacements for shoulders, elbows, finger joints, and ankles, with varying success.

Other operations may be performed too. Someone with RA might have an operation to repair damaged tendons, release a trapped nerve, or a 'synovectomy' (removal of an inflamed synovial membrane, aimed at reducing pain and swelling), or an 'arthrodesis' (fixation of a joint, eg ankle, thumb, wrist, elbow, aimed at removing pain and correcting instability).

ARC's *Arthritis Today* magazine often has articles on different surgical procedures and is an excellent way of keeping up-to-date with developments.

To operate or not to operate?

Stories of the miraculous relief an operation can bring make it all too easy to get carried away and think surgery must be the answer to all your problems. But surgery should be a last resort, with the pros *and* cons considered very carefully, only after everything else has been tried. Don't ever try to over-persuade a surgeon to operate against his better judgement. Be wary, for instance, of pressing for an operation to make deformed hands look more attractive, if there's a danger of losing function. One YPA, who regretted the particular operation she had, wrote in *In Contact*:

"My suggestion to anyone considering surgery is remember, it's your body – make sure it's absolutely necessary, ask questions like: 'What if any are the drawbacks', 'are there any risks', 'is there an alternative?' then if you are satisfied with the answers you can go ahead in the knowledge that you are well prepared for any eventuality."

Listen to orthopaedic surgeon Denys Wainwright in his book *Arthritis and Rheumatism* (Elliott Right Way Books, 1985):

"The decision as to whether an operation is advisable in treating arthritic joints is never easy and it is essential for you to be fully informed about the chances of success and the possible risks of any procedure. You, in turn, must carefully assess the degree of pain and disability from which you are suffering.

"An intermittent ache and the necessity to use a stick when walking any distance are not disabilities requiring surgery and operations are only considered when suffering intractable pain unrelieved by analgesics and physical treatment, particularly if sleep is constantly interrupted. Replacement arthroplasty of the hip is particularly successful in restoring almost normal function to a stiff deformed joint but it is a major operation with a small but significant rate of complications. You should bear this possibility, however remote, in mind. Clotting of the big veins of the leg, infection of the wound and loosening of the components of the joint all occur in a small percentage of cases but if

the alternative is a life of serious invalidism these are risks worth taking...

"Discuss the matter with relatives and the family doctor and then consult a surgeon familiar with these operations, but the ultimate decision rests with you. Never be too influenced by other people who have had replacement operations because no two cases are identical and some joints are more difficult to restore than others."

There's often a gap between our expectations of surgery and the reality, and in a perceptive article in *In Contact* one YPA pinpointed some of the problems:

"There is the problem of role perception. People going to see a surgeon often think of it as 'going to see the doctor'. Surgeons, however, it seems to me, have a much narrower view of their role, and confine it to whether or not to operate. Thus, if you ask a surgeon what he thinks should be done for you, he will come up with a surgical answer. This does not necessarily mean that you need (ie must have) an operation, but rather that, if what you are complaining of is a big enough nuisance, he will obligingly try to do something to help you. I think older people, in particular, find this confusing. They expect to have 'the doctor' tell them what they need. Many patients, it seems to me (after seventeen years of out-patients' clinics) fail to see that the surgeon is offering his considered professional advice which they are free to accept, discuss or (politely!) reject.

"Second, there is a semantic problem. I don't know how people feel about having a 'new' hip, but I don't feel I have a 'new' knee. I'm glad I had the old one replaced, it restored my mobility and independence and got me out of a wheelchair – but, I repeat, what I have is not a new knee. This may sound petty, but...the general public are of the impression that you go into hospital, get a new joint or two and come out of hospital fully mobile and without pain.

"In consequence, if you come out of hospital (particularly if you come out to live on your own) with a large wound, a very awkward joint, a lot of pain, and face two or three months of coping for yourself with great difficulty, spending sleepless nights when you have to get up and around on sticks to ease the 'discomfort' – it's very hard to be told on all sides that it must be wonderful now you've got your new joint and there's no pain any more, and asked when you'll be running down the High Street. At this stage, the reality of your op may seem to you to fall far short of your expectations."

She included several tips about going to see the surgeon. There won't be a lot of time to discuss all the pros and cons, so do your homework, and go prepared:

"Try to think of what he might suggest doing, and write down questions as they occur. Surgeons are so used to doing operations that they often forget to mention little practical details like how long you will be in plaster, or the likely length of your hospital stay, or what you will be able to do on discharge and so on. Take your list of questions with you, wait till he has finished and then say politely that you have things to ask..."

Always remember you don't have to agree there and then. You could, if you want, go away and discuss things in more detail with your GP and rheumatologist.

Total hip replacement (THR) in younger patients

I hope you haven't been completely put off. Many YPAs, including me, have benefited immeasurably from THR surgery. I had both done in 1976, with a three month gap in between. The effect was miraculous, banishing the utterly intolerable pain and restoring mobility to hip joints which had almost completely locked in their sockets, so great was the damage. Afterwards, life was worth living again.

Another YPA enthused, too: *"my new hip joints, [gave] me a new lease of life for without them I would have been bed-ridden at the age of 28."* Janet Mason had a special worry: *"the first thing I asked when they suggested doing my hips was will I still be able to have babies? I was reassured."* For Anne R: *"there is no doubt the replacements are super and can revolutionise the condition, and give you heart and energy to go on fighting."*

But do, *please*, think twice (and more than twice) before agitating for an operation. There are, alas, still problems and drawbacks, especially for younger patients, so try everything else first. 'Everything else' includes all methods of pain control (drug and non-drug methods), reorganising your life to lessen strain on the joint, reducing weight (if you're overweight), keeping your muscles in trim, getting a firmer bed if necessary, and swallowing your pride sufficiently to use one (or two) sticks. Do listen to a surgeon who advises you to try these less dramatic remedies first, hard though it may seem. He's only being cruel to be kind, and really does have your best interests at heart.

How does a hip replacement work? What *can* go wrong? The hip's a ball-and-socket joint. The surgeon replaces the 'ball' (the femoral head) with a metal (usually stainless steel) implant (or 'prosthesis') which looks vaguely like a sort of upside-down very oddly shaped golf club with a round head. Attached to the 'ball' is a long 'stem' which the surgeon inserts and fixes in the leg bone (femur). The socket (acetabulum) is replaced with a special sort of plastic (polyethylene). Both the steel prosthesis and plastic acetabulum are fixed in place with a special sort of 'cement' (or a cement-free technique is used).

Wonderful though the op is, there are two main possible complications – infection and loosening of the components. The problem of infection's been reduced to 1% or less. Loosening of the components remains the major problem and the major reason, alas, why surgeons still hesitate to operate in younger patients. One of Britain's leading orthopaedic surgeons explained:

> *"The frequency with which components loosen depends upon the prosthesis in question, the activity of the patient, the technique used for its implantation and a number of other factors, not all of which are fully understood...*
>
> *"Because of the very satisfactory clinical results obtained in the elderly, and because a number of patients below the age of 60, even in their 20s, may become crippled by hip disease, attempts have been made to replace the hip in younger age groups. It is difficult to summarise the results of these attempts to date except to say that the operation is very much less successful and technically significantly more demanding in younger adults. So marked is this difference that it is the author's opinion that no procedure available today should be used in the osteoarthrosic hip of a patient in their 20s. In the 30s and 40s special techniques of fixation are under evaluation, whilst in the 50s improved cementing techniques may make the outcome similar to that to be expected of someone in their 60s or 70s."* (In *ARC magazine*, 1986)

Sorry if I've upset you. I don't want to put you off completely, nor alarm anyone who's already had it done. The hip op *is* wonderful, but I do want you to know the facts. My medical team were very careful to make me aware of the drawbacks before I had my ops. For me they really were a last resort, and I went in 'with my eyes open' (figuratively speaking!). Though they were likely to be successful, there could still be problems, but I knew none of those problems could put me in a worse position than I was. Anything had to be better than that pre-op hell.

Life was certainly well worth living again afterwards, but in time loosening and pain did occur. I've had to have a 'revision op' on one hip already, and the other has partly loosened. I know that if a 'revision' is not successful I'd end up with a 'girdlestone', where there's no 'ball-and-socket' hip joint at all (see page 62). Meanwhile I have to be extremely careful with The Hips, though the advantages for me still outweigh the disadvantages.

Going ahead with a hip op

If, after full consideration, you and your surgeon do decide to go ahead, I wish you the very best of luck, and as much relief as I and other YPAs have experienced. Your surgeon will be your main source of information, of course. Some publications may help too:

–   ARC's factsheet *A New Hip Joint* (free, but send an SAE to ARC)
–   Two cheap but very informative guides, both available by post: the College of

Health's *Guide to Hip-Replacement Operations*, and the Health Information Network Ltd's *Total Hip Replacement*, written by Mr J M H Paterson FRCS
- You can also phone the College of Health's confidential Healthline (081 681 3311) between 4pm and 8pm and ask to hear the recorded tape *Hip Replacement Operation*
- *Hip Replacement, The Facts* by Professor Kevin Hardinge, MCGOH, FRCS, MChOrth (Oxford University Press, 1983) is worth looking at if you want to go into detail.

Recovery times differ from person to person, and you'll need to be extra careful for several weeks or months after the op, while everything settles into place. You might feel so good that you want to rush around madly at once. I know the feeling! But *don't* if you want the op to be a success. *Do* take things carefully. Listen to your surgeon, physio, OT and the nurses and don't rush off for the nearest mountain or enter yourself for Wimbledon in your heady exhilaration.

Don't cross your legs. Do sleep on your back. Get your chair and bed at home raised to avoid straining the new hip, and ask the OT about raising the height of the loo seat. See about raising any frequently-used electric sockets (see page 162). Avoid strain too by using an easyreach gadget, a stocking puller-on, etc. The OT will advise on all these. Ask the physio or OT to measure the length of your legs after the op. If one's slightly shorter than the other an extra shoe heel-piece or two that side might help avoid strain. After a few weeks you'll be able to drive a car again, though get advice from physio/OT on getting in and out safely. After a few weeks too you'll be able to resume your sex life. Ask your healthcare team for advice on long-term aftercare of your new pride-and-joy. In general:

- 'Bionic' hip joints don't bend as far as 'normal' hip joints, so don't force them further than they want to go.
- Do regularly the gentle exercises taught by your physio to keep the muscles in shape. Strong muscles help bionic joints 'take the strain'.
- Keep your weight down. Being overweight strains the joint.
- Avoid any sort of repetitive jogging, jarring, jumping or twisting movement, which could loosen the joint. Avoid games like soccer, badminton, and squash. Opt for gentler sports like golf or croquet or swimming or gentle cycling. As the College of Health guide says: *"It's wise not to be too ambitious. Nine holes of golf rather than eighteen; gentle gardening instead of digging up all the flower beds; and a stroll rather than an ascent on Mount Snowdon."*
- Avoid low seats, low beds and low cars. Getting up from these puts stress on bionic joints. Ask for help in getting up if you forget to avoid them. *Don't* strain your joint by being too proud to ask for help.
- Treat your bionic joint with great respect, but do, do enjoy your new-found mobility and freedom from pain.

Knee replacement

Get ARC's booklet on *Knee Replacement* (free, but send an SAE), and/or the Health Information Network's cheap but informative *Total Knee Replacement*, written by Mr S Canon FRCS. Several YPAs have had total knee replacements, with varying degrees of success. My friend Ken, in Ireland, had his done in 1976, the same year as my hip ops. The Knee has its off-days, it's not as agile as a 'normal' knee joint and he limps slightly, but it's still going strong and letting him lead a full life, working, socialising, and regularly cycling through France on his annual holiday.

Similar warnings apply as for the hip op – think twice and twice again, several times over. Try everything else first and think of the knee op as only a last resort. Be sure you're not going to end up saying 'if only I hadn't had it done' if there are drawbacks afterwards.

Professor Hardinge includes knee replacements in his book on hip operations:

> *"If the function in a normal knee is called 100 per cent, the best knee replacements are at present offering about 80 to 85 per cent of normal function – this normal function including pain relief, stability, and movement. This is to be contrasted to the total hip replacement, which being a simpler universal ball and socket joint is much simpler mechanically and probably gives 90 to 95 per cent of 'normal' function...*
>
> *"Doctors hesitate to offer total knee replacement to younger patients because they don't know how stable such replacements are over a lifetime, and how the cement-bone bond will behave over such a period. The percentages quoted above are a rough guide to function, but to gain the worthwhile overall benefit of total joint replacement, a patient with a painful knee has to be marginally worse off before the operation than a patient with a painful hip."* (In *Hip Replacement, The Facts*, OUP 1983)

Ankle operations

Ankle replacement joints have been developed but present problems. The design and function of a normal ankle joint is more complex than a hip joint and therefore much more difficult to reproduce artificially. An alternative is an 'arthrodesis' where the surgeon 'fuses' or 'fixates' the joint, to stop the pain that movement causes. Convalescence takes a long time, at least three months in plaster, as bones have to fuse together and you need to be a *very* patient patient! I had a partial arthrodesis, as a last resort in the face of unbearable pain day in day out. I was off work for four months and spent most of that time sitting in a chair or on my bed in plaster feeling *very* helpless and *longing* for a bath. But ultimately it was worth it, and it's been wonderful to get rid of the pain. The limited joint movement doesn't make as much difference as I'd feared, though it's slightly more awkward now going up stairs; but I try to avoid them anyway for the sake of my hips.

The girdlestone

I mentioned this before, as you might hear it proposed as a last resort if a hip replacement op isn't possible for some reason. The 'ball' of the femur is removed and nothing put in its place. As time goes by, fibrous body tissue grows into the 'space', forming a 'girdlestone'. Janet Mason, now 29, who's had JCA since she was four, ended up with a girdlestone on both sides:

> *"I was waiting to go in and have my hips re-replaced. Well I got in, I had to, I was so bad in the end I couldn't move at all. It turns out I had an infection in my hips. I don't know how it happened but I was quite ill. Anyway they had to remove my hips and get rid of the infection. It's been a long job but I think I'm back on the road to recovery at last...I didn't think I would be able to do it but I am actually managing to walk without my hips in, using 'gutter crutches'. It's not as bad as I thought it would be. It's just my muscles and my knees which have stiffened up with not being used, but I am slowly improving."*

Four years later, Janet's still using gutter crutches, but *"I feel fitter than I have in a long time"* and she's busy beavering away as a Young Arthritis Care Contact. Someone else had a girdlestone on only one side:

> *"I had this operation (right leg) in 1968. The following year I had a hip replacement in my left leg which was completely successful. That meant that I had one good artificial hip and, on the other side one grow-it-yourself fibrous tissue arrangement linking hip to femur. Since then I have had practically no pain. I can walk easily on crutches. The shortened leg is dealt with satisfactorily by a built-up shoe. I can cope with most domestic activities."* (Writer to 'Dr Grosvenor', in *Arthritis News*, winter 1986/87)

Going private and/or considering going abroad for treatment

If you're tempted to go private, and have the means to do so, make sure you know exactly what you're letting yourself in for, and discuss it all thoroughly with your doctor first. Check whether the estimate covers *everything*, including medication costs and cost of the hospital stay. What happens if there are complications? Will you still have enough money to pay?

One way of arranging private care is to go through an organisation like the Surgical Advisory Service, who can negotiate a whole package for you so you know exactly where you are. Another scheme, Epidaurus, is run by Western Provident Association Ltd, a UK health insurance company and Mondial Assistance, an international medical assistance group. For a fee, the scheme offers patients three quotations for an operation − one for a hospital near home, one for another hospital in the UK, and a third for a European hospital. Patients must be under specialist care or on an NHS waiting list.

We sometimes hear about people who have operations abroad, paid for by the NHS. This is rare, and even if agreed, has drawbacks, eg what happens if there are complications? If you want to find out more you'll need to get leaflet E112 (from DSS Overseas Branch). The scheme considers applications 'when inadequate facilities exist in the UK or when care can't be provided within the normal time for obtaining treatment' and requires a specialist's referral and agreement by the patient's health authority to pay the cost. In 1990, 449 applications were made to the Department of Health and 261 were agreed.

Chapter nine

DIET AND ARTHRITIS

"What about diet?" is often one of the first questions that comes to mind when you're wondering what on earth you can do about your arthritis. Alas, there's no magical dietary 'cure', though some publications may give that impression. Some people do seem to benefit from looking at their diet and making changes, though 'one man's meat is another man's poison', and what works for one person might not work for someone else.

What should you do if you're wondering whether dietary changes might help *you*? As always, see what your doctor thinks first. Do some background reading too. I hope the list at the end of this chapter will help you find out more, from reputable, rather than 'quack' sources. *Nutritional Medicine* and *The Food Intolerance Diet Book*, for instance, are both written by reputably qualified medics with special knowledge of diet and health.

Why do some doctors give dusty rebuffs to questions about diet and arthritis?
Well – the study of nutrition still plays only a small part in a medical student's curriculum, and orthodox medicine has traditionally been suspicious of claims that diet might have a part to play in either the cause or treatment of inflammatory arthritis.

However that hasn't stopped many desperate sufferers trying out all sorts of diets, some more weird and wonderful than others. And it's left many desperate people at the mercy of unscrupulous 'quacks' whose bank accounts have benefited considerably more than their victims, thus making many caring, orthodox doctors even more suspicious, even angry, at the question "What about diet?".

Fortunately, at last, food sensitivity and dietary therapy *are* being studied in an orthodox manner, as carefully as any other new forms of treatment (though research on diet and arthritis specifically is still at an early stage). So, instead of being at the mercy of any Tom, Dick or Harriet Quack, and instead of the dismissive rebuffs we get from some doctors to questions about diet, hopefully we should soon find a more open-minded reaction, like that of one rheumatologist:

> "*I have no objection to my patients having a special diet if they feel it does them good, provided it does not produce a deficiency. Some diets may do this. I do, however, provide patients with a diet sheet containing the type of diet which would benefit anyone, entitled* Eating Your Way to Good Health." (*ARC Magazine*, 1985)

Either of the two booklets mentioned on page 69, *Guide to Healthy Eating* and *Eating Well on a Budget*, or the *Manual of Nutrition* would help you plan a healthy, balanced diet. But what if you want to try a 'special diet', or to try to identify any individual problem food? You want to be sure that what you do isn't going to do any harm, or produce any dietary deficiency, even if it doesn't actually help. Explain to the doctor this is where you'd welcome his or her support. S/he might even be able to refer you to a dietitian for advice.

Is there anything doctors can say for sure about diet and arthritis?
There are three things. Firstly, attacks of gout may be brought on by excess alcohol or foods like liver, kidney or fish roes, rich in 'purines'. Secondly, being overweight puts unnecessary strains on already suffering joints and muscles. Someone with OA of the hip or knee for instance should find that taking off excess weight will make a difference. The other thing doctors can say for sure is that you should aim for a 'healthy well-balanced diet'. – If arthritis creates problems with mobility and cooking and shopping and finances

it's all too easy to rely on an unhealthy diet of endless bread and jam and cups of tea and to give up trying to eat properly, but we must try.

Why there are no easy shortcuts?

Nutrition in general is a tricky enough topic even before you start to bring arthritis and its eccentricities into the picture. Not suprising when you consider that in addition to carbohydrates, fats, and proteins, there are known to be some 45 nutrients (eg vitamins, minerals, others like fibre, oxygen, water) essential for human life. Too little of any particular one and deficiency symptoms result. Too much, and toxic (poisonous) symptoms occur. Even the happy medium can't be precisely defined, as many other factors have to be taken into account too, like the quality and quantity of the food we eat, the efficiency of the digestive system, plus each person's unique nutritional requirements ('one man's meat, etc') and age, growth, sex, pregnancy and breast-feeding, illness, stress, activity level, genetics, possible interactions with medicines or alcohol, smoking, etc!

Good books on nutritional medicine in general, written by reputable medical experts are few and far between. Dr Stephen Davies and Dr Alan Stewart's *Nutritional Medicine* (Pan, 1987), is written for professionals but isn't *too* technical for laypeople too. One drawback alas – though it's a paperback, it's a very thick one, unwieldy for arthritic fingers. It's the sort of book you could try (tactfully!) lending your doctor if s/he's high in sympathy but low in information. It includes items on rheumatic disorders such as RA, OA, osteoporosis, and psoriasis. The authors are founder members of the British Society for Nutritional Medicine, set up in mid-1984 by orthodox doctors.

The book's a fascinating insight into just how intricate a balancing act has to be performed when designing a healthy diet for anyone even before you begin to look at special diets for special needs. Experts tend to agree that in the West we need to cut down our intake of fat, sugar and salt, and increase fibre. But *too much* fibre stops you absorbing calcium, crucial for good bones, and essential zinc and iron, too. (Fresh fruit and vegetables are a better source of fibre than adding lots of bran to a junk-food diet.) If you cut out citrus fruits and/or potatoes you need to substitute another source of vitamin C. If you cut out milk you need another source of calcium.

It's all a highly complicated balancing act, and certainly explains why it's not a good idea to try DIY special diets without expert advice.

Could an allergy testing service help you find out if you have a 'food allergy'?

No! Outside orthodox medicine there are a lot of dubious and unscientific 'allergy testing' services, keen to part you from your money – don't be misled into using them. *Which?* magazine and Guy's Hospital put five commercial allergy testing clinics to the test. The clinics didn't reliably identify fish allergies in patients known to have them, they gave different results for the same person, and they often gave dubious and risky dietary advice (*Which?* report, January 1987).

There's no easy shortcut like this to finding out whether you have a food 'allergy'. In any case, doctors prefer to make a distinction between the terms food allergy and food intolerance (or sensitivity). It's usually more correct to use the term intolerance or sensitivity rather than allergy in someone who's looking for, or finds, a link between what they eat and their arthritis.

The Royal College of Physicians defines food allergy as 'an abnormal immunological reaction to the food'. Allergy is for life: once identified, the cause must be avoided rigorously and always. In true food allergy, the body produces excessive amounts of immunoglobulin E antibodies to fight a particular food which it considers a foreign invader: symptoms may vary from wheezing and a runny nose, for example, to extremely serious problems. Food intolerance is usually unconnected with the immunoglobulin E system, and produces a more delayed reaction, builing up over a period of time.

Finding out if you have a particular food intolerance/sensitivity

A small number of people find that a particular food or drink (eg wheat, beef, milk, coffee, tea) does cause an allergic reaction directly affecting their arthritis. In 1981 a report in the British Medical Journal described a woman with RA whose illness was made worse by cheese. Someone I know finds that strawberries activate her RA symptoms even before she's finished eating a bowlful! However that doesn't mean cheese or any other food is necessarily harmful to *you*, just that *some* people may have that particular food sensitivity.

Perfect food intolerance tests don't exist and it's not easy to work out whether or not *your* symptoms might be linked to something you eat/drink. Bear in mind too that arthritis could be activated by something totally different, such as hormonal changes after childbirth, or some sort of viral infection. However if you think your aches and pains do have a specific pattern in relation to something you eat or drink, trial and error might help you work out what suspect 'trigger' to avoid. One YPA wrote in *In Contact*:

> *"I decided that I'd do a small experiment, after all, I had nothing to lose. So I cut apples out of my diet for about five days, then I ate one. The effect was amazing. I had the apple in the afternoon, the next morning I was incredibly stiff. Coincidence, I thought, so I did it again, five days with no apple, waking up with only a slight stiffness and getting better every day, then I ate an apple, same response as before. I cut apples out of my diet entirely. Since then I have found that all fruit (except strawberries for some reason) affect me in the same way, though I haven't tried melons, kiwi fruit and all the more exotic fruit. Tomatoes are included in this."*

She doesn't say how she makes up for the essential vitamins and minerals she isn't now getting from fruit, but it's crucial she still gets all she needs. She needs to avoid ending up with scurvy, for instance, through not getting vitamin C, to say nothing of many other possible deficiency problems.

If, with your doctor's agreement, you want to try to identify any food intolerance you may have, you could look at *The Food Intolerance Diet Book* by Workman, Jones and Hunter (Macdonald Optima). The writers are at Addenbrooke's Hospital, Cambridge. Elizabeth Workman is a state registered dietitian and Dr Hunter a consultant physician and recognised authority on the subject of food allergy and intolerance. They describe an exclusion diet you can use for testing different foods, and include lots of tempting recipes. On the topic of diet and RA they comment:

> *"Several different diets have been promoted by doctors and herbalists, but unfortunately none has proved to be entirely successful...The role of diet in arthritis is far from established. Although a number of doctors have reported they have a few patients with RA who have found that foods have definitely caused their problems, a large number do seem to improve for a short time only because of the placebo effect – if they think the treatment is doing them good, it will.*
>
> *"However, we are now treating people with an exclusion diet specially adapted for arthritis, and we have been successful in relieving symptoms in seven out of twelve people..."*

Davies' and Stewart's *Nutritional Medicine* also describes the exclusion diet approach to discovering which food(s), if any, might be causing particular symptoms. They include the well-known 'lamb and pears and mineral water' diet, and stress that such diets are best followed under the guidance of someone experienced in the field, eg a doctor, dietitian or nutritionist, who's aware of the problems and pitfalls that can occur.

Whatever you try, do stick to orthodox medicine and practitioners.

Research into specific diets for people with arthritis

The first difficulty researchers face is that something like RA waxes and wanes so unpredictably anyway that it's difficult to say whether any improvement is due to a particular diet, or whether it might have happened anyway. A second difficulty is the placebo effect (see page 80) – something may seem to do you good simply because you *believe* it's going to do you good. Even coloured water can work this way. Thirdly, it's difficult to get people to follow a diet experiment exactly when it involves changing tastes and habits of a lifetime and avoiding all temptation to go astray...

Some researches on diet and RA have suggested that low-fat diets (cutting out red meat, full-fat milk, butter, biscuits, cakes made with butter) may help *some* people, in the short term, anyway. Dr Gail Darlington is a consultant physician and rheumatologist who's been studying diet and RA:

"Speculation about food intolerance in rheumatology dates from the early part of the century but it was not until 1979, when Sköldstam and his co-workers showed improvement among rheumatoid patients partially fasted for seven to ten days, that interest was rekindled and a series of papers on the subject have been published recently.

"In 1983, Panush et al in Florida undertook a ten week, controlled, trial in 26 patients to investigate the Dong diet for rheumatoid arthritis. This is a popular diet free from additives, preservatives, fruit, red meat, herbs and dairy produce. Panush et al stated that their study failed to provide evidence of overall benefit for the diet but felt that the results were consistent with the possibility that individualised dietary changes might be beneficial for some patients with rheumatoid arthritis.

"In 1984, Kroker and his colleagues described a study in which there was improvement in 43 patients with rheumatoid arthritis who underwent a water fast lasting for one week under controlled environmental conditions.

"In January 1985, Kremer and his colleagues described their manipulation of diet in patients with rheumatoid arthritis by giving them a diet high in polyunsaturated fat with a fish oil supplement and these patients were compared with a group of patients on an ordinary, comntrolled diet. The results favoured the experimental group at 12 weeks and after stopping the diet the experimental group deteriorated. The coverage of Kremer's paper by the media led to the name of the 'Eskimo Diet' being given to the reduction in dairy produce and animal fat in the study and the use of a diet rich in fish and fish oil.

"In 1985, Dr Ramsay, Dr Mansfield and I completed our placebo controlled study of dietary therapy in patients with rheumatoid disease and this showed significant benefit for the patients receiving dietary therapy. There are a number of possible reasons for this improvement and it would take considerably more research before the role of dietary therapy in some patients with rheumatoid arthritis is fully explained. Nonetheless, there are a number of very interesting explanations being tested at present.

"Not all patients respond to dietary therapy but the treatment is safe when supervised and its relevance to any particular patient can be determined in about six weeks. It certainly appears to help at least a sub-group of patients with rheumatoid arthritis. It should, however, always be undertaken under medical supervision."

Dr Darlington's 1985 study was reported in the *Lancet* (February 1st, 1986, 236); the Kremer study in the *Lancet* (1985, volume 1, 8422, pages 184 – 187).

Fish and fish-oil were significant in the Kremer low-fat diet and scientific research has been looking at how and why they might be beneficial. What most definitely does *not* happen is what many quacks suggest, ie that fish oil or olive oil is absorbed and 'acts as a lubricant in the joint'. That's quite impossible, as the oil is broken down in the gut before being absorbed. Instead, researchers have discovered that fish oils contain chemicals which thin the blood and make it less likely to clot. Dr Tony Smith, Deputy Editor, *British Medical Journal*, described the findings in *Self Health* (no.11, June 1986):

"In practice the diet also lowers the blood pressure – and may be of benefit to victims of chronic inflammation causing arthritis, skin disorders, such as psoriasis, and some forms of kidney disease. In the words of the Harvard Medical School Health Letter *the*

'fish oil story seems almost too good to be true'."

Because of its properties however, people with blood disorders or bleeding problems should take fish oil *only* under strict medical supervision, something a quack is unlikely to warn you about.

YPA Julie McKechnie found the Dong diet suited her:

"..after only a few weeks I began to feel the benefits resulting from a complete change in my eating habits. Inflammation and swellings were reduced, aches and pains were less and tiredness down to a minimum and believe me, with a lively two year old to look after, that was an added bonus. Then, after a couple of months, with my doctor's advice, I was able to reduce my cortisone level by 1 mg. I know it doesn't sound a lot but arthritics on cortisone will know how hard it is to drop just that tiny bit..." (*In Contact*)

Some scientists believe that a diet low in certain carbohydrates (especially starches and flour products) and high in protein may benefit some people. This follows research by Dr Ebringer at the Middlesex Hospital in London, which has been exploring the relationship between HLA B27 (in AS) and the micro-organism Klebsiella. Along with other micro-organisms, it enters the gut with food, but is present in increased numbers in the gut during a flare-up of AS. A team of scientists in Finland agrees with Dr Ebringer's findings, though other researchers elsewhere don't! The spring/summer 1989 newsletter of NASS (National Ankylosing Spondylitis Society), included the diet guidelines, and an article on the research. It may be that there is also a relationship between rheumatoid arthritis and the micro-organism Proteus in the gut, and this may be a mechanism by which dietary treatment works.

Arthritis drugs and diet

It's crucial you don't mess around with your anti-arthritic drugs without first consulting your doctor. Davies and Stewart say there's no reason why the nutritional approaches recommended in their book (*Nutritional Medicine*) shouldn't be combined with the use of painkillers and anti-inflammatory, anti-arthritic drugs.

They also point out that some of the drugs used to treat RA may actually necessitate an increased intake of some nutrients, for instance long-term use of penicillamine and steroids can produce zinc deficiency. The BMA *Guide to Medicines and Drugs* includes an A to Z of vitamins and minerals, and gives dietary advice for individual drugs where appropriate, eg prolonged use of penicillamine may deplete pyridoxine (vitamin B_6) and iron; sulphasalazine may reduce absorption of folic acid from the intestine, so plenty of green vegetables should be eaten and at least 1.5 litres of fluid a day should be drunk.

Summary of dos and don'ts

1 Remember we're all different. A diet that seems to work for one person may not work or could even be harmful for someone else.

2 Do talk to your doctor. With a bit of luck s/he might realise that an open-minded, supportive approach is more helpful than an attitude which sends you scuttling off in search of the nearest quack remedy. Explain that you'd like support in making sure that any diet you try is sufficiently well-balanced not to do you any *harm*, whether or not it helps your arthritis. If s/he's supportive but feels s/he doesn't know enough about it, try suggesting a look at the books I mentioned earlier, or referral to a dietitian, or suggest s/he writes to the British Society for Nutritional Medicine for information (point out membership's limited to bona fide orthodox professionals, eg GPs).

3 If your doctor's unhelpful *do* be wary of rejecting his/her trusted remedy in favour of what could be a restricted and unbalanced diet. Avoid 'miracle cures' and fad diets which claim to 'eliminate noxious acids' or 'boost lubrication', etc.

4 You don't necessarily have to embark on a complicated trial of every food under the sun. Some people, like the YPA quoted on page 66, find that just one or two particular types of food make their arthritis worse. If so, with your doctor's agreement, eliminate that particular bugbear from your diet.

5 Even if you don't want to be bothered with 'special' diets, do keep an eye on your eating and drinking habits. It's all too easy to put on excess weight, especially if you can't take much exercise. Aim for a sensible, well-balanced diet (see booklets below). And remember diet's not the only essential for good health; others include taking regular 'mental exercise' (eg reading, writing, creative arts, hobbies); having goals; cutting down on avoidable stresses; finding something to enjoy in life; not smoking (apart from causing cancers and respiratory and circulatory illnesses, did you know smoking also has a powerful anti-vitamin C effect, and inhibits the workings of the pancreas, essential to good digestion?).

6 Sometimes minor dietary changes like cutting down or cutting out caffeine-containing tea, coffee and cola drinks and chocolate may be helpful. An average cup of strong tea contains 50mg of caffeine, coffee 100 mg, though it varies a lot. Caffeine's a stimulant and a diuretic (increases your need to pass urine), so you might find you sleep better and don't waste so much precious energy on journeys to and from the loo! Tea and coffee also inhibit the absorption of iron and zinc, and have other sometimes surprising adverse effects, listed by Davies and Stewart. Incidentally, cutting out caffeine may cause withdrawal symptoms at first, eg headaches, but these do pass.

Further information

- Both ARC and Arthritis Care publish information sheets (free, but send SAE).
- Two booklets on healthy eating in general: *Eating Well on a Budget* (Age Concern); and *Guide to Healthy Eating* (free from the Health Education Authority).
- *The Manual of Nutrition* (HMSO), produced by the Ministry of Agriculture, Fisheries and Food, and regularly updated, is packed with fascinating food facts.
- *The Food Intolerance Diet Book* by E Workman, SRD, Dr V Alun Jones, and Dr J Hunter (Macdonald Optima 1986)
- *Nutritional Medicine* by Dr Stephen Davies & Dr Alan Stewart (Pan, 1987).
- *The Complete Guide to Food Allergy and Intolerance* by Dr Jonathan Brostoff and Linda Gamlin (Bloomsbury). Dr Brostoff runs an allergy clinic at the Middlesex Hospital in London.
- *Food Allergies and Intolerance* by Professor M Lessof, who started the Allergy Unit at Guy's Hospital (one of the low-cost Health Information Network series).
- On slimming, look at the British Medical Association's *BMA Slimmers' Guide*.

Some other books you might come across; opinions vary on how helpful they may be:
- Collin H Dong and Jane Banks' *The Arthritic's Cookbook* (Granada)
- Mary Laver and Margaret Smith's *Diet for Life: Cookbook for Arthritics* (Pan). Mary Laver's RA was first diagnosed when she was 26, recently married, and working as a traffic warden. Margaret Smith is a Member of the Association of Home Economists. The book uses Dong diet principles.
- *The Arthritis Diet Cookbook* (Victor Gollancz), by Michael McIlwraith, fellow of the Hotel Catering & Institutional Management Association. Foreword's by Mollie Hunter, who has RA and writes award-winning books for children and young adults.

Chapter ten

ALTERNATIVE/COMPLEMENTARY MEDICINE

"I've tried various treatments in the past in my determination to beat Mr 'Itis' (I'm not fond enough of Arthur to call him by his first name!). Let's see, I've had acupuncture, both oriental and English, hypnotherapy (that was a rip-off), osteopathy, a 'miracle machine' called EMMA, herbal remedies, diets and even foreign mussels with green lips would you believe?!" (Marilyn S, in her 30s, with psoriatic arthritis)

For centuries there have been hundreds of 'alternative' remedies claiming miraculous cures for rheumatic and other disorders, and we continue today to be bombarded by media and friends with tales of miracle treatments. A lot of these are just a waste of time and money; others are potentially harmful. But is there any truth in any of the tales? Might there be *something* in it for us? How are we to know? How can we avoid rip-offs and quacks, keen to make money out of other people's despair and misery?

First of all, don't, for goodness sake, turn your back on orthodox medicine. Though it can't yet produce a cure, it can do a tremendous amount to treat rheumatic disorders. Orthodox doctors are highly skilled, work to a high code of ethics, and aren't out to fleece you of all your money. Try not to get downhearted if finding the right treatment takes time and a trial-and-error approach, but keep at it, and give orthodox medicine a fair chance.

'Good' practitioners of alternative medicine will also usually encourage you not to turn your back on orthodox medicine, but to look on their treatment as 'complementary' rather than as a substitute ('alternative'). Rheumatic disorders are complicated, and it's essential to have correct diagnosis and management by orthodox doctors.

'Bad' practitioners of alternative medicine might well prescribe treatment that's actually harmful to you, besides lining their pockets at your expense. For instance forceful manipulation of the neck in someone with RA could very seriously damage the spinal cord and nerve. Herbal remedies aren't as harmless as often thought: like orthodox prescribed medicines they can sometimes produce unwanted side effects and drug interactions yet they're not subject to the same strict testing and licensing controls as orthodox drugs. Nutritional deficiency problems can result from some 'alternative' diets. Bear in mind too that unorthodox practitioners aren't legally obliged to take out insurance, and you might not be able to get compensation if anything goes wrong.

If you want to try complementary medicine, do first talk to your doctor. Ok, s/he may pour cold water on the idea, but don't be put off mentioning it. Explain that you're asking because you want to know if it will do you any harm or will conflict with your orthodox treatment. It's important to check, *whatever* it is, whether a physical treatment, an external preparation, a tonic, a herb/plant remedy or whatever. Here's what one orthodox doctor has to say: Dr J T Scott, Consultant Physician, Charing Cross Hospital, London and Honorary Physician, Kennedy Institute of Rheumatology:

"Patients are often embarrassed to mention [this], fearing the wrath that may fall upon them when it is learnt that they have strayed from the paths of medical orthodoxy. This should not be the case, however, and doctors are often interested to hear the results: knowing our limitations, we can hardly blame the patient for trying something new...But some of these [alternative practitioners] are not exactly generous with their skills, and anger is an understandable reaction when one hears that a patient with RA has been persuaded to spend large sums of money which she can ill afford, on worthless bits of

quackery." (In his *Arthritis and Rheumatism. The Facts*, Oxford University Press, 1980)
Your doctor might surprise you by *not* scorning your enquiry. Some have become more open-minded towards complementary medicine, and interested in its uses in treating chronic illnesses. They feel that any treatment with few or no side-effects which might help patients is worth investigating scientifically. Professor Malcolm Jayson, Head of the Rheumatic Diseases Centre at Manchester's Hope Hospital, for example, uses acupuncture for treating certain types of back pain. Bart's hospital in London uses acupuncture for some patients with RA and OA. Spiritual healing is used in Liverpool's Walton Hospital Pain Management Programme and for arthritis patients at Leeds General Infirmary.

Dr J Kenyon MD, MB, ChB, and Dr G T Lewith, MA, MRCP, MRCGP are doctors who established 'The Centre for the Study of Complementary Medicine' in Southampton:

"in the profound belief that treatments such as acupuncture and homeopathy have much to offer mankind and that research and education within these areas were both essential and long overdue...It seems to me that some of the more exciting and potentially useful concepts within medicine exist in the philosophies of the various alternative therapies. Many of these ideas will prove to be false, but if some could be verified and formulated in a more specific and practical manner, then we might reap untold rewards..." (In *Alternative Therapies*, ed G T Lewith, Heinemann, 1985)

Since 1977 GPs have been allowed by the General Medical Council to refer patients to an alternative practitioner, provided they maintain overall responsibility for the patient. So it's worth asking whether your GP knows of someone suitable. Besides talking to your doctor, find out as much as you can yourself about any therapy that interests you. Look, for instance, at the publications on page 75.

Dr Lewith's *Alternative Therapies*, mentioned above, is aimed at orthodox health professionals, and deals with acupuncture and transcutaneous nerve stimulation (TENS), manipulation, biofeedback and meditation, homeopathic medicine, and clinical ecology (food sensitivity). It might be worth mentioning to your doctor if s/he's interested but admits to not being terribly well-informed. Though the book contains some difficult medical jargon, some of it's readable by a layperson, eg the chapter on homeopathy.

Bear in mind that what seems to work for someone else won't necessarily work for you. Firstly, because each person's body is different. Secondly, because a characteristic of most chronic inflammatory rheumatic disorders is that they are 'episodic', coming and going unpredictably; so an improvement might have happened anyway. Thirdly, improvement might be due to the placebo effect (see page 80): if people believe a treatment will do them good, then some 20 – 30% will actually experience an improvement, even if they're being treated with dummy medicines or non-functioning apparatus.

Be wary of being taken for a ride simply to line someone else's pocket. When you come across an advert for a new product or form of treatment, avoid especially those which use words like 'miracle', 'cure', or 'breakthrough'; those which claim to have support from unnamed or suspect 'experts', include testimonials from people who were 'cured', and make vague references to 'published research'.

The best way to find an alternative therapist is on the personal recommendation of your doctor, or, with your doctor's approval, on the recommendation of a friend. Don't be fooled by impressive-looking letters after a therapist's name. Outside orthodox medicine anyone can stick letters after their name and set up as a homeopath, herbalist, or whatever with no qualifications and little or no knowledge of their subject. Find out what the letters stand for, and whether the therapist belongs to one of the well-established professional organisations concerned with training and upholding high codes of practice amongst members.

The British Holistic Medical Association will supply a list of medically qualified practitioners who are also skilled in acupuncture, homeopathy, osteopathy, chiropractic, herbal medicine, breathing and relaxation, meditation, visualisation, exercise, diet, autogenic training, biofeedback, and naturopathy. 'Holistic medicine' means replacing mechanistic approaches to medicine with approaches which respond to a person as a whole within the environment, a person composed of mind, body and spirit. See the BHMA's free leaflet *What is Holistic Medicine?* Membership of the BHMA is open to orthodox healthcare professionals and members of the public too.

The BHMA also sells self-help tapes on subjects such as *Healthy Eating, Introduction to Meditation, The Breath of Life, Undoing Muscular Tension*, and *Skills in Self-Care*, and produces a low-cost helpful reading list of over 100 books on all aspects of 'whole person' health. Topics covered include taking care of yourself – general principles, mind-body relationship, relaxation/stress management, diet, anxiety and depression, families, spirit/inspiration: relationships/personal growth.

The Institute for Complementary Medicine runs a computerised library service about practitioners, research documents and books on homeopathy, acupuncture, herbalism, chiropractic and osteopathy, and produces an annual directory of UK practices and therapies. Practitioners listed have undergone a professional (usually three years) training, subscribe to a code of professional ethics, and are fully insured. The Institute can supply information on other therapies, and has 72 volunteer-staffed local Public Information Points (PIPs).

Some Complementary Therapies

Acupuncture, TENS treatment, homeopathy, spiritual healing, osteopathy/chiropractic/ manipulation, and herbal medicine are dealt with here. For dietary therapy see chapter 9, for meditation and relaxation techniques see chapter 14.

Acupuncture and TENS

Acupuncture's been used in traditional Chinese medicine for more than 2,000 years. It can't cure rheumatic disorders or repair damaged joints, but some people find it relieves pain, though usually only temporarily, lasting anything from a few hours to a few weeks or months. Some patients react by temporarily becoming a little worse after the first or perhaps second acupuncture treatment.

An acupuncturist aims to restore health through restoring 'bodily harmony', by inserting fine, hairlike needles at key acupuncture points found on invisible channels on the body called meridians. There are over 350 key points on the body, but usually only about 8 to 12 are used at any one time. Theories suggest that acupuncture may work by stimulating the release of the brain's own pain-killing substances 'endorphins', or by modifying pain messages being sent from damaged tissues to the brain. (See page 79).

Most acupuncturists in Britain practise privately. Acupuncture for pain control is used to a very limited extent in the NHS, for instance a few physios now use it, some hospital pain clinics, and a few consultants, like, for instance Professor Jayson (page 71).

Three main professional bodies provide training courses for acupuncturists, including the British Acupuncture Association, which runs postgraduate courses for registered medical practitioners, dentists, paramedics. All three bodies are represented on the Council for Acupuncture, which publishes a Combined Register of British Acupuncturists and sets professional standards. Members aren't allowed to advertise. In addition, the British Medical Acupuncture Society is an organisation of registered orthodox medical and dental practitioners, all practising acupuncturists, to whom referral is possible through your own doctor. For ethical reasons the Society can't send the list of its members direct to the public. But they can send the list in a sealed envelope for you to give your GP!

Transcutaneous electrical nerve stimulation (TENS) is an adaptation of acupuncture, which uses electrical instead of manual stimulation, and works through surface rubber electrodes instead of acupuncture needles. The patient feels a tingling sensation around the electrodes. Apparently the Romans used electric eels to provide similar treatment for people with arthritis!

TENS *doesn't* work for everyone, and like acupuncture, pain relief is usually temporary, but it's convenient and portable (a small box), though expensive. TENS machines aren't generally available on the NHS, though some GPs have bought their own machines, and lend them out to patients to try. An improvement, if there's going to be one, should have started appearing in some two to three weeks. TENS *shouldn't* be used by anyone who has a cardiac pacemaker, or while operating heavy machinery or driving a car.

Dr Lewith mentions a number of controlled studies of TENS treatment used for people with low back pain, phantom limb pain, pain caused by osteoarthritis of the knee, and pain caused by RA:

"All these show that...the treatment is effective in approximately 45 – 50% of patients depending on the condition studied.

"...TENS is now used...in pain clinics, and is generally available in physiotherapy departments throughout the United Kingdom, but there are only a few general practitioners in the United Kingdom who are using this therapy. In my opinion it would be extremely valuable to use TENS as an equivalent therapy to analgesics and non-steroidal anti-inflammatory agents for chronic pain, in the context of general practice, particularly in view of its minimal side-effects..." (In *Alternative Therapies*)

Homeopathy

Homeopathy is based on the principle that in certain illnesses 'like cures like'. In a healthy person, for instance, the plant belladonna produces a headache, but a minute controlled dose would be prescribed to treat certain types of headache. Quinine taken by a healthy person produces malarial symptoms, but is used to treat someone ill with malaria.

The founder of homeopathy, Samuel Hahnemann, believed it was possible to treat a patient effectively and avoid side-effects by giving only a microscopic amount of a remedy, known as the 'minimum dose'. Looked at scientifically, it's difficult to see how this can work, for these remedies (known as 'potencies') are prepared by being diluted to an incredible extent. Sceptics believe there may be a placebo effect.

As in orthodox medicine, the homeopath takes a history of the illness, and examines the patient physically. Choice of remedy is based on a detailed holistic assessment of the patient's personality as a whole, family and social circumstances, and the way s/he reacts to the illness. The homeopathic remedy used for one person might be totally different from that prescribed to treat the same illness in a different person.

In *Alternative Therapies*, Dr Lewith looks at alternative theories and describes research investigating how homeopathy might work. Few strictly controlled trials have been carried out, but he describes one on some RA patients, reported in 1980 (Gibson R G, Gibson S L M, MacNeill A D, Watson Buchanan W: 'Homeopathic therapy in rheumatoid arthritis: evaluation by double-blind clinical therapeutic trial': *British Journal of Clinical Pharmacology*, 9: 453 – 9):

"[The trial] made a rigid comparison between one group of 23 patients on orthodox first-line anti-inflammatory treatment plus homeopathy and a second group of 23 patients on orthodox first-line treatment plus an inert preparation. There was a significant improvement in the subjective pain, articular index, stiffness and grip strength in those patients receiving homeopathic remedies, and no significant change in the patients who received placebo. Both groups were seen by the same two physicians and the experiment was done under double-blind conditions."

Where appropriate, reputable homeopaths will prescribe conventional drugs (undiluted), as well as or instead of homeopathic remedies. Dr Lewith stresses that homeopathy should be regarded as a complement to conventional therapies, and not as a substitute:

"In certain cases both types of therapy may be used to complement each other. A patient with severe rheumatoid arthritis may still require an analgesic or non-steroidal anti-rheumatic drug as well as his homeopathic remedies, or an asthmatic patient may require inhalers. But with successful homeopathic prescribing it may be possible to reduce other medication and to stop administration of drugs which cause unpleasant side-effects.

"Advanced cases of rheumatoid arthritis or osteoarthritis can be alleviated, but may require additional conventional drugs...The patient's well-being and ability to cope with the disease are often markedly improved, and some relief of pain and stiffness obtained."

However, in a chronic disorder, ongoing treatment's required and a response, if any, may be slow in coming. In the early days, the symptoms may even be worsened temporarily, 'the homeopathic aggravation' or 'healing crisis', though homeopaths usually take this as a sign that improvement will follow.

Many people don't realise that homeopathy is available on the NHS (in theory, anyway), and the remedies used are prescribable in hospital or by GPs in the same way as conventional drugs. In practice however there aren't many homeopathically qualified doctors around, and most are in private practice. There are five homeopathic hospitals in Britain (Royal London, Glasgow, Liverpool, Bristol, and Tunbridge Wells). For information about medically qualified homeopaths and homeopathy, contact the British Homeopathic Association.

Spiritual healing

Over the last few years the Confederation of Healing Organisations (CHO), an umbrella body of 15 healing organisations, has set up trials in hospitals to try to prove the value of spiritual healing. It's being tested in use alongside orthodox treatment for conditions like AIDS, cancer, and even arthritis, for instance in London and outside, at hospitals like the Walton in Liverpool (in its self-help course for people with chronic pain) and at Leeds General Infirmary (for people with arthritis). It's even being tested on horses.

Responsible spiritual healers, belonging to the CHO, don't claim that it will produce instant 'miracle cures', and stress that *"healing must be seen as strictly complementary to orthodox medicine...Registered healers are forbidden to indulge in medical diagnosis, manipulation, the prescribing of drugs, or to interfere in the medical regime".*

Though spiritual healing may not cure, many people do feel better mentally and spiritually, and better able to cope with physical pain, even if it doesn't go away. How healing may work is a mystery, but healers themselves believe they act as a channel for energy from some outside force, which they pass on and which stimulates the patient's own healing powers. Surprisingly, you don't usually have to be religious to try spiritual healing; you just need to have a strong desire to feel better. YPA Janet Flower contacted a healer:

"I had an open mind as to what would happen and didn't expect miracles, nor on the other hand did I think it would be a useless exercise. I suppose I didn't feel I was really the right sort of recipient, not 'worthy' of receiving healing. I have my own sort of 'faith', and don't go to church; perhaps I felt a bit hypocritical.

"Anyway, Carol reassured me and during the healing session all worries fell away. My mind was completely calm, but also very alert. I definitely felt some kind of 'sensation', which varied on some joints and limbs. Normally, if a joint is playing me up I tend to ignore it as much as possible. During the healing sessions, I was very aware of each joint, and without changing my lifestyle or routines at all, seemed to know whether a joint pain needed rest or exercise. Perhaps I was more able to relax and ease a joint than before − I used to be more inclined either to try to force a joint or just ignore it, neither of which helped! Coupled with a greater awareness of my joints and muscles, I felt a

marvellous inner peace (difficult to describe) and at times a kind of glow (like ET?).

"Perhaps it's all due to my vivid imagination but since I've been receiving healing I've felt so much better inside. The feeling I get from each healer is different but it's always gentle, soothing but also invigorating. Like having your batteries charged. I wouldn't claim to be terribly better physically but nevertheless, I'm stronger mentally and spiritually; which makes my physical problems seem to lessen and fade." (*In Contact*)

For more information contact the Confederation of Healing Organisations (CHO), or the National Federation of Spiritual Healers (NFSH). Payment to part-time healers (who have other jobs to support themselves financially) is usually a small donation. Full-time healers charge fees for sessions which may last 20 minutes to an hour.

Osteopathy, Chiropractic and Manipulation

Each of these treatments uses a degree of controlled force to move a joint. Although in some conditions such treatment may be helpful, that does *not* usually apply to us, younger people with the inflammatory types of arthritis. As the ARC leaflet on alternative medicine emphasises: *"Given to the wrong patient or in the wrong way, it can be disastrous - particularly when applied to the neck."*

So do *not*, ever, try these treatments unless your doctor has specifically agreed. If s/he ever prescribes any form of manipulation for you, it should be undertaken only by physios or doctors specially trained in the technique, and fully briefed on your medical history.

Herbal Medicine

Because herbal and plant remedies are so readily available, many people believe they're harmless, but that's not true, so beware. They can be poisonous, and cause unwanted side-effects, just like any other drugs, and most haven't undergone the same stringent clinical trials as orthodox drugs to test for safety and long-term effects. Comfrey, for instance, traditionally used as a remedy to promote healing of wounds, ulcers, bone fractures and bronchitis, is potentially poisonous to the liver; feverfew can cause ulceration of the mouth and tongue.

The Medicines Control Authority (MCA) issues product licences to medicines it has approved for use. The letters PL, followed by a number, on a herbal remedy label, indicate that it's intended as a medicine, has been assessed by the MCA, and given a product licence. The MCA specifically says that sassafras, comfrey, mistletoe, broom and senecio aureus are *not* safe for use in herbal remedies, and very many herbs should specifically *not* be taken in pregnancy, including feverfew, parsley seeds, sage, pennyroyal, black cohosh, berberis, blue cohosh, bloodroot, fumaria, helonias, hydrastis, juniper, kelp, mugwort.

So for goodness sake check with your doctor before trying any herbal remedy, whether purchased or home-made. *The Dictionary of Modern Herbalism* (Thorsons), includes possible adverse effects. It's by Simon Mills, joint director of the Centre for Complementary Health Studies at Exeter University. His *Out of the Earth* (Viking, 1992, pricey) examines herbal medicine and its safety in detail. Professor David Phillipson, professor of pharmacognosy (the study of herbal products!) at London University's School of Pharmacy, is currently compiling information on adverse effects.

Further information

- ARC's *Alternative Medicine in the Rheumatic Diseases* (free, but send SAE)
- The College of Health's low-cost *Guide to Alternative Medicine*
- Dr A Stanway's *Alternative Medicine: A Guide to the Natural Therapies* (Penguin)
- *Reader's Digest Family Guide to Alternative Medicine* (Reader's Digest)
- Look too at the publications on the British Holistic Medical Association's low-cost reading list (see page 72).

Chapter eleven

THE PAIN DRAIN

The chronic pain of inflammatory arthritis is very different from acute pain, as Mary*, aged 30, with RA, knew only too well:

"I want to talk about pain. I'm in constant pain day in, day out, sometimes better, sometimes worse, but always there. If it were just the occasional pain one could talk about it openly but, understandably, no one wants to hear a constant moan about aches and pains, so the tendency is to say nothing lest you say too much, until a barrier develops and eventually you find you can no longer talk about it to anyone. Even when someone specifically asks how you are you never admit to pain. 'I'm fine' means 'I'm not too bad', 'I'm not too bad' means 'I'm not very good' and 'It comes and it goes' means it's come – with a vengeance. In the end you become isolated with your pain, locked in a world which no others are allowed to enter. It becomes very lonely. Pain is central to my whole existence yet I can't talk about it. So there is a large chunk of my life that I'm unable to share with others. There's a large chunk of me that I'm unable to share with others."

Fourteen or so years later Mary* re-read what she'd written:

"I was astonished to re-read my own comments and realise how bad things were, or could be, at the time. Perhaps you could add a note to your book, reminding folk that it does get better. Nowadays there's nowhere near as much actual pain unless I've been stupidly overdoing it which, being inherently stupid, I often choose to do."

Let's look back, for a moment, to experiences of chronic pain when it's at its worst. What happens and how do we start dealing with it? It can drain you not just physically, but psychologically and emotionally too.

"Acute pain may be a life saver but chronic pain...turns strong individuals into weak, nervous folk. It turns the affable into the irritable; it makes cowards of the brave...

"The sufferer from persistent or recurrent pain cannot sleep or rest; his hopes will be built up repeatedly and then quickly dashed; he will often find it difficult to explain to others the extent of his pain and suffering. However bizarre they may seem, he will explore all potential possibilities for relief and understanding, support and sympathy. He will struggle to understand what purpose his pain can serve. He will be depressed and discouraged no matter how often he is given hope and encouragement." (Dr Vernon Coleman, *Natural Pain Control*, Century Arrow, 1986)

A bleak picture. But wait. The darkest hour is just before the dawn. The enemy is Arthur Itis. His most vicious weapon is chronic pain. But we can fight back. Even if we can't eliminate him completely (not just yet, anyway) we *can* weaken his hold over us. As in any battle, sometimes he'll have the upper hand despite our most valiant efforts. But the tide will turn, and we and our weapons can always be ready and waiting to take the advantage.

A good General finds out as much as possible about the enemy before planning his strategy and marching into battle. I think we too can fight better if we first understand what pain is and how 'pain-control' works. The first step is to understand more about how pain can be both a physical and a psychological experience.

The *cause* of pain in inflammatory arthritis is physical. It's a warning signal that your joints are having a bad time; something's not as it should be. If you touch a hot stove, or hit your thumb with a hammer, you can respond to the pain warning signal, and stop the cause of the pain ('acute' pain) at once. Easy. *Not* so easy with RA and its cousins. The pain signals just go on and on and *on*, *long* after you've got the message and want it to shut up ('chronic' pain). But you can't remove the cause (yet), so instead, to quieten the signals you've got to use pain-control (drugs or non-drug methods or a mixture).

Most people who've never suffered chronic pain can't begin to understand what it can do to you. It's especially hard for them to understand how something apparently so invisible and so physical in its cause can also have such a huge psychological, emotional and social impact. Someone who does understand is Connie Peck. She's Senior Lecturer in the Department of Psychology at La Trobe University in Australia, and a member of the International Association for the Study of Pain. In *Controlling Chronic Pain* (Harper-Collins Publishers Ltd) she wrote:

"When pain becomes a chronic condition, a predictable set of problems are likely to befall those who suffer from it. Some of these problems can, in turn, further aggravate the pain, eventually creating a vicious downward spiral of compounding pain and complex new sets of problems. Such complications can take many forms. The most common involves trying one unsuccessful treatment after another; losing faith in doctors; taking too many drugs or too much alcohol; worrying about drug dependency; giving up activities from which pleasure and mastery were previously achieved; pain and illness becoming the focus in one's conversation and thoughts; depression; marital discord; feelings of anger, guilt and anxiety; and finally low self-esteem. All of these add up to what will be called the Chronic Pain Trap.

"Simply understanding the process as an identifiable syndrome is often comforting to the chronic pain sufferer; since the knowledge helps him to combat the feeling that he is alone with his problem and that no one else understands what is happening to him. Families, doctors and friends sometimes express doubts about the reality of a chronic pain sufferer's experience, implying that they are wondering if, perhaps, the pain is really exaggerated or imagined. Such misunderstanding of the problem only serves to aggravate the condition of the pain sufferer, to make him feel angry with others and eventually to cause him to have negative thoughts about himself...."

Whew! Please don't get too depressed at all this. – Plenty of tips on *how* to get out of the Chronic Pain Trap come later.

Talking about chronic pain as a *psychological* experience is tricky, and all too easily misinterpreted to mean 'it's all in the mind, so it doesn't exist', which is definitely *not* so. The pain of inflammatory arthritis is definitely *not* 'all in the mind'. It's very real.

Some theories about the cause of some types of inflammatory arthritis suggest emotional stress might be one of many possible 'trigger factors' but since there's no proof, and since that theory can so easily be misunderstood, let's stick here to what we do know for sure.

We need to distinguish between *cause* and *symptoms*, because the mind most definitely has a large part to play in how we react to the symptoms. A person's psychological response and the physical pain experienced are closely interlinked. In recent years much has been learnt about how pain works and how it can best be controlled, even if it can't be cured. Scientists have been trying to understand, for instance, how a large percentage of even seriously injured accident victims don't feel immediate pain: the experience of the heroic policeman in the Kings Cross Underground fire in November 1987, for instance. His hands were critically and horrifically burnt, yet he said he wasn't aware of any pain at the time. He was too busy thinking of getting people out, and thinking of his family. Incredible. No painkillers, yet he wasn't aware of the pain. How? Why? How could the mind shut out pain like that? Is it a skill people could learn to turn on at will?

The mind and how we feel can certainly make pain *worse*. Chronic pain can lead to anxiety and misery and fear of yet more pain. And the more we worry about pain the worse it seems to get:

"The way we respond to pain is influenced by our mood..If you're feeling unhappy and

you hit your thumb then the pain will stay with you all day long. Indeed, the pain may well exacerbate your depression, with the inevitable result that you become locked in a vicious circle. Your pain will make your depression worse; your depression will make you more susceptible to pain, and as your pain threshold is lowered so your depression will be deepened. " (Dr Vernon Coleman, *Natural Pain Control*, Century Arrow, 1986))

Resentment of pain, the 'why-did-it-have-to-happen-to-me?' angry response can aggravate it too, whereas faith in the Almighty, doctor, physio, or anyone else may help pain tolerance. Fortunately, though mind and body often seem to conspire together in a vicious circle, they *can* also work together to *break* and reverse the circle, as healthcare professionals and we old-handers have long recognised. One rheumatologist summed it up nicely:

"An occupied mind in a relaxed and happy person needs fewer pain pills to get through the day than an unhappy person with no mental distractions, even though both have the same amount of painful arthritis." (*ARC magazine*, autumn 1983)

Easier said than done, I hear you say. True! But how? Easy enough to prescribe painkiller drugs, and they do have their part to play, but in moderation when possible. Can non-drug painkillers really work too? How might they work? What are they? Before we start the pain-control and repair work let's try to understand recent researches into the workings of pain. No point in trying to repair the car if we don't understand how it works in the first place.

How our bodies 'feel' pain, and 'block' pain

A network of nerve fibres in the body busily transmits messages (eg heat, cold, touch) to and from the brain, via the spinal cord. Nerve endings are highly sensitive to pain and soon alert the brain that all is not well in an arthriticky joint.

You might have come across the 'gate control theory' of pain, a theory put forward by Ronald Melzack and Patrick Wall in the 1960s. Basically, this suggests that only a certain volume of messages can be processed by the nervous system at a time, and a 'gate' in the spinal cord controls the flow.

Some nerve fibres are thick, some thin. Some convey messages quickly, some slowly. Some fibres (called C fibres and A-delta fibres) carry pain messages. Other fibres (A-beta) carry non-painful messages. Messages move along the A-beta fibres very quickly, and they're thicker than C and A-delta fibres. The theory suggests that one way pain control works is by increasing the A-beta (non-painful) messages so much that they block pain messages travelling along the other fibres.

Apparently C fibres (painful messages) can regrow if damaged, but A fibres can't, and also tend to decrease in number as you get older. Maybe there's a tiny note of encouragement there for us younger people with arthritis? Youth and arthritis are nasty bedfellows, but at least we should have a good network of A-beta fibres (non-painful messages) to help 'block' pain.

There are basically two ways of blocking pain. First, at the site of the pain, you can interfere with the release of chemicals which trigger the nerve endings into dispatching a pain message to the brain. These chemicals are called kinins and protaglandins. The prostaglandins also increase the flow of blood to the site of tissue damage, inflaming the site and making it red and swollen, and they also make the pain receptors on the nerve endings even more sensitive, wickedly increasing the sensation of pain. Painkillers like aspirin (the 'non-narcotic painkillers' mentioned on page 45) and the anti-inflammatory drugs ('NSAIDs', also page 45) are 'anti-prostaglandins' which work to stop pain messages ever starting their journey to the brain, by interfering with the manufacture of prostaglandins.

You can also block pain messages at the site of the pain by increasing the flow of alternative messages to the brain along the non-painful A-beta fibres. For instance, if you bang your thigh, the natural reaction is to rub it better. The 'rub message' helps block out, or reduce, the volume of pain messages getting to the brain. Similarly, RA aches and pains in a thigh can seem less if you cuddle a warm comforting hot-water bottle.

The second basic way of blocking pain is to let the pain messages travel along the nerve network, but to stop the brain recognising them. Drugs that work this way are the 'narcotic analgesics' like codeine and morphine (see page 45). Something like morphine seems to work by mimicking chemicals called 'endorphins'. Research has shown that the body can actually produce its own endorphins (inner pain-killing chemicals), in the brain and spinal cord. They can switch off the body's pain alarm system by fitting into special receptors on nerve cells.

Doctors from Newcastle General Hospital investigated why healthy men in the annual Tyneside half-marathon fun run went on until they collapsed in confusion without first feeling intolerable pain. In their report in the *British Medical Journal* (April 1987) the doctors reported that all the runners had more than three times as much 'natural painkiller' in their blood as before, but those who collapsed had on average four times as much as those who didn't. Endorphins suppressed the pain, produced 'feelings of well-being', and meant that the runners pushed themselves much further than if they'd felt pain.

Hearty exercise is the one thing we YPAs can't really indulge in to stop the pain (though maybe sometimes swimming works? And laughter's been called 'stationary jogging'!). However, endorphins also seem to be produced if you're busy doing something really important to you, more important than 'pain'. An occupied mind helps stop the brain recognising pain messages. If you busy yourself with an enjoyable chat with friends the pain seems less than when you sit alone, feeling sorry for yourself, letting the pain messages rush around the body unhindered. Try to flood your mind with pain-blocking activity so there's little or no room left for pain and misery messages. Tips to help follow in later chapters. Dr Sampson Lipton wrote:

"What is allowed to rise into your mind depends on what you are doing at the time, how much you are concentrating on something else and how important this information is to you.

"If you have severe chronic pain, you can learn to use this modulation to your advantage. By immersing yourself in work, exciting games, books and films or by just watching an interesting programme on television, you can distract your conscious mind from recognising pain. One famous actress was able to make the pain of arthritis vanish while absorbed in performing her role on stage, and dentists have found that their patients bear the pain of drilling much better if they are listening to music they enjoy."
(*Conquering Pain*, Macdonald Optima, 1984)

Other non-drug methods of controlling pain messages include methods used and taught by physios, such as massage, heat treatment, ice treatment; or simple anti-stress techniques like those described in chapter 14 (eg meditation, relaxation methods, laughter or talking therapy); or the use of counter-irritants (liniments rubbed into the skin, for instance). Some people find something like acupuncture or the use of a TENS machine, as described in chapter 10, helps. Other chapters suggest ways of cutting down on pain-causing activity or stress, and ways of 'being positive' and distracting your mind from recognising pain.

What's meant by the pain 'threshold' and pain 'tolerance' level?

How someone feels pain is influenced by his or her pain threshold and pain tolerance level. The pain threshold is the point at which you first feel pain. Above this level you'll still be able to stand increasing pain, until your pain tolerance level is reached, when it becomes simply too much to bear.

Just as some people's eyesight is better than others, some people are able to stand more pain than others. Social conditioning, learned behaviour, and personality all play their part. If a child making a fuss about a pain finds he's rewarded with attention and affection which he wouldn't otherwise get, then his pain tolerance level may decrease to ensure more of this welcome attention. If pain brings 'rewards' why bother to fight it?

That's why people around the child, or around someone in chronic pain should make a special point of showing attention and affection at other times too, as rewards for things *other* than the expression of pain. That *doesn't* mean ignoring somebody in pain: support and comfort *are* needed, especially when it's severe, but they should try to give even *more* encouragement to efforts to fight the pain and efforts to take an interest in other things. In *Conquering Pain* Dr Lipton explains:

"The realisation of how your behaviour may be affecting how much you are feeling pain can go a long way towards making you more able to deal with it."

Mind and body: What is the 'placebo effect'?

We've looked at some of the ways the mind can influence the body in its response to pain. Isn't it amazing too how the very act of doing something to help yourself can make you feel good? And how the belief that someone or something is going to do you good sometimes seems to have the same effect?

This fascinating influence of mind on body is seen when new drugs are tested on patients who've agreed to take part in 'clinical trials'. Half the patients are given 'placebos' (dummy drugs), while the others are given the real drug to be tested. Incredibly, on average, about a third of patients respond to placebos, though the results vary widely. In a trial conducted in 1984 on patients suffering from Crohn's disease (which causes irritation of the gut and bowel) 25 to 40% of the patients who were on placebo treatment improved enough to be considered to have had a remission.

However, though placebos seem sometimes to help in relieving symptoms, there's still no evidence to suggest that they can cure a disease. Researchers still have a long long way to go before understanding all the whys and wherefores.

The placebo effect may be one reason why sometimes strange remedies seem to work for some people with a rheumatic disorder. Another reason is that natural remissions are unpredictable anyway, and sometimes just happen to coincide with a particular treatment. However, *provided* a placebo does no *harm* to you or to your pocket, and *provided* you've got your doctor's agreement, why scorn something which makes the most of the magical power of the mind?

What is 'referred pain'?

Some of us with hip trouble have been surprised to experience pain in the knee, and find it hard to understand how the doctor's so confident the trouble hasn't actually spread to the knee! What we're feeling is 'referred pain' – pain that doesn't actually arise where we seem to feel it. It's all to do with the arrangement of nerve fibres.

Sciatica is another type of referred pain. The pain actually arises in a prolapsed disc in the back, but is referred down the *leg*, down the back of the thigh and part of the calf. (It's called sciatica from the name of the nerve involved).

Developing your own pain-control programme

I hope all this helps you understand how pain 'works' and, more important, understand how drug and non-drug methods of pain-control can work. I hope this helps you as you develop your personal 'Outwit Arthritis Kit', your self-care programme worked out to meet your own very individual needs.

Remember, you're not a failure if the pain's still there, and if there still seem more downs than ups. Sometimes the arthritis just refuses to let you even begin to take control of your life. In those bleak times don't hesitate to let the doctor help you take the strain with whatever treatment helps, and *don't* feel somehow you're to blame for the pain. You're not. Just hang on in there till the better times arrive.

Ideas in this book will help you develop your self-care programme. Your personality, your family and friends and your healthcare team will all play their part too in helping (or hindering!) you along the way. Remember it may be a slow process, and a lot of it done subconsciously.

Some of the arthritis books on page 16 have helpful ideas too, especially Dr Dudley Hart's *Overcoming Arthritis* and Dr Vernon Coleman's *Arthritis*, which includes what he calls an 'Arthritis Control Programme'. Some people under 45 may find helpful the Personal Development Courses run by Young Arthritis Care (page 123).

You might also like to read other books dealing specifically with pain, and pain-control. Some of what they contain isn't relevant to someone with an inflammatory arthritis like RA or AS, but a lot is, and can give you helpful ideas. Personally I find it helpful just reading the words of someone who understands what it's like to 'live with a chronic disorder'.

– Dr Sampson Lipton's *Conquering Pain* (Macdonald Optima, 1984) is written by a professional in language readable by non-medical people, with lots of colour illustrations and diagrams. Dr Lipton was Director of the Centre for Pain Relief at Walton Hospital, Liverpool, for many years before his retirement. He's edited and contributed to many medical books, and his own books include *The Control of Chronic Pain*.

– Dr Vernon Coleman's *Natural Pain Control*, subtitled *A new and positive approach to the problem of persistent and recurrent pain* (Century Arrow, 1986) examines the whole subject of pain, and talks you through his 'Pain Control Programme'.

– Connie Peck's *Controlling Chronic Pain* (HarperCollins Publishers Ltd) is another general book which may give you ideas. The foreword is by Professor Patrick Wall who with Ronald Melzack put forward the 'gate control theory' I mentioned on page 78. Generally speaking, her advice on coping *psychologically* is more relevant than her advice on coping physically. Some of what she writes *isn't* relevant to someone with RA and its cousins, for instance 'How to resume more normal activity' and 'Controlling the painkillers'. If in doubt, try to persuade your doctor to read it and to guide you on dos and don'ts specific to you. (As an incentive to the doctor – there's a good appendix of 'References for Professional Readers').

Chapter twelve

PSYCHOLOGICAL AND EMOTIONAL REACTIONS 1:
The dark side of the hill

Medical books on rheumatic disorders like RA, AS, etc, tend to say very little about their psychological and emotional impact, and yet for me and, I know, for many other people, this is sometimes as hard to cope with as the physical symptoms.

"Generally speaking, I think I needed help to adjust to my illness emotionally and psychologically, more than just practical treatment. I hope you will be able to cover this aspect in your book and, perhaps, convince new sufferers, that it needn't be the end of the world." (Marilyn S, who has psoriatic arthritis)

"I suffered bouts of intense depression and how my poor husband put up with me at the time I don't know...I battled on accepting the physical pain but still not mentally adjusting to my insidious limitations. I would get so annoyed and frustrated at not being able to do things such as washing and dressing and being an independent person by nature – even stubborn! – this made things doubly difficult – result more bouts of depression and so the vicious circle continued and my joints deteriorated.." (Carol J, who has RA)

Grace Stuart developed RA when she was 19 and in her 50s wrote about her experiences (*Private World of Pain*, Allen and Unwin, 1953, now out of print, alas):

"..one can be stupid with pain, stupid, so that thinking grows inept and feeling harsh and out of tune...those of us who are badly hurt can hate, we can be jealous and bitter and destructive; hurting that which is free from pain, because on somebody we must revenge our own..

"With every year that I live...I become more profoundly convinced that...the situation should be met both psychologically and physically. I put the psychological aspect first, for I believe that upon the health of the ego, the self, may depend much of the virtue of the physical treatment...I believe...the training of the self to a now 'different' kind of life, [is] not at all to be done hastily but with as long and as great a skill as that demanded by the physical machine."

The next two diary extracts might sound as if they were written by two different people, but they're both by Mary*, who has RA. First, a very bad day:

"Sometimes, just occasionally. I get bloody sick of the whole business of arthritis. I get sick of smiling and gritting my teeth and making jokes. I want to cry my eyes out or, alternatively, kick someone's teeth in. I'm sick of the pain – pain in my hands as I write; pain in my knees, my feet, my shoulders. I want to stand up straight with no bent, aching knees. I want to climb up the stairs the normal way instead of one step at a time. I want to go to bed when I feel tired instead of delaying the process for half an hour because I can't face the pain involved in getting upstairs. I want to go upstairs to bed without biting my lips all the way to stop the grunts of pain from slipping out. I'm sick of pain. I'm sick of being silent and playing it down and pretending it doesn't matter. It does. It's a bloody awful, painful pain and it's there day in, day out...I want to talk about it; to tell someone of it but who'd want to listen? I want to cry and be comforted like a child. Pain is such a lonely business."

Hard to believe that Mary* is also a pretty active, optimistic person, who runs a household of two energetic sons and a husband, organises swimming sessions and does voluntary work. Here she is again, this time reminding us that there are good times too:

"Today I feel absolutely great, bursting with health and dying to tell the world. Even my knee is slightly improved and the rainy weather doesn't seem to have had its usual effect on me. There's no describing the relief and joy when it does let up for a while...Just 24 hours gives you a breather, a chance to pick yourself up off the floor and prepare to do battle again. There's just no words to describe it. You suddenly become aware of the absence of pain as the mother of a young child can suddenly become aware of the absence of noise. It ought to be a negative thing but it isn't because, where once there was pain, there is now not emptiness but triumph, exhilaration. You've got it on the run even if it is only for a few hours. Of course it doesn't go completely. There is still pain but just a gentle, achey background sort of pain, one you can virtually ignore."

Some 14 years and two knee joints later, Mary* was astonished to re-read her 'bad day' diary extract (see her more recent comments on page 76).

Back to the early reactions. Most of us blissfully take our good health for granted until one day it's not there. It's a particular shock when you're young or youngish and suddenly find you're imprisoned in a body which not only refuses to do just what you want when you want, but also inexplicably and unpredictably produces alarming aches and pains, which no one else seems able to understand; worse still, may even disbelieve.

Coping emotionally when you're young is, I think, especially difficult. You're at an age when life is making peak demands on you and your friends. Finding a job, getting married, having a family, finding somewhere to live, getting enough money, etc – there's quite enough to sort out as it is. But usually your friends are working their way through similar situations too, which helps. That's not usually the case with something like RA or AS, and that in itself can be frightening and isolating.

However, you're *not* alone. Many of us out here also know the disconcerting ups and downs of 'living with arthritis'. Most important, though, we *can* tell you there *is* light at the end of the tunnel; spring does follow winter. Somehow, 'good' or 'better' days do come, hard though it may sometimes be to believe that in the gloomiest depths. It does become possible to count blessings and to stop the arthritis dominating life completely. You'll discover plenty of ways of coping and adapting and outwitting the arthritis. People like us *do* manage to hold down a job, raise a family, find a purpose in living, enhance other people's lives, 'do our bit' for society, and find happiness in life.

By the way, if you've only mild inflammatory arthritis, please don't alarm yourself by thinking gloom is necessarily in store for *you*. It *ain't* necessarily so – you might well remain only mildly affected, like one YPA in his 20s:

"I have had RA since I was 14...The only problem I have is that I cannot run very fast and am weaker than most people. I have hardly any real pain and my illness is quite stable...I can't forget arthritis, but I can ignore it."

or like another YPA, writing to *In Contact*:

"...I have mild RA and take tablets daily, and apart from being a bit careful I lead a normal life with isolated bad patches. However, I do find the limitations of the disease frustrating at times especially when basic things like hair-washing, housework, and outings with the children are affected. I'm sure others will agree...that explaining to other people why you can disco dance one evening and yet barely walk short distances another, is a very difficult task. I no longer try since I have come to terms with the situation and I have so much love and support from my husband and family, who understand and could not be more helpful."

If you too have only mild arthritis, and wonder what on earth I'm going on about at such length, do please feel free to ignore the rest of this chapter!

Understanding stress in general

'Stress' has become a fashionable concern nowadays, featuring widely in the media. Chronic inflammatory arthritis (CIA for short?) is a particularly nasty source of stress. Understanding stress can help you start to deal with CIA. It can help you break the vicious pain circle (worry about pain = more pain = more worry = more pain) and help you adjust to the whole unwanted shenanigan.

It's interesting to see that research in the new area of psychoneuroimmunology (!) is now showing scientifically that the body's immune system responds to how stressed we are. Disorders like RA and lupus are auto-immune disorders, where for some unknown reason the immune system malfunctions. Might stress play some part in what happens?

We all experience some sort of stress (or tension) in life. Stress is the way your body tries to adapt to deal with challenges at work, or to stop your child doing something dangerous, or, on a simpler level, to answer an unexpected doorbell ring. Stress isn't necessarily harmful, it can be stimulating too. Some people, racing drivers, politicians, daredevils, seek out stress and thrive on it. And most of us enjoy the thrilling tension of an exciting game or film.

How does the body react to stress? Faced with an outside threat, our primitive ancestors needed bodies that would let them either *fight*, or take *flight*. Even nowadays, faced with some sort of 'threat', our bodies react the same way.

The body responds by instantly preparing itself for fight or flight. Muscles tense, ready for action. Heart rate and breathing speed up, blood pressure rises, and adrenalin surges into the blood so that extra sugar is produced to feed working muscles. They need extra oxygen too so blood is diverted from other areas to bring it, thus draining smaller blood vessels leaving them 'white' (hence 'white with fear'). Other body systems, like the digestive system, slow down or stop. Skin sweats, to cool overheating muscles.

These reactions are fine if vigorous physical activity *is* needed to fight or escape from a stress situation, but they aren't appropriate for so many of the situations we twentieth-century humans find ourselves in, like coping with a difficult child, an unreasonable boss, time pressures, overcrowded trains, moving house, unemployment. And they're definitely inappropriate for coping with chronic inflammatory arthritis. In an inappropriate situation the body's fight or flight reaction can actually make coping *more* difficult.

Continued chronic stress, if unrelieved, can lead to health problems. Continued high blood pressure, continued strain on the digestive system, continued muscle tension, etc, can all cause physical problems well worth avoiding if possible. Some of the psychological effects were described by psychologist Jane Firbank in *Practical Health* Aug/Sept 1987:

> *"It's the result of destructive pressures involving constant, unresolved frustration and conflict. It is about a growing, pervasive sense of helplessness and failure which saps your will and energy, which can send you going round in circles..A major component in distress is* helplessness, *not feeling in control of your own life. Thus stress symptoms are common among the unemployed and among mothers of small children."*

Does any of this ring true with you? It's hardly suprising that someone coping with the strains of chronic arthritis might feel this way too.

The particular stress of chronic arthritis

Chronic arthritis can set up a vicious circle of pain and stress. It's a circle that *can* be broken, but if unbroken reads something like this: arthritis = pain = stress = more pain = perhaps more stress in other areas (eg social, financial, work) = worse arthritis...

Stiffness and pain and the fight or flight stress response make muscles become tight and tense, worsening joint movement and increasing frustration and anxiety and fatigue. In turn your pain tolerance level is lowered and pain increases. Pain increases stress and stress increases pain. Prolonged stress and muscle tension can leave the healthiest body feeling exhausted so it's not surprising if your poor 'old' arthriticky body feels as if someone's been over it with a steamroller. In the early days, or during the worse spells of living with arthritis, it's all too easy to feel overwhelmed by the helplessness and 'not feeling in control' which Jane Firbanks described.

Some sources of unwanted stress in life can be removed. Arthritis is one which can't. Not yet, anyway, though medical treatment can bring relief. What we *can* change is how we react to it, and to other unwanted stresses in our lives. For example, if you're helplessly stuck in a traffic jam is it better to torture your poor body with ranting and raving and raised blood pressure, or to take stock of what can and can't be done and then try making the best of it − sing songs, tell jokes, listen to the radio, read a book, or whatever?

In the words of Hans Selye, the endocrinologist who first explained stress: *"It is not so much what happens to you that matters, but how you take it. "*

How you react to the arthritis and how you set about breaking the vicious circle of pain and stress depends on all sorts of things. On your personality of course, and on outside factors too (eg doctor, family, social, financial circumstances). There are simple self-help anti-stress techniques you can learn, too (see chapter 14), plus plenty of ways of tackling stressful emotional and practical situations.

As I said, stress has become a fashionable topic nowadays, so take note of what's said and written about it by reputably qualified, responsible people. Some of what's said *won't* be relevant, but keep an eye open for ideas that could be helpful. OK, so you can't deal with *your* stress by jogging, or running a four minute mile, but breathing exercises or relaxation techniques or swimming or self-organisation techniques or 'talking therapy' can help. So too can tackling practical and relationship problems, taking up an absorbing hobby or occupation, and trying to 'think positive'. I hope the ideas in chapters 13 and 14, and the rest of the book will help too. Even if the arthritis doesn't seem to benefit directly, cultivating a healthier, less stressed body will at least help you cope better.

Keep in mind as your guideline the 'Serenity Prayer':
"Grant me the serenity to accept the things I cannot change,
The courage to change the things I can,
And the wisdom to know the difference. "

Understanding negative emotional reactions

WARNING: Please don't be depressed by the list of 'downs' that follows. We need to understand them first, before we can get to work on increasing the 'ups' in life.

I don't want to spend too much time dwelling on disheartening aspects of chronic arthritis, but I do think it helps to understand something of what can happen, and to know that you're not alone. Self-knowledge is an important item in your Outwit Arthritis Kit. Before we can 'think positive' I do think we need to understand 'the negative'. Heather Unsworth (In *Coping with Rheumatoid Arthritis*, Chambers) quotes a young housewife with RA:
"Most people can cope with a situation if given the facts, but my biggest problem initially was feeling guilty and thinking that as a mother and wife I had let the family down. This depression and frustration was very difficult to handle as I had led a very active life... 25 years later, I would advise any new sufferer that a positive attitude is most important − and the ability to live one day at a time will get you through. "
Chapters 13 and 14 will get you started on maximising the ups and minimising any of these downs in your life, and help you start to take control of your life again. Some of the strains of coping with chronic arthritis come in our relationships with other people, and I hope chapter 25, and others, will be of special help there.

Fear is common. Fear of the unknown. Fear of the future. Fear of the illness's effect on you, on your life, on your family, on your finances, on your work, on your social life, etc.

With fear there's also *anxiety*.

Start to cope with the fear and anxiety by listing all the things you're afraid of. Then by yourself, or with someone else's help, plan what you could do about them. Maybe you're afraid of ending up wheelchair-bound? Resolve to ask your doctor what the chances are; explain your fears. Find out the statistical likelihood of this happening. In fact the chances are much higher that you *won't* end up as a full-time wheelchair user. So is it really worth wasting your limited time and energy worrying about something that may never happen? Concentrate on reality rather than fiction. Even if a wheelchair does become necessary, that *isn't* the end of the world:

> *"To most people, going into a wheelchair is the last straw and the passport for giving up. To me it was the opposite, after struggling with Zimmers and sticks, etc, each step feeling you had walked miles. To be able to sit in a wheelchair and go about your jobs is heaven."* (A YPA, writing in *ARC magazine*, 1987)

You might find helpful MIND's low-cost leaflet *Understanding Anxiety* even though it's not specifically for people with arthritis or chronic illness. In *Private World of Pain* Grace Stuart described how she dealt sensibly with another common fear:

> *"...fear that if one does not go on and on one will do, not less, but nothing at all, just be stuck. It takes perhaps more effort to conserve effort than to overspend it, but it is certainly worth the effort, to have less pain and, generally speaking, to live more pleasantly."*

You may experience **anger**, too. Perhaps anger that there's no instant cure. Anger at your doctor. Anger at people who don't understand. Anger at a world that seems wilfully and constantly to thrust obstacles in your way. Anger at your uncooperative joints. Anger that you take out on your nearest and dearest. Anger at being left to fend for yourself too much or anger at being too mollycoddled. Anger at 'just everything' – that you vent on the nearest scapegoat in a desperate attempt to blame someone or something for what's happened. Anger's a natural reaction, but it has to be handled carefully. In his book *Coping with Lupus*, psychologist Robert Phillips compared anger to a stick of dynamite:

> *"Anger is a form of energy, and the more physical energy that builds up in the body because of anger, the more necessary it is for you to release that energy. The energy cannot be destroyed, so if it is not released in some constructive manner, it will eventually come out in some other, less desirable way. Imagine the energy from anger as a stick of dynamite, all ready to explode. If you can get rid of it, it will explode away from you. It may cause some damage, but damage that will not hurt you internally as much as if you swallowed the dynamite to keep others from being hurt. Obviously, the ideal solution is not to throw that stick of dynamite, and not to swallow it, but...to try and de-fuse the dynamite!..."* (Avery Publishing, Garden City Park, New York, USA.)

Anger, expressed or unexpressed, can be a real pain in personal relationships, and needs handling extra-carefully. More about that in chapter 26.

Start to cope with the anger by turning it to positive uses – eg by doing things to change society's attitudes (eg by joining a group, or by writing letters to newspapers, calling a radio phone-in). Instead of shouting your anger at someone, use the thought-stopping technique: picture a big red 'stop' sign and do something to divert your anger, eg count to five; imagine yourself in the other person's shoes; if you then still need to express anger, do it calmly and clearly, 'talk not bite'. Try too reducing a heated argument by

> *"complimenting a person or looking for positive things in what that person is saying to you, even if you're angry. This works in two ways. One, it will probably surprise the person, and two, you will be focusing on words or thoughts which are more constructive, rather than letting yourself get angry because of what's being said to you. Calmly restate your feelings."* (Dr Phillips again.)

Avoid blaming someone else if the real culprit is the arthritis. Some people find it helpful to personify the arthritis, as a villain named Arthur Itis. You then have a named scapegoat you can blame, and complain about, instead of blaming yourself or someone else.

Try to find harmless outlets for anger, or express it in a controlled way. Play an exciting, tense, stimulating game, read a gripping book, watch an exciting film or TV programme, to help release pent-up emotion and anger. Playwrights and the ancient Greeks called this technique 'catharsis'. Rather than expressing anger aggressively and destructively, learn to be *assertive*, instead. Look for instance at Gael Lindenfield's *Assert Yourself* (Thorsons, 1986) and Anne Dickson's *A Woman in Your Own Right* (Quartet, 1982). Young Arthritis Care's Personal Development Courses (see page 123) include assertiveness and confidence training.

Maybe **guilt** is something you feel? Guilt that the housework's not getting done. Guilt that your family's suffering. Guilt that you can't keep up high standards at work. Guilt at taking out your misery or anger on your nearest and dearest. Guilt at complaining at all when 'there's others worse off than you'. Feeling somehow responsible for what's happened, and for what the arthritis makes you unable to do. Some people even have a strange guilt feeling that they've caused the RA or whatever themselves – but that's impossible – it's certainly *not* something self-inflictable like smoking-induced illness, for instance.

Start to eliminate the guilt by accepting that the arthritis is in no way your fault. So stop feeling guilty. Instead concentrate on what you *can* do. Accept what your body won't let you do. Stop worrying about the can't dos. Either forget them completely, or use your brain (and other people's) to find alternatives. Eliminate 'should thoughts' ('I should have been able to do the housework today'). Give yourself more realistic goals instead.

Exhaustion, fatigue Sheer inability to keep going. That devilish old crony of Arthur Itis nicknamed 'General Malaise'. Exhaustion from battling with pain and frustrations galore. Feeling physically and emotionally shattered. Fatigue which may lead to other problems, eg at work, or with lively youngsters, or with your sex life.

Start to cope with the fatigue by learning your limitations and planning a rest and exercise routine to suit your body; by 'budgeting' your energy and eliminating all non-essential demands on it; by asking for help with what can't be eliminated; by using all possible labour-saving gadgets and techniques. Keep your energy rations for what gives you a boost and makes you feel good.

Frustration Frustration at the constant conflict between mind and body, between what *you* want to do and what your uncooperative body wants to do (or not to do). Someone said she felt as if she was constantly trying to struggle through thick mud. Maybe non-arthritic people get an inkling of our frustrations when they try something like learning to ski or skate – but it's only a tiny inkling, because the big difference is that they're doing what they want to do, *choosing* to struggle, not fighting against pain to do so. And *their* frustration doesn't go on and on.

Frustration at a world suddenly full of obstacles so that tiny molehills become mountains. Simply making a cup of tea can involve so many struggles that we give up altogether, or spend so much time and effort on it there's none left for anything else. The tiniest achievements may become a luxury. No wonder we get tetchy when a non-arthritic person unthinkingly puts away the saucepan of water we've just spent hours getting out and filling! Frustration that no one seems to understand, or care. Frustration at losing independence. Frustration at not being in control. Frustration at losing the joy of being able to be spontaneous.

Start to cope with the frustration by learning how to be independent where possible. Get over the 'invisibility barrier' by communicating, explaining; by identifying escape valves for pent-up frustrations; by giving yourself a sense of purpose and vowing to control what can be controlled in your life. Planning ahead is a good way of cutting down on some frustrations. Try not to dwell on the can't dos but remind yourself of all your can dos and work at increasing them.

Bewilderment   The search for a reason why? Why has it happened? What have you done to deserve it? Hard to accept that we *don't* know why, and that we most definitely have *not* done anything to deserve it. Bewilderment at uncertainty and insecurity, not knowing how we'll be tomorrow, or next week, let alone next year, or even later the same day. Bewilderment at simply not knowing what to do for the best. Why won't my pathetic body do what I want? Why can't I just *do* things like I used to – bop happily for hours at a party, go off for a walk with the kids, window-shop for hours, just get on a bus for a ride? Bewilderment at what Grace Stuart, talking about RA, calls:

"the strange powerlessness...of the arthritic joint, so well known to the arthritic and so little known to anyone else...Beyond a certain point in this disease there is no question of endurance. You may endure all the pain you can or will, but if your wrist, lifting the teapot, gives way, you spill the tea or drop the pot. There is no argument! Only acquiescence! Useless to lift teapots!" (In *Private World of Pain*)

Depression   Not surprisingly, a build-up of fear and frustration, of unrelieved stress, and setback after setback may leave you feeling depressed, especially in the early days, before your Outwit Arthritis Kit begins to work. Physical and emotional 'bruising' may turn the liveliest extrovert into an introvert:

"You may feel that everything is hopeless, that life as you know it may never be the same again. Is it even worth carrying on? Is your life going to be so miserable that you cannot face it? You may be in a trough of despair and just don't know how to start climbing out. Of course, your family, friends, and doctors will all be helping you as much as they can and when you begin to get some relief of pain due to treatment this will make you feel better." (YPA Sue Gunn, writing in *In Contact*)

Maybe it helps to remember that a million and one 'life-events' can bring on depression in anyone, not just you. Chronic inflammatory arthritis just happens to be a particularly beastly life-event, beastly in itself, and beastly in the way it magnifies other setbacks. It's hardly suprising if you feel depressed instead of gleefully shouting yippee.

Starting to cope. Sometimes you can weather the storm yourself, sometimes you need help (the right sort) from others. At one extreme a depression may be so intense that you need medical help to get out of it. Don't hesitate to see your doctor for help if you feel imprisoned in a black depression that just seems to go on and on. Talk to the Samaritans, too. Remember they're there not just to help people on the verge of suicide, but always ready to help *anyone* feeling particularly miserable. The counsellors on the Wyeth helpline at Arthritis Care (see page 112), and Young Arthritis Care Contacts are always ready, too, to lend an understanding and friendly ear.

Good family relationships and a close reliable friend or two are worth their weight in gold. Some people understandably may find it difficult to know how to react, either trying too hard to be reassuring or giving you the 'pull yourself together' routine. Try showing them bits of this book, to help them understand. Try too to explain that simply 'just being there' may often be their best approach, as psychiatrist Robin Skynner and comedian/writer John Cleese explain:

JC: Sometimes just being with someone we like and trust helps us in a way that's slightly different from either rest or reassurance.

> RS: *I think that's right. It's easy to remember to do the shopping for people under stress, to take around some food, or share experience, but sometimes we forget that just sticking around, just 'being there' also helps enormously. Even though it doesn't feel as though we're doing much...*
>
> JC:...*I don't think it had ever occurred to me that you could quite simply sit with someone and say, 'Yes this is very difficult for you and you have some unpleasant feelings to cope with. So I'll just sit here and be with you while that's going on.'*
>
> (*Families and How to Survive Them*, Methuen London)

As time goes by you'll build up a repertoire of ways of either avoiding black and gloomy times or ways of at least living through them, knowing there'll be light at the end of the tunnel. Sue Stephenson (with JCA) learnt the value of 'talking to someone' after problems when she started a secretarial course:

> "*By this time my arthritis was pretty bad, so having to walk around the college and climb all the stairs eventually put a strain on myself and my work. Being an idiot, I didn't try to talk to anyone about it, so as my work suffered and my health, I got more and more depressed. I let it go on for a long time. That was my first big mistake...Now I know to try to talk to someone, get it off your chest. When I did talk to my college tutor about the problem, she immediately saw to it that I had my hours spent at college reduced by half. The other half I was able to work at home. My work improved in no time at all. I still did the same amount of work, but by working partly at home, I didn't get half as tired as I did before. If only I'd talked to someone earlier I would have saved all that misery...*" (*In Contact*)

Again, later, Sue lost hope, and for two years just watched TV and read books all day. Eventually she realised she just couldn't go on like that. Step by step she started to get out and about and to get over embarrassment at her arthritis. She began to enjoy herself and meet people, and eventually her future husband:

> "...*people are more than willing to help if you ask, but initially it is down to you to do something about it. Don't think you won't ever get out of your depression, or you can't have a normal life. You will, and you can! I thought like that too, but look at me now...Fight it, there is a life after depression you know! Only don't leave it too long, like I did. With fight in you, and the help of other people, who says you can't do it?*"

Look at the section on 'talking therapy' on page 110. You might find helpful a couple of general publications: MIND's low-cost booklet *Understanding Depression* or the British Holistic Medical Association's paperback *Overcoming Depression* (Dorling Kindersley, 1987), by Dr Richard Gillett, British psychiatrist and psychotherapist.

The **uncertainty** and **unpredictability** of something like RA takes some adjusting to – what someone described as being 'up and down like a perishing yo-yo'. Not knowing what's going to happen. Not knowing what to do for the best at any one time. Wondering which body part is going to let you down next. Sociologist Carolyn L Wiener (University of California) analysed the socio-psychological aspects in an article, *The Burden of Rheumatoid Arthritis: Tolerating the Uncertainty* (*Soc Sci & Med*, Vol 9, Pergamon Press 1975). Sorry about the jargon but it's a fair insight nevertheless:

> "*The variability of progression, severity and areas of involvement cannot be stressed enough. For example, an arthritic may have reduced mobility but no impairment of skill, reduced energy but no interference with mobility, reduced energy one day and renewed energy the next and so on. Loss of skill will remain fairly constant if it is caused by deformity, but it is variable if caused by swelling; the other resources, mobility and energy, can fluctuate. There is uncertainty about: (1) whether there will be any pain, swelling or stiffness; (2) the area of involvement; (3) the intensity of the disability; whether the onset will be gradual or sudden; (5) how long it will last; and (6) how frequently flare-ups will occur...*"

The person with RA lives in a state of 'variable uncertainty', she says, where on the one hand pain and disability and on the other the need to keep going are in constant competition with each other, 'like two runners in a nightmare race'.

"In tolerating the uncertainty, the arthritic is engaged in a precarious balancing of options – options somewhat limited because of already reduced resources of mobility, skill, strength and energy. Indeed, a balancing is involved in all of the pacing decisions (weighing the potential benefit of acupuncture against the climb up two flights of stairs 'that will just about kill me', the potential withdrawal from church activity against the loss of social interaction). The options are constantly presenting themselves, each to be met with an ad hoc response: whether to cover-up and risk inability to justify inaction when needed; whether to keep-up and suffer the increased pain and fatigue; whether to elicit help and risk loss of normalizing, whether to re-normalize and decrease the need for covering-up and keeping-up. Furthermore...there exists a constant balancing of the hope of relief and/or remission against the dread of progression."

By 'normalization' she means social strategies used to keep up a 'normal' life, eg covering-up and keeping-up, and by 're-normalization' she means adjusting to reduced activities. Pacing is a practical strategy – identifying which activities you're able to do, how often, and under what circumstances, and budgeting your limited energy accordingly. Hope is a psychological strategy we use to keep going. Though all humans live in a state of some uncertainty, we YPAs experience it in an exaggerated form and with limited options.

Start to cope. Use the information here and elsewhere to help you make the most of limited options. Accept physical limitations which are realistic but don't add others by giving-up or over-doing. Resolve to extend what you can do in every way possible that doesn't harm your fragile joints. Keep going mentally, but with the brakes on physically.

In some ways it's like learning to live on a limited budget. Overspending's dangerous; it's more intelligent to learn how best to live within your budget. The learning process takes time and effort, and unfortunately the size of the budget may suddenly change, but coping's still possible, even so.

Self-pity, self-hate, apathy, lethargy, bitterness, resentment, envy, jealousy – are some of the other unhelpful negative reactions which may dog our paths, but I think we've already looked at enough, and need to start looking towards the positive!

Ways of understanding why arthritis may cause these negative reactions

One way of understanding is to see what's happened as a sort of bereavement. Losing your good health is a shock to the system, like losing someone close to you through death. It's all the more of a shock when it's so unexpected. But like a bereavement, with time and support, information and motivation, you can come to terms with what can't be changed, and can change what can be.

The best description of this 'bereavement effect' I've come across is by psychiatrist Alexander (Sandy) Burnfield. He's lived with a chronic illness, too, for 20 years, since his days as a medical student. His condition, multiple sclerosis (MS), is medically very different from RA and its cousins. But they're all 'chronic disorders', all as yet without a cure and unpredictable, and emotional reactions can be similar:

"...instead of having lost a loved one through death, we have lost our good health through illness. We have in fact lost a part of ourselves which we loved very much and we must instead take on a different identity as 'a person who has MS' or as 'a disabled person'. It is necessary to mourn our loss if we are to make a good adjustment in the end, and this process cannot be avoided or rushed.

"When we lose a loved one through death, it may take months or even years, before we can accept our loss. This is also true for MS, but not quite so straightforward and

clear cut. We lose our good health gradually and slowly and we can never be sure how final the loss will be. We might be restored to health completely, sometimes partially but perhaps not at all, and this insecurity is hard to bear. We may hardly have become used to one new self-image when we must abandon it and take on a different one.

"...It is not surprising that we must go through a period of sadness and grief. This is usually mixed with feelings of anger, and we may deny both to ourselves and others that we have the disease at all. Like the bereaved, a person who has MS must come to terms with his or her condition and learn to value himself or herself again and to enjoy living. This will take time, perhaps several years, but much less time for some people than for others.

"It seems that we have to experience shock, anger and sadness over and over again before we can become inwardly strong enough to be open and realistic about our limitations. When this stage is reached we shall have begun to come to terms with MS. Some people will be able to start leading a life just as fulfilling as before, a life that may be given more meaning by the experience of illness and suffering...We can emerge from fear and depression when we have first accepted these feelings and been able to express them to ourselves and others.

"Relatives also experience similar feelings of grief when someone in the family develops MS. Coupled with their grief, they may have complicated feelings of guilt, and frustration, as well as a desire to be strong and supportive. When the whole family is faced with these complex feelings, they may not be able to support each other. They may require help from someone outside the family for a while, perhaps for a long time.

"The emotional strain...can cause even more suffering than the physical effects of the disease. This is true both for the person who has MS and for those close to him or her. The psychological process of adjusting to new identities, new roles and a new lifestyle is often long and complicated. For many, however, there will be unexpected rewards and fulfilment. Life sometimes appears as a random and purposeless experience from which we are asked to create meaning. For those of us with MS, and for our relatives, this is our particular challenge." (In *Multiple Sclerosis: A Personal Exploration*, Souvenir)

Sandy Burnfield reminds us of something it's easy to forget. That those close to us may 'suffer' too and may also need to adjust psychologically. They too may feel hopeless, helpless, wanting to help yet not knowing how to. They too may feel angry, frustrated, fearful, and miserable. Some may seek a way out of their dilemma by turning away. Others realise that both of you need time and perseverance and help to work through problems.

Relationships with outsiders may be affected, too, in the same way as bereaved or divorced people may find other people act oddly towards them. Usually it's because the latter don't know how to handle the situation, but this can often be overcome (chapter 25).

Another way of understanding our emotional reactions is described by John Cleese and Robin Skynner. Like babies and children, in the early days someone faced with a stressful 'life change' may need 'looking after', 'mothering', like a baby or a child:

John Cleese: "..to summarize, to handle change we need: one, to be shielded from usual demands so we can rest; two, information to reassure anxieties and help us to cope; and three, emotional support." (*Families and How to Survive Them*, Methuen London)

But just like children, as we learn the skills of coping, so we can 'grow up' and learn to stand, psychologically speaking, at least, on our own two feet again. Our nearest and dearest have to learn to let go too, to 'let us grow up' just as parents with their children. Though some support is welcome, *over*-protection stops us learning how to cope. Even if some physical dependence remains we can still become psychologically independent.

A particular bugbear of something like RA is that it's not usually a static condition, and so the 'readjusting' and 'learning to cope' process may have to happen more than once, as Sue Gunn (with RA) described:

"There is a marked difference between this and something like an amputation or spinal

injury. Once that has happened you have to work through the stages to accepting it but once you're there, that's it. You are not likely to change. With arthritis you just get to accept your present situation when it changes again. Perhaps another joint becomes involved and you have to go through the stages again and again.

"I see my life as a steeplechase. I can be running (!) along quite happily and steadily when suddenly I hit an obstacle. I then have to go through the various stages in order to climb up and over that obstacle. Depending on the obstacle's size it varies how quickly I can overcome it. When I've gone through all that then I can get back on an even footing...

"What I am trying to say is that 'acceptance' is an ongoing thing with arthritis. At each setback you may have to go through the stages [again] to accept your new situation. It is a little like grieving for each loss of ability or each new joint affected. If your Grandmother dies, that grief process does not suffice to keep you going if your Mother dies. You have to start again. " (In Contact)

True, though you don't always need to go right back to square one. Every bit of wisdom and information you gather to deal with one setback gives you that much better a start in adjusting to the next, *if* it comes.

What does it all add up to?

Learning to cope with a chronic inflammatory arthritis *is* difficult. It's not surprising we (and our nearest and dearest) may go through some bad emotional times, especially in the early days, maybe longer. Just take it a day at a time. Please don't feel so overwhelmed that you forget to be hopeful and to keep yourself looking forward. Work your way slowly towards the light at the end of the tunnel, keeping firmly in your mind the reassurance that despite everything we do work out ways of coping and of enjoying life. Try to avoid drowning in self-pity and vow instead to make the best of the life you've got. Look back at the serenity prayer (page 85) and ponder these thoughts:

- *Despair is easy but it doesn't lead to action. - Determination is difficult but it leads to solutions.* (Sorry, I can't remember where I read that.)
- *The best thing about the future is that it only comes one day at a time.* (Dean Atcheson)
- *Not everything that is faced can be changed – but nothing can be changed until it is faced.* (James Baldwin)
- *My mind is free and it walks for me* (words of a song sung by actress and TV presenter Elly Wilkie, who had cerebral palsy)

Some important things to keep in mind
- Importance of **YOU** – you're the one who can do most to help yourself
- Importance of **friendship and support** – from family, friends, doctor and the rest of the healthcare team, from support groups, and from other YPAs
- Importance of a **sense of humour** – and keeping things in perspective.
- Importance of **stabilisers** in your life – eg people, home, job, religion.
- Importance of **minimising stress** elsewhere – ie non-arthritic stress.
- Importance of **information** – so limited options are kept as wide as possible.
- Importance of **escape valves** – for anger, frustration, misery, etc
- Importance of **time** – time to adjust, to learn new skills, to work out ways of coping, and readjusting relationships and responsibilities.

Like many younger people with arthritis, I've been to hell and back more than once; the crucial thing to remember is the 'and back'. Things do get better again, things do change. Perspectives change. You change. Your attitudes and abilities change. And Dame Fortune waves a magic wand at the most unexpected times.

Chapter thirteen

PSYCHOLOGICAL AND EMOTIONAL REACTIONS 2:
Working towards a positive philosophy: The brighter side of the hill

---

"Though much is taken, much abides and tho'
We are not now that strength that in old days
Moved earth and heaven: that which we are, we are;
One equal temper of heroic hearts,
Made weak by time and fate, but strong in will
To strive, to seek, to find, and not to yield."
from Alfred, Lord Tennyson's *Ulysses*

Coping with arthritis is a balancing act; but there's a lot you can do to tip the balance in your favour. Don't worry if it takes ages. Learning any new skills takes time. *"Make up your mind that there is one hell of an adapting job to be done, but that the end result is well worth adapting to"* (Corbet Woodall, in *A Disjointed Life*, Heinemann). Be encouraged by Dr Coleman:

"If you do what you can to control your own destiny and make a genuine effort to take a positive and aggressive part in your own treatment and future, you will benefit enormously. By remaining active and determined you will reduce the level of pain. And by remaining positive you will weaken your illness and strengthen yourself." (*Natural Pain Control*, Century Arrow)

Some of the best tips can be picked up from talking and listening to a sensible, thoughtful person who's been through similar experiences, for instance in a self-help group like Arthritis Care, or Young Arthritis Care. Best if you share the same type of arthritis. Avoid the sort of person who has, say, rheumaticky twinges in one hand who assumes they can pronounce authoritatively on *any* rheumatic disorder! Concentrate on the non-medical aspects: bodies and symptoms differ so much. Specific medical advice is best left to the experts.

Books can give you ideas too, for instance those in chapter 29, and ARC and Arthritis Care publications. People's feelings about having arthritis are described in autobiographies, but are usually mentioned only briefly in other books on arthritis.

Learning to adapt to and to outwit the arthritis means rethinking your lifestyle where necessary. It means counterbalancing the uncertainty of RA and its cousins by introducing as much certainty and stability as possible in other areas of your life. It means *reducing* other stresses, controlling what you *can* control, leaving you with more physical and emotional strength to cope with the uncontrollable. It means *accentuating* the can dos and keeping the can't dos in perspective. It means working on *increasing* your inner resources, restoring any lost self-confidence, and building up reserves of courage, motivation and wisdom, a resilient sense of humour, and various self-help skills.

Facing up to smaller problems can help you deal with larger ones *if* they come, in the same way as vaccinations prepare the body to defend itself against a major invasion by germs. Avoid 'crutches' like alcohol, smoking, or too many tranquillisers. They only postpone the day you need to face up to problems: worse, they may even add new ones.

Work on non-physical abilities and skills. Brain not brawn! When you were physically fit, there were masses of ways to let off steam at difficult times. Playing football or going for a long country walk are wonderful ways of working off angers and frustrations if you're fit. When arthritis is around there may still be some physical outlets open to you, such as swimming, or gentle exercise, or making love, or gentle dancing, but you'll need specially to build up your *non*-physical skills and interests.

Be patient with yourself. Give yourself plenty of praise and encouragement as you learn to live with the arthritis. Your self-confidence and self-esteem may need rebuilding. Above all, give yourself time. Don't give up, just keep working slowly in the right direction. Don't blame yourself or feel guilty if it's easier said than done. On a bad day, *any* achievement deserves a medal. Simply struggling out of bed to face another day can be the equivalent of a fit person scaling Mount Everest.

Encouragement from some YPAs

J's in her 20s, with JCA since her early years:

"Just because you have arthritis life doesn't have to be too bad. You just have to take things a bit easier and carry on, after all life is what you make it. I try to keep happy. I get on with a lot of people but like everyone I have my off days, but family and friends close to you understand and get used to your moods. The pain isn't always bad although it's always there."

Anne Ryman's had RA for several years:

"One thing that keeps me going on a bad day is that 'nothing lasts for ever, not even rheumatoid pain', which is true. My advice is never to give up, do as much as you can each day, according to how you feel, no one else, and instead of saying I can't do this, etc, start from the other end and catalogue all the things you can do. You will be surprised how they all add up.

"Even if one is unable to do anything, on a bad day when the pain is just flowing over you, you are still able to listen to other people. Often a sympathetic ear is much appreciated by someone caught up in the hurly burly of life with no one who has the time to listen."

Carol J's married and in her 40s:

"I contracted RA severely at the age of 21 and it undoubtedly changed my life but despite all the traumas of those early years I believe I have emerged as a much stronger person, more compassionate towards other people's problems, more patient, more tolerant and above all more positive.

"My maxim being accept what you can't do and enjoy to the full that which you can do! Each one of us has something to offer, some interest we can pursue, no matter what disabilities we may have. Don't dwell on the disabilities. They are not what's important, it's the person that counts, the individual, and each of us has something to give."

Marilyn S is married, in her 30s, and has had psoriatic arthritis for a few years:

"I feel more in control now – of my feelings, my actions, my whole life really. Do I sound weird? I suppose I'm just more relaxed – just taking each day at a time and doing what I can with it. If the weather is nice, I can sit in the garden, or even go for a short stroll. If not, I can get a book from the library, or try a bit of cookery or whatever."

1 Understand your particular rheumatic disorder

Better the devil you know, and try to understand, than the devil you don't. Reduce fears and anxieties by finding out facts; why waste energy worrying about fiction? You need that valuable energy to make life easier, not more troublesome. I do believe the more you understand what's going on in your body, the more in control you'll feel, and the less you'll worry unnecessarily.

Ask your doctor and other members of your healthcare team to explain your illness to you. Each viewpoint may differ slightly, but each will add to your understanding. Don't expect to be told or to understand everything at once – the rheumatic disorders are mighty complicated, and even the experts are still learning. So be prepared for some irritating answers that begin 'it's possible that', 'it's difficult to say whether', 'you might or might not find that'...Most frustrating of all, there's unlikely to be any clear answer to the most important question of all – what's going to happen to *you*?

Jacqueline S's questions met with a very helpful response:

"After the operation to replace my left hip joint I badgered the consultant for more information so that I could help myself more. He and his staff produced a booklet they'd been working on, full of hints and written in a light-hearted manner which has proved very popular and useful to anyone with difficulties of everyday living."

Read up about your disorder too, preferably in publications recommended by your doctor and those on page 16. Make sure what you're reading is by someone reputable, medically qualified and up-to-date. Medical knowledge changes so rapidly. Beware of the dangers of half-knowledge. If you don't understand, or are worried by what you read, ask for an explanation. Get worries off your chest by talking to a member of your team. As you do your reading you'll pick up some medical lingo too, helpful in understanding doctors!

Don't fall into the trap of believing everything you read will necessarily happen to *you*. Remember no two of us share precisely the same body and symptoms, so even an illness with the same name will behave differently from person to person. There are similarities, as there are in makes of car, but the variations on a theme are vast.

Don't depress yourself by reading too many books and listening to too many people who go on about the don't dos and the can't dos. Go for the dos and the can dos!

2 Take an active part in your treatment

The doctor's spent years learning his/her skills, so too has the rest of your healthcare team. But don't expect *them* to do all the work! Learn how to make the most of their skills to help you help yourself.

The doctor may prescribe pills for you, but that's only step number one. The next steps are your responsibility – for instance taking the tablets in the right dose at the right time, noting their effects, and watching out for side-effects, not fearfully, but realistically. Similarly with other treatments: the doctor may recommend physiotherapy and the physio may show you exercises – but then it's up to you to do the exercises, to give the prescribed treatment a fair and honest trial. If it doesn't work, at least you'll have tried. What you try next could be the winner.

Use the team's expertise to help you work out ways of coping physically, ways of avoiding or at least controlling pain. Learn about joint care, pacing and energy conservation, helpful exercises, medication, ways of balancing exercise and rest, and how to recognise and respond to your body signals. Don't be disappointed if they don't lay down hard and fast rules ('do this and such-and-such will happen'): although they know masses about their speciality they're only newcomers to your particular body. So for starters they'll be making 'informed suggestions'. You and they will then have to see how your body responds.

Build up other 'patient/health consumer skills' to help you negotiate your way through the NHS maze. Find out who does what, and how, when and where. Make sure you, at least, are efficient – in remembering appointments, for instance, and making the most of limited time available – the sort of thing chapter 4 deals with. Don't assume everything will be done *for* you – for instance if you're told you'll need to go into hospital, you're the only person who knows what problems that'll create, so start planning right away – and seek help early, if necessary.

3 Overcome the information barrier

Leave no stone unturned in your quest for information! You'll solve problems and feel more in control. Sharpen your detective skills. So many opportunities are overlooked simply through not knowing what exists to help or challenge us. Arthritis may impose limits, true, but the information barrier is one we can certainly overcome.

One of the keys to successful coping is knowledge, and one of the main aims of this book is to share it. However immobile, you can do plenty of detection from your own armchair through reading, writing, telephoning, talking to people, and using the media. Ferret out information on medical, practical, financial, personal and emotional matters.

You need to know where to ask for help, and when, and what sort of questions to ask. I hope chapter 15 will help get you started. Seeking help in one area may help you in another. For instance finding out about special gadgets may also help you cope emotionally, by cutting down on frustrations which take their toll on you and yours. So − happy hunting.

4 Get yourself organised!

Good planning and organisation can reduce unnecessary stresses and strains and help you feel more in control in at least some areas of your life. Someone who makes a list before going shopping can ensure they buy everything in one go, with less problems to sort out than someone who doesn't make a list but buys on impulse. A motorist who keeps the car serviced and the petrol tank filled has fewer unexpected breakdowns than a disorganised motorist.

OK, so the unpredictability of arthritis doesn't exactly make planning easy, but use your brain to keep one step ahead. Plan your life and pace yourself so as to make the most of what energy and abilities you have.

Keep notebooks and lists of what needs to be done. Then when you have a good/better day look at your lists and instantly get cracking! They'll also help you avoid forgetting things, and taking two journeys to do what might be achieved in one. Make notes too on what you need to ask other people to help with, so you're ready instantly to take advantage of any kind offers.

Halve lists and halve them again to eliminate inessentials. You don't need to serve 'cordon bleu' meals to your family, don't need to wash the bedlinen quite so often, don't need to put yourself out for guests. Cut out most of your ironing, and bedmaking, and save energy too by doing some shopping by post. Eliminate or delegate or facilitate each task, ie cut it out, get someone else to do it (paid or unpaid), or find an easier way of doing it yourself. Break down heavy tasks into smaller, easier tasks, if possible (eg clean only one room or half a room at a time). Here are some general guidelines. Look too at page 158.

- Get yourself organised − but avoid being a perfectionist. What matters more, a bit of dust, or your health? Why should 'your way of doing things' be the one and only way?!
- Organise home, surroundings and people around you (with help if necessary) to minimise stress on you and your joints and your nearest and dearest.
- Set yourself up with a Medikit (see page 33), and an Infokit (see page 112).
- Don't leave everything until the last minute − that increases stress. Think ahead. Before you get out of your chair to go to the loo, think how else you can use the journey. Can you avoid having to get up again two minutes later to fetch a book, or to turn the oven on?
- Don't try to do too much. Decide on your priorities in life and save your energy rations for them.
- Learn to say 'no' (sometimes at least) and mean it!
- Pace yourself, and think 'energy conservation'.
- List practical problems so you can put satisfying ticks alongside as you find solutions.

Here's how Sue Gunn organises her life:

"*Organisation   All my days have to be organised well in advance if I am to maintain my independence. For instance, when I do my washing my husband has to get out the linen basket, washing powder, clothes horse, etc. If there are any heavy items he has to load and unload the machine for me. I have to decide well in advance what we're having for dinner so he can get anything out of the freezer or cupboard that I need. If we are having visitors for a weekend, for example, I have to know a good couple of weeks in advance so that I can plan the shopping and cooking etc, so that I have very little to do when they are actually here. Only then can I ensure I have enough energy for entertaining...*

"*Spontaneity   I think one of the major effects of being disabled is that you cannot be spontaneous. I would love to be able to get up at weekends and suddenly decide to go out for the day... I know that if I have a busy day, I am going to be extremely stiff and tired the following day. This doesn't stop me going out but I do have to plan my timetable very carefully. If I am going out, I make sure I can rest the next day. Hence if I feel like going out on the spur of the moment, I have to check my commitments for the following few days. This also puts a restraint on my husband especially as he is very active and has got plenty of energy. Often he will go ahead and play golf or squash while I rest at home. There are, of course, occasions when I ignore sense and go ahead and suffer the consequences later!*" (*In Contact*)

5 Reduce other stresses in your life

What other unwanted stresses are there in your life besides the arthritis? Try not to blame the arthritis for everything, though it's a great temptation. Can you cut down on any other stresses, eg at home, at work, in your leisure activities, personal relationships, finance?

- Some stresses can be relieved by changing the way you do or think about things. For instance do you get landed with doing too much for other people − should you learn to say 'no' more often? Do you blame other people for problems of your own making, forgetting they can't mind read? I do! Work on skills of communication, and skills of avoiding misunderstandings.
- You may need help. − Use this book to work out where to get it from, and try your healthcare team too. Don't let lethargy create additional stress. Resolve to crack those problems which *can* be solved, eg practical problems of reaching and bending. Don't wait for help to come to you. − Seek it out.
- To help you cope less stressfully with things that simply can't be changed see chapter 14 for starters.
- Learn to accept comfort, help and support, gracefully, if the going gets too tough to cope alone, but avoid being over-demanding when there's no need.
- Find for you the best way of 'standing back' from stress and gaining a different perspective, so things will seem more manageable when you 'return' (eg relaxation, meditation, purposeful daydreaming, a holiday break, sitting in a beautiful garden, praying/religion). Set yourself a regular time for standing back and switching off.
- Counterbalance *un*wanted stresses of feeling overstretched or under-appreciated with wanted stresses, ie seek challenges to stimulate you, something you *can* control and seek success in. Maybe you feel you haven't the energy for anything, but it'll come, eventually, if you try, and if necessary, try, try, try again.
- Seek creative outlets for energy and frustrations, for instance in art or poetry or writing or music or singing. (See chapter 35.)

Try to avoid inviting too many 'controllable stresses' into your life at once. For instance, moving house, getting married, giving up smoking, starting a new job, having a baby, are each individually stressful experiences − if you have the choice, avoid taking on more than one at a time! Try to stabilise what Dr Vernon Coleman calls the 'four cornerstones of life'

− family, work, leisure, friends.

Some further reading might help (though none's specifically about arthritis/chronic disorders):

−   Dr Vernon Coleman's *Overcoming Stress* (Sheldon, 1988)
−   Alex Kirsta's *The Book of Stress Survival* (Unwin)
−   *Living with Stress* (Consumers' Association)
−   *WOMAN* magazine and the College of Health both have book lists on stress. So too does Relate (*Books with Care*). Books listed, including the Coleman and Kirsta books mentioned above, can be bought by post from Relate.

6 Make the most of your can-dos

OK, so maybe your bones, joints, muscles, etc are pretty dodgy. But what about your brain, your voice, the richness of all your senses? Your brain hasn't got arthritis. Make the most of it! Researches show we use only a fraction of the brain's abilities. You don't need paper qualifications; just keep your brain active. Look at how apathetic so many 'fit' people can be − we can outshine so many of them simply by being mentally active.

Learn new skills, for pleasure or for a purpose: for instance lots of YPAs now drive cars or wrestle with computers and word processors. Shut pain-awareness out as much as possible. Look on a problem as a challenge. Remember what fun a child has faced with a problem. Relish the sense of achievement when you solve a problem (however small) and reward yourself with a gold star and big pat-on-the-back.

If you can't do something such as getting a bowl off a low shelf in the fridge, get the brain working! My solution was to use a clean long-handled dustpan and easyreach gadget. My brain told me that if I couldn't get a dish of food out by *lifting* it, I should try the opposite, and *lower* it − on to the dustpan. Raising it up was then a simple matter. ('Thinking of opposites' is a useful problem-solving trick.)

In the office, if you've got six different things to do, eg photocopying, collecting mail, consulting someone about figures, going to the loo, looking in a reference book, don't make six separate journeys − instead get the brain to plan one journey to achieve all six aims. Similarly if you've got to go upstairs, or into the garden. Use a book like Edward De Bono's *The Uses of Lateral Thinking* to stimulate the old brain cells.

Use all your senses, *really* use them − eyes, ears, nose, sense of taste, and touch. Incredible how many people don't. Incredible for instance how many people walk straight into things: they may claim it's because they're concentrating on something else, but it's just lazy eyes. If bumping into things causes pain, you soon train your eyes to notice obstacles and avoid them, while *still* concentrating on what's for dinner or the end-of-the-month financial returns. Occasionally some types of chronic arthritis affect the eyes − if so, concentrate on sharpening the other senses.

Make your ears work for you. Learn for instance to tell from your armchair how the cooking's going using your ears and nose (long before the burning stage). A pre-boiling pan of water sounds quite different from a boiling pan.

Use your senses for pleasure, too. Really revel in a beautiful sunset, sharpen your ears to hear birdsong, train your nose to tell you what's going on around you, make a meal a taste-experience not a frantic gobble to quieten hunger-pangs. And marvel at the infinite variety of touch experiences. Train yourself by making a long, slow, total sense experience out of eating a strawberry. I worked so hard on my 'senses' I was a semi-finalist in a Great Gourmet competition, identifying gloriously mysterious foods by taste, smell and sight, and I was very nearly a finalist!

Your voice is an incredible tool, for work and pleasure. Make the most of it. Use it to influence other people's reactions to you. Does a harsh, grating voice, or a whining voice, make you want to listen to someone, or help them? No? What sort of voice *does*? Learn to sing, or debate. Use your voice to find things out, to 'educate' people to help not hinder you (and the rest of us YPAs too), and to persuade and cajole people. Use it effectively in your job and on the telephone. Use it to help other people, to praise them, to make them feel good, to tell jokes, to spread a little happiness and help the world go round.

That's only for starters. I haven't even touched on a sense of humour yet – and *that*'s worth a good million or two.

A dodgy body can achieve the unimaginable, given ingenuity, motivation, and luck. Renoir painted masterpieces from his wheelchair though the paintbrushes had to be tied into his gnarled hands. Modern technology helps us too. – With phones, TVs, computers and modems the world comes to *us* increasingly. Stuck here convalescing for three months my typewriter, cordless phone, remote control TV, radio and vacuum flask kept me still reasonably sane and in touch with the outside world.

7 Give yourself goals, and a sense of purpose

It's all too easy to sink into a sea of self-pity and lethargy. Why bother trying to do *anything?* Understandable, especially in the early days, but if you let that continue, things will just get worse. Instead, start picking yourself up. Motivate yourself, little by little, and you'll start to have good feelings again, less time to feel pain and misery, and to feel worthless and uninteresting. Choose realistic goals, so you don't risk the disappointment of failing to achieve them.

Give yourself things to look forward to, even if it's only the next episode of a radio or TV series, or follow the progress of a football or cricket team regularly, week by week, for example. Don't just sit mesmerized by the TV screen regardless of what's on. Instead get the Radio or TV Times magazines, and have a forward planning session, circling in red anything of special interest. Switch on only for those. Use programmes as inspiration for further reading, studying, and developing hobbies. Keep your eyes open for anything of interest to friends: they'll appreciate being told about something they might not have noticed themselves.

Continue with your interests and hobbies, or develop new ones. See later chapters for plenty of ideas. They'll not only give you a sense of purpose, but also something to chat about, a welcome change of topic from arthritis. Don't waste energy moaning if physical activities like gardening or sport are out. – Why not become an expert armchair gardener, traveller, or sportsperson, accumulating a wealth of ideas and information that many physically active people don't have time to accumulate?

Going in for competitions (see page 291) is a fun hobby that's stimulating and definitely keeps you looking forward. Who knows, you could even win prizes. I've notched up quite a few paper-and-pencil competition wins (nothing really big – well not yet) – also third prize for apples in the Flower Show and first prize (more than once!) for best fruit flan. Other YPAs have triumphed in singing contests, bridge competitions, art shows, etc.

Many people find a fulfilling sense of purpose in working for a cause of some sort, for instance by becoming a Contact for Young Arthritis Care, or working to raise money for arthritis welfare (Arthritis Care) or arthritis medical research (ARC), or by working for a local voluntary organisation like Sue G. RA stopped Sue practising as an OT, but she used her knowledge working for the local DIAL Group. Or you might want to get involved in some local action group or with the local church. (See chapter 33 on voluntary work.)

If your arthritis is too unpredictable you might prefer to avoid committing yourself to any specific task, but there's still lots you can do. If nothing else, do make 'educating' other people about arthritis your cause! Goodness knows they do *need* educating! Sitting here with my ankle in plaster I've managed to have a go or two at that – taking part in a radio phone-in, writing letters to newspapers, etc.

A good job's another way of achieving a sense of purpose. Read chapters 31 and 32 on employment to see what you can do to find a job, or change jobs, or to keep your existing job. People with children have another good 'reason to keep going', even though they can be such hard work, arthritis or no arthritis.

Learn new skills, by doing an OU or other correspondence/distance learning course if you can't get out and about (see chapter 30). If you can get about then the possibilities are vast – evening classes, residential weekends, etc. Who knows what your new-found skills may lead to. – Marie Joseph taught herself to type, and became a successful novelist; Ann McFarlane enjoyed cooking as a hobby, and has published a cookery book. So get cracking!

8 Balance the 'giving' and the 'taking'

"One cannot write a prescription which says that so-and-so, being much injured, will need much loving and much opportunity to love." (In *Private World of Pain*)

So wrote Grace Stuart, with feeling, after many years of living with RA. 'Wounded', physically and emotionally, we do need much loving. Living with a chronic disorder does seem to mean doing a lot of 'taking' from people, taking their time, help, and love. But grateful though we may be, we do also need the 'opportunity to love', and opportunity to 'give' too. Being on the receiving end is lovely for a while, but if it goes on too long it reinforces feelings of uselessness and being a helpless invalid. Instead, 'giving' instead of constantly 'taking' can be a real morale-booster.

If only more of those who so kindly offer help would realise how much they could help by simply allowing *us* to do some 'giving' too. Friends, for instance, who so kindly help you to get to the pub, but then refuse to let you buy a round – something you definitely *could* do! However good their intentions, they're adding to your mobility disabilities by *dis*abling your self-esteem and pride.

Surprisingly, sometimes our *accepting* help gracefully is actually a form of 'giving'. Many people do have a great need to feel needed – and so though you may *seem* to be on the receiving end, you're actually doing *them* a favour (but keep it quiet or you'll spoil the effect). So much the better if their need and yours coincide, for instance if a friend offers to look after your children for an hour or two, just when you could do with a really welcome breather, or a friend who loves window-shopping can be commissioned to report back on what's available in the shops, or friends going sightseeing can be commissioned to assess access for you.

You *can* 'give', in lots of ways, however bad your arthritis. You can still keep up or make friendships, by giving people time, by listening to them (a rare treat nowadays), even giving them a shoulder to lean on (metaphorically at any rate). Some YPAs have become Samaritans. You can be that rare friend who always remembers birthdays and special occasions with a card. Keep in touch by phone, cassette, or letter if physical outings are difficult. And you can still share love, and a sense of humour, corny jokes, funny stories, even a zest for life, with people, however bad the arthritis. After experiences of pain and physical frustrations, simpler things in life take on new values; this enrichment can in turn enrich relationships with other people.

Maybe you can't take the children off for a walk, or play football, but you can read or sing to them, and give them time and emotional support. You can 'always be there' for them. Too many children lose out on these precious gifts.

A good way to enjoy 'giving' instead of constantly 'taking' is to have a pet, especially if you live alone. A pet can make you feel needed, and loved, and offers you ample opportunity to love in return. If you have a pet yourself, do be sure you can cope with it physically of course. No sense getting a dog which needs lots of exercise. Try a bird, or a gerbil or a guinea pig, or a cat which looks after itself. Or take an interest in a neighbour's pet, or 'adopt' an animal at the local zoo. – Choose carefully: you can't pet a lion!

There's a lot of medical support for the belief that stroking an animal is soothing and can reduce blood pressure and stressed feelings. A US study of coronary sufferers discovered that survival during the first 12 months after a heart attack was strongly related to the patient being a pet owner. Even if you don't own a pet yourself, there's a nationwide charity, the PAT Dogs Scheme, whereby friendly and well-adjusted dogs are taken by their owners, registered volunteers, to visit someone 'in need' in hospital or at home – a real morale-booster when you're feeling unloved and low. You might prefer to be a volunteer yourself if you own a gentle and friendly dog. Another charity, Dogs for the Disabled, trains dogs to be useful companions, like Elton, the labrador, whose many skills include bringing in post and newspapers, even the milk (in a special padded carrying case).

9 Be kind to yourself

Chronic arthritis can undermine self-confidence. Try hard not to add to the problem with guilt, self-criticism, or self-pity. Instead, work on morale-boosters.

Try to be comfortable with the arthritic changes in your body that can't be altered. Try not to waste time and energy asking 'why me?' That leads to self-pity and bitterness, unhelpful to you, and unattractive to other people. It's not a punishment for something, it's just the way things happen to have turned out for *you*. Other people have other crosses to bear.

A poor self-image is understandable; it's not always easy to come to terms with twisted hands or knees, or a clumsy body you'd happily step out of if you could, especially in a world which worships perfect youth and beauty. But try. Attractiveness really does lie in your personality and in how comfortable you can learn to feel with yourself and your body. Other people may withdraw from someone, *not* because of the way they look, but because that person's discomfort makes them uncomfortable, or because that person tries too hard to *over*compensate for a poor self-image, and in a craving for reassurance makes too many emotional demands on others.

Don't get obsessed about your appearance, but don't neglect it, either. Emphasise the good points, and say to hell with the bad points. An ugly person who's at ease with himself is more attractive than a handsome or beautiful person who's obsessively narcissistic or self-critical.

Encourage yourself to keep going. Remind yourself of your good points, and work on them. Do what you do do well. Don't feel guilty about what can't be changed. If you're a man with arthritis, maybe you and your wife have to swap roles, with her going out to work as the wage-earner and you staying at home. Well, instead of telling yourself you're a failure, try making a good job of it (hopefully with encouragement). No need to be a perfectionist, but reapply work skills to managing a household. If you can't do practical things, then do paperwork and brainwork and things which require less physical effort.

Be patient with yourself. Live one day at a time, and make the most of the good times. Too few of us learn to enjoy the moment and really appreciate the happy times. Like any other skill, you can develop that of savouring each and every good moment, so that in the bad times you look back not with regret, but with the tonic of remembered pleasure.

Make the most of the *absence* of pain. *Relish* a better day, don't waste it worrying about the next day. On a bad day pain can dominate your existence – well, on a good day, really let the *absence* of pain dominate you instead!

Why shun praise and encouragement from other people? Accept it, quietly. You deserve it, for it's a real achievement to 'keep going'. And as Pamela says: *"When you know that other people admire your 'pluck' you begin to develop some self-respect."*

Have faith in yourself, and the courage to be different, if necessary. Be considerate of others, but don't worry too much about what people think. It's not always easy to be self-confident when you're already laid low emotionally and physically, and long to be that weird and wonderful thing 'normal'. But *you're* the expert about what's right for you. For instance, living together may be a better option for some people than marrying, choosing *not* to have a baby better than choosing to have one, even though marrying or having a baby might make you seem 'more normal'. (Vice versa too, people may think you shouldn't get married or have a baby 'because you're disabled'.) It's not 'what other people think' that's important – the choice and the responsibility for making that choice is *yours* alone. Don't let other people organise your life for you.

In its Personal Development Courses, Young Arthritis Care includes help with developing self-esteem skills, and raising confidence:

> *"Taking a deep breath, crossing your fingers and hoping that a potential employer won't ask awkward questions about your arthritis at a job interview is all very well but the ability to deflect such questions or answer them to your own advantage is a skill which can be learned. Having the confidence to remain seated at a wedding when everyone stands up to toast the couple is a skill which can be learned. Having the confidence to close conversations about arthritis or open them up when it suits you is a skill which can be learned."* (*Young Arthritis News*)

Finally, keep things in perspective. Count your blessings – a cliché, but good advice. Make the most of your sense of humour. Dig it out *now* if you've buried it somewhere. No excuses. Don't be too serious and sensible about it all. Give yourself occasional treats. As Sandy Burnfield advises, from his own experiences of living with a chronic illness: *"Moderation is the key to leading a full and happy life, but occasionally, extremes give spice."* True!

10 Escape valves

Fit or unfit, we all need some form of escape from stress, and some way of recharging our batteries. Nothing like a good holiday, for instance, (though also potentially stress-causing if the wrong sort!). Or simply a day off, enjoying the countryside or watching a sport or whatever.

Be wary of 'bogus' escape valves that may appear helpful in the short term, but could create additional problems in the long run. Alcohol, tobacco, illegal mood-altering drugs won't solve problems. Prescribed tranquillisers or sleeping pills won't solve them either, though may help you cope *briefly* at a time of crisis (see page 48 for more about them).

Be wary too of quack remedies and therapies which promise to solve all your problems at great expense. Try not to seek comfort and solutions in over-eating. Putting on weight only increases stress on weak joints. Watch your consumption of tea, coffee and cola drinks. They all contain caffeine which produces tension symptoms of headaches, nervousness and anxiety (and makes you go to the loo very frequently!).

We YPAs need better ways of 'escaping' from our stresses. A permanent transplant into a new, perfect, body, or at the very least, a rest from time to time outside my body is, alas, totally unrealistic, at the moment, anyway!

Let's be realistic. What 'escape valves' might suit you?. What helps you let off steam, recharging the batteries so you return to the fight with renewed vigour? Use a diary, a good friend, a Young Arthritis Care Contact, the Wyeth helpline (see page 112) as an uncritical ear for your moans and· groans, and see 'Talking therapy' (page 110). Or pour out frustrations on paper and later, when you feel better, tear it up and forget it: preferable to a snappy remark that lingers in other people's memories. Write stories about the intruder in your life called Arthur Itis. Use the anti-stress techniques in chapter 14, like relaxation, meditation. Above all, use 'laughter therapy'! Make the most of your sense of humour. Laugh and the world laughs with you. Wonderful medicine.

Daydreaming can be a helpful escape valve. – Usually it just happens, but Dr Vernon Coleman, in *Natural Pain Control* and in *Arthritis* describes how you can use it consciously, to help control pain. Ordinary dreams can help too – amazing what ambitions and what recreational and sexual fantasies you can fulfil in your dream body – enjoy them. Music, religion, a romantic novel or gripping detective mystery, even watching TV can be good escapes, too, provided you're not storing up long-term problems by totally ignoring your family or partner!

Do something so absorbing that problems can't intrude, or train yourself to 'switch off' for a while at least. Or try the opposite, but in a controlled way: schedule for yourself a regular 'worry half-hour' or so, when you can worry as much as you like but allow yourself *no* worrying outside that time.

Silence, solitude, or sleep, can be blissful escapes. – Make time for them in your life, and get the family to understand and cooperate. They'll benefit too.

11 Learning to live with the minding

"We ought, of course, to stop minding, but we are only human, after all. And another picture rises before my mind's eye. A sunny tennis lawn where I watched 'the others' playing and a friend who said to me, apropos the arthritis, 'Of course, you've got over minding this!' But I was young and I hadn't – though I smiled and said that I had. For to people who guess as badly as that one never tells the truth; any more than one tells it to those who guess well, for they have known it all the time! No, I hadn't stopped minding, and I have tried to learn, too, not to let it weigh too heavily on those friends ..who must leave me out or behind. And that, I think, is the best one can do, for not to mind at all might be nearer to masochism than to merit." (Grace Stuart, in *Private World of Pain*, Allen and Unwin).

Alas, 'minding' is hard. It can easily become jealousy, envy, hatred, bitterness, which gnaw at the soul, using up already depleted emotional energy reserves, and which may add to problems, by turning other people away. Minding doesn't go away, but it can be lived with.

Audrey Shepherd found one way of living with the minding:

"I believe that an important part of being made whole involves learning to absorb suffering instead of passing it on in another form.....Suffering comes to us in the forms of pain, frustration, ill-health or unhappiness, and we take our part in the vicious circle of never-ending suffering by passing it on to other people in the forms of irritability, resentment, bitterness or cynicism. But hope for mankind will only come when we cease to do this, when we absorb the suffering that comes our way and render it powerless by our refusal to pass it on to other people in some other guise. Seen in this light, suffering is robbed of its most unbearable feature, the sense that it is futile and meaningless. It is seen instead as a challenge, not in a pious but in quite a practical way. To say that suffering is no longer meaningless is not to say that it ceases to be inexplicable. It remains, or much of it remains, a mystery." (In Paul Hunt's *Stigma*, Geoffrey Chapman.)

Where to start? Instead of envying someone doing what you wish you could still do – mountain climbing, travelling to exotic far-off lands, or just tramping around the sales, take an interest. Difficult but rewarding. That person will be attracted by your interest rather than repelled by envy. And instead of wasting the time they're away letting the envy gnaw away, do something interesting yourself, if only watching a film on TV or listening to a radio programme. Something you can talk to them about later, maybe. And train yourself to enjoy listening to what they've been up to – with practice it becomes a genuine pleasure. (Even if it doesn't come automatically at first.)

Minding about being dependent is hard, too, minding about having to swallow your pride and ask for help. As Sue Gunn says:

"..I don't like other people being in control of my actions. Of course, I am dependent on my husband, family and friends for a lot of things. And, if there is no way I can be independent in something then I don't think it is worth worrying about it. The main

thing is that I remain as independent as I possibly can. I prefer to take my time to do something I want to do than let someone else do it for me in half the time. At the same time, if it takes half an hour to put my stockings on then I prefer my husband to do it, so I can save my energy for something more important!" (In Contact)

True. And also, don't forget that with a gadget here, or a nifty bit of brain-work there, you can achieve unimagined independence.

Minding about other people's attitudes can be tackled in various ways (see chapter 25). 'Invisible' symptoms can lead to embarrassment, to misunderstandings, just as much as 'visible' disabilities. Don't be demoralised by people who would 'segregate' and 'discriminate' (however subconsciously) against someone with a chronic disorder/disability. Counter-attack instead by 'melting the ICE block' (see page 104). Unjust though it may at first seem, learn to take the initiative *yourself* in getting over any unease/misunderstanding/prejudice. You are the expert, after all, and that way you'll show you're not a 'victim', but very much in control.

One of the most valuable things each of us can do, I believe, is to be an ambassador for the rest of us with arthritis or other disabilities. For instance, by graciously accepting even unneeded help from other people remember you're doing your bit to encourage them to help again when that help may actually be needed. And the able-bodied of today may be the disabled of tomorrow.

From time to time, if 'minding' does become overwhelming, don't feel guilty about giving in to it. As one YPA put it:

"The struggle goes on and I think we should feel free to allow ourselves some days of weakness, self-pity and self-indulgence in order to keep the battle going − we want to win the war not just every battle..."

Allowing yourself the right to half an hour's snivel is important. A good cry, alone, or on someone's shoulder is very therapeutic. Or you could follow PB's example:

"I consulted a good friend and arranged with her that...I would phone her any time I felt the need to relieve my pent-up frustration and aggression by delivering to her a stream of abuse..."

12 Melt the ICE block

ICE stands for the 'information, communication, education' block, between those who know about younger people with arthritis and what it means, and those who don't. We can all help melt the ICE block. You'll feel you're doing something constructive. It can even be fun and lead to all sorts of unexpected happenings, like being interviewed on local radio!

On page 120 one YPA describes how she, as a local Councillor, was educating the Chief Executive of her local council about arthritis. Peter Nightingale was a manager with his local council. He found that melting the ICE became an important part of his job. An OT put his name forward to take part in a discussion on access for people with disabilities. Soon he was asked to join a local union group called Workers with Disabilities, became its Secretary, and member of a working party on equal opportunities policy:

"So there you are, get arthritis and see the world. I would not have had it by choice but it has given me experiences and led me to gain knowledge I would not otherwise have had. People notice that you have it. A few years ago the Council decided to introduce specially designed public toilets for disabled people. The Engineering Department got involved. I was asked, being 'disabled', if I would liaise with Social Services and with RADAR to promote the National Key Scheme in the borough. I did some of the publicity, a report to committee, and handed the whole thing over to the Hammersmith and Fulham Action on Disabled..."

At home, at work, at play, every day and everywhere each of us can do something, however small. Let people know we exist, let them know our needs, our hopes and fears, but don't forget to ram home the message too that we're all individuals and have plenty of talents and abilities. Project a positive image so we get away from stereotyped views. It's good therapy, too, to feel you're actually doing something positive.

Use newspapers and magazines, radio and TV programmes and phone-ins, to speak up. Don't go just for 'disabled' items. Try consumer programmes, too, and write in or telephone with comments on new developments in your area (what are the architects doing about access, disabled loos, etc?), parking regulations (have we been forgotten?), hospital and healthcare developments (have they remembered the 'young chronic sick', who *don't* have private medical insurance, *can't* walk miles to get prescriptions?). Write to manufacturers about packages you can't open, new ideas for gadgets in the kitchen, home, garage, garden, etc. Point out that what helps us YPAs often helps others too, eg young mums with prams and heavy shopping, old people, and other people with disabilities.

Amazing what you can do simply sitting in your armchair. Laid up after an op, I telephoned the Jimmy Young show after the doctor had answered a question about lupus. He hadn't mentioned the lupus support group so I phoned to publicise it, and ten minutes later the nation (well, the JY show audience, anyway) knew all about it.

Fund-raising, selling raffle tickets, charity Christmas cards, getting people to collect stamps for charity, are other ways of publicising your 'cause', and making other people feel they're doing something to help. I put a notice in the office bulletin asking people for coffee labels. These raised funds for the Raynaud's Association, helped publicise Raynaud's, *and* helped explain to colleagues about one of my 'problems'.

Look on things like a stick, or a wheelchair, or electric scoota or even an ARC or Arthritis Care badge as bridgebuilders in the way that a baby or pet is often a bridgebuilder, something to melt the ICE between you and Joe Public. My yellow scoota gets admiring glances, especially from children, and comments. A smile from me lets people feel they can ask questions and find out a little about me and being a YPA.

Join groups of people who share your interests. Melt the ICE block through groups directly connected with arthritis or healthcare (Arthritis Care, ARC, the Community Health Council or local access or disability group). Or through something totally unconnected, like Hadyn Martin (see page 290), playing pétanque. People who meet him see and learn not only that he has RA, but is 'normal' too, and talented!

Play your part in democracy. Get a postal vote if you can't get out to vote (see page 122). Keep your councillors and MP informed of your views on what needs doing or undoing to help YPAs.

Endpiece

I'll end by letting Sandy Burnfield summarise how he aims for a positive philosophy in living with his chronic illness:

"The German poet... Goethe wrote the following: 'It is in self-limitation that a master first shows himself'...Once I can accept these limitations, then I can go on to find some sort of meaning and satisfaction in life in spite of them, and perhaps even because of them. " (In *Multiple Sclerosis: A Personal Exploration*, Souvenir Press)

Chapter fourteen

SOME SIMPLE SELF-HELP ANTI-STRESS TECHNIQUES

Simple anti-stress techniques won't, alas, cure arthritis, but do help some people cope better with it. Before you try these techniques, do first share any worries with your doctor. S/he may be able to help. Medical support's especially essential if you find you're sinking into a continuing depression, with relentless feelings of despair and lethargy.

Relaxation

The right sort of relaxation is a harmless anti-stress device worth trying by anyone, and in some people may even help reduce pain, anxiety, and disease activity, as suggested in a randomised controlled study of 53 patients in America (Bradley L A, Young, L D, Anderson K O, et al, 'Effects of psychological therapy on pain behavior of rheumatoid arthritis patients', in *Arthritis and Rheumatism* 1987; 30; 1105 − 14, see page 294).

Jane Madders, qualified physiotherapist, lecturer in health education and author of *Stress and Relaxation* (Macdonald Optima), says:

"Relaxation can counteract the effects of high levels of arousal and the stress disorders these generate, it can dispel the fatigue and aches that are caused by prolonged muscle tension, it can help you tolerate pain, make personal relationships easier and give feelings of well being and aid restorative sleep.

"There are, of course, some things relaxation cannot do. It is no cure for conditions that require medical or surgical treatment, though it may well help them, and will be of great benefit in the recovery period. Relaxation cannot remove personal or work problems but you can learn to diminish your reaction to them and this in itself may go part of the way towards solving them. When you are more relaxed, it is easier to talk over your problems with someone else."

She explains, too, that good circulation and muscle relaxation help reduce the build-up of lactic acid in the joints. Lactic acid is a waste product resulting (with carbon dioxide) from the energy-generating breakdown of sugar and oxygen in the muscles. Normally muscle action would keep the blood flow pumping and taking away excess lactic acid, but with unrelieved muscular tension, lactic acid build-up in even healthy joints that are tense can lead to pain, stiffness and physical fatigue.

Here's a beautifully simple relaxation technique, Robert H Phillips' 'Quick Release' method (from his *Coping with Lupus*, 1984, Avery Publishing, Garden City Pk, New York):

"First read the directions and then try it. Close your eyes, take a deep breath, and hold it while you tense or tighten every muscle in your body that you can think of (your fists, arms, legs, stomach, neck, buttocks, etc). Hold your breath and muscle tension for about six seconds. Then let your breath out in a whoosh, and let your body go limp. Keep your eyes closed, and breathe rhythmically in and out for about 20 seconds. Repeat this tension/relaxation cycle three times, and by the end of the third repetition, you'll probably feel a lot more relaxed."

In London the Royal Free Hospital has been trying out a non-drug pain control and relaxation self-help technique devised by Ursula Fleming. It's used especially for patients with chronic pain or an incurable illness. *Woman* magazine (15 February 1986) featured three readers who'd benefited too, one with severe back problems, one with pre-menstrual tension, and the third, a professional pianist, with RA:

"I was immensely interested when I first heard about Ursula Fleming...as she used to be a pianist, which is my own profession. I have had an arthritic hip for several years and know I'm making the problem worse by tensing up in expectation of the pain. I find it almost impossible to relax. At first, the tape didn't seem to be doing me any good. But now I'm finding that the muscles really are less tense and, as a result, the pain has lessened...

"Normally, I do think I am a fairly relaxed sort of person, but once the pain starts, a vicious circle builds up. I've been taking lots of treatment for arthritis, including homeopathic medicine, and there's no conventional medicine I haven't tried. I've had every kind of pill there is.

"I know that relaxation will never cure arthritis, but I've been anxious to cut down the many pills I've been taking and to avoid major surgery. Already, the arthritis in my fingers has gone. For a time, it stopped me playing the piano, but I can play perfectly well again now."

Laura Mitchell was a qualified physiotherapist, who taught at St Thomas' Hospital, London and the London School of Occupational Therapy. She also suffered from OA:

"...I have an arthritic spine, an arthroplasty of one hip joint, and removal of the other hip joint, plus a shortened leg bone, a built up shoe, a crutch and very shaky balance. I therefore know that having any disability means a continuous battle. Patience one can learn, but frustration always remains. Getting in or out of the car is a major event, and carrying a tray a difficulty."

That quotation is from her book *Simple Relaxation*, (John Murray, 1987). It's very readable, but with plenty of 'professional references' too. She explains how muscles work, what can go wrong, how tension builds up, and then goes on to explain her method of controlling tension and changing it, at will, to break the vicious circle of stress and tension.

The British Holistic Medical Association (see page 71) has a self-help tape, *The Breath of Life, Undoing Muscular Tension*, by Dr Patrick Pietroni, which explains how breathing correctly can help, plus information on relaxation and body awareness.

Some people find relaxation techniques easier to learn with the help of a teacher. One way of avoiding expensive fees is to find out about classes run locally by The Look After Yourself Project. The Project gives guidance on safe exercise, understanding nutrition, and dealing with stress (which includes relaxation techniques). For the address of your local Project contact the main office of The Look After Yourself Project.

You could also send an SAE to 'Relaxation for Living' for a list of leaflets, books and cassettes on relaxation. The organisation has a countrywide network of teachers who give guidance on reducing tension and understanding stress. Fees vary. Tuition's not specifically aimed at people with a chronic illness, so find out about its methods first and seek your doctor's agreement before embarking on anything.

Meditation

Meditation's a technique anyone, however uncooperative their body, can use to develop inner resources to cope more effectively with stress and problems like a chronic disease. You don't have to shave your head or get involved with strange religions. You don't have to join an organisation, buy any equipment, attend any course, or even leave your home. It's easy and it's free.

Meditation's a way of calming the mind and making you feel good. It's not a cure, but a way of strengthening ourselves to help us deal with difficulties. It's a useful natural, non-drug technique we can call on to help us deal with stress and pain. If you're in pain, it's very comforting to have a way of creating an 'inner retreat' away from jagged nerves.

Psychiatrist Dr Sandy Burnfield, affirms:

"The effects will be beneficial and will lead to better concentration and memory, as well

as a general improvement in relaxation and self-confidence. Eventually you will be able to use this technique in all sorts of situations, from waiting on a station platform to travelling in a bus. Some people find that they can regain peace and tranquillity through this technique if they are upset, anxious or angry about something. Others find that it helps them to get their lives in perspective, and some use it as prelude to sleep." (*Multiple Sclerosis: A Personal Exploration*, Souvenir Press).

I find the 'inner break' it gives me helpful at work, for instance, to relax me at lunchtime, when I can't get out for a change of scene, to relax me when I get home after a hard day at work, and to calm me if I wake in the middle of the night with a churning mindful of worries.

Some of the body's responses to meditation have been scientifically measured. It can induce what Dr Herbert Benson, of the Harvard Medical School, called 'The Relaxation Response', the opposite of the fight-or-flight response to the threat of danger or stress (page 84). The heart rate decreases, so does the rate of breathing, and the body's metabolic rate. Blood lactate goes down: high levels are associated with attacks of anxiety. Dr Benson found that meditation can reduce high blood pressure in some people, and it can produce slower brain waves, indicative of a state of relaxation.

'Counting the breath'
This is the simplest method to start with.

1 *Preparation*
- Aim for a mood of quiet contentment.
- Pain may make meditation difficult, so try to time your session for when your pain's at its least intense. If you take painkillers time your session for when they start to work.
- After a warming bath or shower might be a good time. Or just refresh your hands and face. Blow your nose. Brush your teeth. Go to the loo.
- Choose a quiet room, and take the telephone off the hook. Make yourself as comfortable as possible. Sitting upright in a straightbacked chair may be better than lying down, but try either. You most definitely do *not* have to contort yourself into the famous 'lotus position' sitting cross-legged on the floor!
- Eyes can be open or closed. Closing them may help cut out distractions.
- Start by practising for five minutes, and extend the time by five minutes as you get used to it. Then set aside maybe 10 to 15 minutes once or twice a day for regular sessions. If you find it difficult to guess the length of time, set a kitchen timer beforehand, provided its noise doesn't distract you.

2 *Counting*
- Don't force anything. Just let things happen quietly and easily. Just 'let it be'. First let your mind focus on your breathing. Take a few slow, regular deep breaths, but don't force your breathing. You can tell if you're relaxed by the way your stomach moves: out as you breathe in, and moving in as you breathe out.
- Then start counting. First − breathe in. Then as you slowly and evenly breathe out count 'one' in your mind. Breathe in again. Without straining, when you next breathe out count 'two'. The next out-breath will be 'three', then 'four'. Then start at one again. And so on... The idea is gently and gradually to train your mind to focus on one thing (ie on the counting), and one thing only, thus refreshing and relaxing it and you.
- Be relaxed about the whole thing. If distracting thoughts and feelings come into your mind, just be aware of them, but let them drift away again, while you concentrate on the counting. Don't criticise yourself or feel you've failed if distractions occur. Self criticism makes matters worse, not better. If you find counting one to four is a distraction, just count 'one' on each out-breath.

● Incredibly, that's all you need to know. It may seem too simple at first and not worth bothering with, but with time and practice you should feel benefits. Once you know how to do it you can use the technique at other times too, to help counteract the build-up of stress.

Finding out more

If you want to read more about different types of meditation, East or West, good introductions are L Le Shan's *How to Meditate* (Thorsons), Simon Court's *The Meditator's Manual* (Thorsons) and James Hewitt's *Teach Yourself Meditation* with useful bibliography (Hodder and Stoughton Teach Yourself Books).

If you'd prefer to learn with help from a teacher, contact the British Holistic Medical Association for details of their regional branches and guidance on finding a teacher. BHMA also produces two self-help tapes: *Seven Days' Meditation*, by Max Mackay-James, and *Introduction to Meditation* by Dr Patrick Pietroni.

Laughter and smile therapy

Laughter has been called stationary jogging, as it provides good exercise for internal body systems. − So it's perfect for the likes of us, and cheap, too. Though it can't *cure* illness, it *can* act as a natural tranquilliser. It has definite beneficial effects, which researchers are at last taking seriously. West Birmingham Health Authority recently opened the first NHS laughter therapy clinic for people undergoing treatment for stress. Many American hospitals already employ humour therapists.

A French doctor, Pierre Vachet, has studied laughter for many years. He's found that it increases oxygen intake, deepens breathing, improves circulation, speeds tissue healing, and strengthens the body against infection. French neurologist Henri Rubinstein says it can reduce the heart rate, stimulate the appetite and improve the digestion too. Apparently it can also boost production of endorphins, the body's natural painkillers and tranquillisers (see page 79). Liz Hodgkinson has written a whole book on *Smile Therapy* (Macdonald, 1987)! She describes some experiments in America:

"In the experiments, a group of actors were asked to simulate a variety of emotions by putting the appropriate expression on their faces. They were asked to smile, to look surprised, angry, disgusted, fearful and sad. As they put on each expression in turn, various bodily functions, such as heart rate, skin temperature and blood pressure were monitored. In every case, smiling was the only expression which served to calm down the body's activity. All the other expressions, which indicated negative emotions, sent heart rate and blood pressure soaring."

She believes that facial expressions do, in time, actually alter emotions. So by first trying to *look* happy, you improve your chances of actually *being* happy, and doing your body good. People who smile and can see the funny side of life actually make other people feel good too. Gloomy faces spread gloom and fear. Fear stops people regaining their health, she believes:

"When we laugh, all our body systems are shaken up and tension is released. Laughter is a relaxing activity in itself, and could do more good than all the exercises, aerobics and mental tricks people are currently using to try and help them to relax...Henri Rubinstein states in his research papers that laughter is the best relaxant there is − as even one minute of laughter can give the body up to 45 minutes of therapeutic relaxation. Laughter, it appears, has much the same effect on the body as regular physical exercise, in that the 'high' produced goes on working long after the exercise is over. Laughter is, after all, another form of bodily exercise."

Having a sense of humour is a vital escape valve from worries and difficulties. Smiles and laughter help get things in perspective again. Replace a miserable expression with a cheerful one and, says Liz Hodgkinson, even though illness or pain may still be present, 'the healing process can actually be set in motion'. Though the illness may not disappear your reactions to it will alter, and make you better able to see solutions and ways of coping.

Liz Hodgkinson quotes Ursula Fleming (mentioned on page 106), who also believes in the value of laughter:

"Laughter is essential to getting well. Each of us has to understand that life has to be laughed at, otherwise it becomes unbearable...People who are afraid cannot laugh, but once they have learned to laugh, they have then triumphed over themselves and their disease...

"The most important aspect of getting well is... to alter the emotions. Only by changing the way you feel can you start to get better. The body responds to positive emotions, and particularly to lightheartedness."

With the support of his doctor, Norman Cousins made 'laughter therapy' a keystone of the treatment programme for his AS, with splendid results. He wrote about it in *Anatomy of an Illness, As Perceived by the Patient* (first published in Britain in 1987, by Bantam, with detailed bibliography and medical references). He reckoned that just as negative emotions can make people ill, so positive emotions ought to help make us well again.

He arranged special laughter sessions for himself, hired a projector and some of his favourite Marx Brothers and Candid Camera comedy films, and read funny books. He laughed so much he was asked to move out of his hospital room because he was disturbing the other patients! He felt less pain (*'ten minutes of genuine belly laughter had an anaesthetic effect and would give me at least two hours of pain-free sleep'*), and his doctor measured beneficial effects in his blood. He took sedimentation rate readings just before as well as several hours after the laughter episodes. Each time there was a drop of at least five points, not massive, but enough, and it was cumulative.

Norman also used, under *strict* medical supervision, ascorbic acid. His physical problems didn't disappear overnight, but in time he recovered sufficiently to go back to his editorial job full-time *'and this was miracle enough for me'*. He became senior lecturer at the School of Medicine, University of California at Los Angeles, and consulting editor of *Man & Medicine*, published at the College of Physicians and Surgeons, Columbia University.

Dr Vernon Coleman prescribes laughter therapy in his book *Natural Pain Control*. He suggests keeping a list of favourite funny films and books and videos that make you laugh out loud. His choice include Jerome K Jerome, James Thurber, Stephen Leacock, Robert Benchley and S J Perelman. My favourite laughter-makers would include the TV *Fawlty Towers* series with John Cleese and Co, Michael Crawford in *Some Mothers Do Have 'Em*, the *Yes, Minister* series, anything with Peter Sellers; radio programmes like Tony Hancock's (eg the *Blood Donor*), the *Round the Horne* series, *I'm Sorry, I'll Read That Again*; and books by Gerald Durrell, James Herriot, Maureen Lipman, Tom Sharpe, and David Niven's *The Moon's a Balloon*. So – start smiling, and try taking the laughter medicine!

Talking therapy

Talking over problems and sharing worries can help enormously with the problems of 'living with arthritis'. Sometimes just putting fears or emotions into words helps get them in perpective and makes them easier to sort out. Perhaps a good friend can help, simply by listening to you, or your local Young Arthritis Care Contact, or phone the Wyeth helpline at Arthritis Care (see page 112). Or try your doctor, or priest, or a counsellor recommended by your doctor. Or the Samaritans, if you're feeling particularly low and unable to talk to anyone else.

The person you talk to needs to be the right sort of person, someone who'll let *you* talk and offload your worries, and clarify your thoughts and feelings, rather than a self-styled expert over-keen to dictate what you should do. Sometimes it helps just to pour out your thoughts and feelings on paper, in a diary or on scrap paper that can be thrown away later. Or write an article (or a book!).

Sometimes it helps to talk to a professional counsellor, someone trained to listen and to offer support and insight. Some can teach helpful skills such as relaxation. GPs may refer people to nurses, social workers, clinical psychologists, psychotherapists or other counsellors for emotional support.

If you'd like first to do some background reading on 'talking therapy', on counselling and psychotherapy, get MIND's low-cost Factsheet 6 *Talking Treatments*. Another readable guide is Lindsay Knight's *Talking to a Stranger. A Consumer's Guide to Therapy* (Fontana, 1986). She shows how different therapies work, who they benefit, what happens, and how long it takes. She stresses that therapy *isn't* just for people diagnosed as mentally ill, or severely distressed: it's for ordinary people with ordinary problems.

Another shorter guide, helpful and clearly written, is Hilary Edwards' *Psychological Problems. Who Can Help?* (Methuen and the British Psychological Society). She explains what sort of help you might expect from a GP, voluntary organisations such as Relate, MIND, and specialist professionals such as a clinical psychologist, a psychiatrist, a community psychiatric nurse, a nurse therapist, and social workers. A community psychiatric nurse explains:

"My work involves counselling, support, and problem-solving. I also give a lot of practical information, such as how to get a home help, or where a lonely person can go to meet people...."

A MIND worker says

"The main things we offer are befriending, counselling, group therapies, help with welfare matters, and general support for people with problems and for their families...Most of our users are self-referred...People who use MIND have a wide range of difficulties. Many are suffering a life trauma, such as job loss, bereavement, the break-up of a relationship, or major illness..."

The British Association for Counselling (BAC) produces a directory of counselling agencies and individual practitioners, most of whom offer general counselling for such problems as anxiety, stress, low self-esteem and relationship difficulties. Some also specialise in a specific area such as careers, redundancy, or mid-life crisis.

Chapter fifteen

OVERCOMING THE INFORMATION BARRIER
Finding help to help yourself
(For the full address of all organisations mentioned
in this chapter, see Appendix 2)

To deal with any new situation you need information, and especially with something like chronic arthritis. Not easy if you don't know anyone else in the same boat, or when your body stops you going where and when you want, or when the world seems full of rules and regulations most decidedly *not* designed for your totally unique situation. Well – get organised, start finding out, and some barriers at least will start to fall. Life should start to get a little easier.

Get two smart foolscap cardboard wallets from a stationer's, or use a couple of large envelopes or cardboard boxes. The first is for your Infokit; the second for your Medikit (look back at page 33). Next get some notepaper, cheap envelopes, and some second class stamps. Also helpful and cheap – ready printed self-stick address labels (eg from Able-Label, Steepleprint Ltd). When writing for information and leaflets (except for government department publications) do enclose a stamped addressed envelope (SAE) or a stamp, at least, to be sure of a reply.

Then start writing and sit back and wait for the goodies to fall through your letter-box!

Your Infokit of low-cost information

1 Useful phone numbers

Keep these all together in your Infokit:

- *0800 289170* – Wyeth Helpline (free), at Arthritis Care, which is staffed by people who have arthritis and are usually from the health professions. You can phone between 1pm and 5pm, on weekdays. (More about Arthritis Care on page 113 and 118.)
- *081 681 3311* – Healthline, at the College of Health. Confidential tape-recorded information on different rheumatic disorders, on hip and knee replacements, etc. You can phone between 4pm and 8pm any weekday. (More about the College on page 119.)
- *0800 666555* – Freeline Social Security (free), for general information on benefits.
- *0800 882200* – BEL, Benefits Enquiry Line (free) for information specific to disabled people. Phone between 9am and 4.30pm, on weekdays. (Northern Ireland: 0800 616757.)
- *Citizens' Advice Bureau.* Find the address and phone number of your local CAB in the phone book or from CAB Headquarters. If you're housebound someone from CAB may be able to visit you. (More about CAB on page 118.)
- *DIAL (Disablement Information and Advice Lines UK).* Look in the phone book, or contact DIAL headquarters for address and phone number of your local DIAL information service. (More about DIAL on page 120.)
- *Other numbers* – Include in your Infokit, too, names, addresses and phone numbers of your MP, your Young Arthritis Care Contact (if you're a member), and local library.

2 Books and booklets

(Mostly free, unless it says otherwise, below, and all full of helpful information)

Arthritis information from the Arthritis and Rheumatism Council (ARC) (see page 118)

ARC concentrates mainly on medical, research, and educational aspects. Send SAE for any of these which sound appropriate, and ask for their up-to-date publications list:

- *Introducing Arthritis*, a general booklet.
- Booklets on *Rheumatoid Arthritis, Osteoarthritis Explained, Gout, Ankylosing Spondylitis, Osteoporosis, Scleroderma, Marriage, Sex and Arthritis, Backache, Pain in the Neck, Your Home and Your Rheumatism, Lupus*, etc.
- Factsheets *Tennis Elbow, A New Hip Joint, Polymyalgia Rheumatica (PMR), Choosing Shoes, Diet, Exercise, Alternative Medicine.*
- Also available, handbooks on *When Your Child Has Arthritis, Are You Sitting Comfortably?* (guide to choosing easy chairs).
- Subscribe to the excellent *Arthritis Today* (colourful, only £2 for three issues a year), written by experts specially for laypeople – news about research, education, treatment.

Arthritis information from Arthritis Care (see page 118)

Concentrates mainly on social, practical and welfare aspects of living with arthritis. Send SAE for any of these:

- Leaflets include *Introducing Arthritis Care (Action for People with Arthritis)*
- *Eating and Moving, Food for Thought*
- *Designed for Living*: catalogue of gadgets on sale by mail-order (send two 1st cl stamps)
- *Arthritis: Some questions answered* – free 20 minute audiocassette (send SAE at least 6" by 9") featuring Barbara Kelly interviewing Dr Andrei Calin, Consultant Rheumatologist at the Royal National Hospital for Rheumatic Diseases at Bath.
- *Arthritis News*, excellent quarterly newspaper, contains news of Arthritis Care activities, rheumatology and healthcare issues, plus cookery and gardening features, and all manner of hints and tips. On subscription, or free to paid-up members.
- *Young Arthritis News*, also excellent regular magazine, produced by and for members of Young Arthritis Care (see page 117 and 123). Free to paid-up members.

For specific information on AS, Lupus, etc

Write to the appropriate self-help group (names in chapter 3, addresses in Appendix 2).

Essential information to make life easier

- *Equipment and Services for Disabled People* (HB6 1990) – essential for your Infokit, and free from the Department of Health.
- *Which Benefit?* (FB2) – your key guide to financial assistance, and *Sick or Disabled?* (FB28). Both free from local social security offices, or by post from DSS Leaflets Unit.)
- *Door-to-Door: A Guide to Transport for People with Disabilities* – indispensable for newcomers and oldhanders alike, however mild or severe your arthritis. Available by post from Department of Transport. Free, no SAE needed.
- *Disability Rights Handbook*, all-purpose rights guide (page 128, £6.95, 1992, inc p&p).

Other low-cost information

Write to these organisations asking for their publications list. Most are charities and on tight budgets, so a stamp or SAE's *essential*.

- Disabled Living Foundation (see pages 121 amd 144)
- RADAR (The Royal Association for Disability and Rehabilitation) (see page 123). Ask for their free booklet *If only I'd Known that a Year Ago...*, and their booklist, too, is a real eye-opener on what's around to make life easier. They also produce a monthly

Bulletin (on subscription) of current disability news and information.

● Healthwise – bookshop of the Family Planning Association, but don't let that put you off! They produce a very good introductory list of books available by post, not just on family planning and sexuality, but also on relationships, and physical and emotional health generally.
● Relate (see also page 217) – excellent booklist on relationships, emotions, etc. Books on the list are available by post.
● British Medical Association – ask for their *Family Doctor Publications* booklist of low-priced booklets covering many topics, eg pregnancy and childbirth, childcare and management, sex education, psychological medicine, and general health.
● British Holistic Medical Association (see page 71) – wide-ranging booklist.
● Write to the commercial suppliers listed on page 144, asking for their catalogues packed with wonderful 'sanity-savers' to make life easier in all sorts of ways.

Adding to your Infokit

Continue to add anything else you come across, eg any specifically local information, like your local access guide. Keep useful newspaper cuttings (regular health pages appear in the *Times*, *Independent*, etc, and in local newspapers and in magazines like *Woman*, *Woman's Own*, *Prima*, *Family Circle*, *Practical Health*, *Living*, *Good Housekeeping*, *Bella*, *Best*). Pick up free leaflets in the post office and chemist's.

Keep up-to-date by listening to radio programmes like *Does He Take Sugar?*, *Medicine Now*, Dr Mike Smith on the Jimmy Young Show on Tuesdays, Dr Michael van Straten on Radio 5, and local radio programmes too. Watch TV programmes like *Link*, *People First*, *One in Four*, *Same Difference*. Jot down useful addresses and books to read.

Disability Now is a well-written monthly newspaper full of useful disability-related updates and information (available by post).

A useful reference book is the *Directory for Disabled People*, compiled by Ann Darnborough and Derek Kinrade, published by Woodhead-Faulkner, in association with RADAR. It's expensive though, so look at it in your local library. Well worth knowing about too is the BMA *Guide to Medicines & Drugs* (see page 49). Your library may have a copy if you prefer not to buy one.

One thing leads to another, and information already in your Infokit will entice you to go after yet more information specific to *you* and *yours*. Eventually you'll have so much clutter you'll wish you'd never started!

Buying and borrowing books

Throughout this book I mention lots of other books worth dipping into. Most of them are paperbacks, so cheapish, but that doesn't mean you have to get them all! You can see many of them in your local library.

As you see new books mentioned on TV and in magazines, make a note in your Infokit (title, author and, ideally, publisher, price and ISBN number) ready for your next visit to the library or bookshop. Good local bookshops will order books for you if not in stock. Some may even post or deliver them to you: try asking.

Other organisations supply books by post. Though you might have to pay post and packing costs, balance that drawback against the exhaustion of trekking from bookshop to bookshop only to find it's out of stock. Many publishers will send books direct. Useful if your bookshop isn't keen to order just one copy. Phone or write to the publishers and ask. Your library can help you track down the address/number – eg in the *Writers' and Artists' Yearbook*.

The Family Planning Association, Relate, and the British Holistic Medical Association will send by post books on their booklists: a specially useful way of getting books you might be too embarrassed to ask for in a bookshop. Other postal sources are *The Good Book Guide* or Waterstone's (see page 281). You can telephone an order to one of Hatchards branches and pay by credit card, cheque, or account (head office number in Appendix 2).

Best of all, for paperbacks only, is the mail-order service I've been using for ages, run by J Barnicoat (Falmouth) Ltd. They stock over 400,000 paperbacks, and reply promptly, usually enclosing two or three publishers' catalogues with my order to tantalise me into wanting yet more books!

Libraries and librarians

Librarians are information specialists, not just issuers and storers of books. Most enjoy being asked to show off their skills, so do ask, not just about books but information of any sort, including local organisations, bus services, evening classes. Every chartered librarian is bound by his or her professional code of ethics to provide information unless that information is restricted by law. Public libraries are free, though there may be a small charge for some special services.

If you can't get there yourself or send anyone on your behalf, then see if the social services or local library can arrange for the visiting library service to call. You can also telephone the library with queries, eg for specific addresses. If at first they're unhelpful, explain you're disabled/have got mobility problems.

If you can get along there yourself, so much the better. What they offer nowadays besides books is amazing – periodicals, newspapers, timetables, maps, talking books, music cassettes, children's stories and activities, and information about other specialised libraries, eg how to get information on a medical matter. Some libraries arrange guided tours to explain what's available. Or you could phone to ask if someone would have time to show you around, explaining you're keen to have help in making the most of your limited ability to walk/get about. Ask where to find, and how to use:

- *The catalogue system*   This might be a card index, or on microfiche (easy to use once you know how). Indexes can be arranged three ways: alphabetical or author index, subject index, and classified index. Books on related subjects are grouped together, using the 'Dewey' system. The classified index will give you the Dewey number for any subject, thus directing you to the right shelf for all the books on that subject.
- *The reference section*   Includes medical dictionaries, drugs guides, medical directory, *Hospital and Health Services Yearbook, Guide to the Social Services, Social Services Yearbook, Charities Digest, Directory of Grant-Making Trusts.*
- *The medical section* in the lending library (Dewey classification 610 +)   You can borrow these books or just browse. RA, AS, and cousins come under 616.7 'Diseases of the musculo-skeletal system'. But look in other areas too, eg the social sciences section (Dewey 361 +), psychology (Dewey 150 +). Books on stress, disability, depression, families, children, budgeting, 'how to' books, biographies, etc may all have helpful nuggets tucked away inside. The Dewey system rather confusingly separates disability-related books (eg Peggy Jay's *Coping with Disability* is classified at 262.4, while the AA's *Travellers Guide for the Disabled* is at 914.2).
- *The reservation service*   If the book you want is in the catalogue but isn't on the shelf, ask if you can reserve it. You'll be asked to write the details on a card, pay a small fee, and will be notified when the book appears in the library. You'll need to collect it within a stated period of time.
- *Inter-library system*   Even if the book you want isn't held by your local library, you can ask to borrow it through the inter-library system. You may need to pay a small fee. Your library will borrow it from another library for you. I've tried this and it works well. Once they told me the book was available at another library not too far away (but too far for me) where I could see it as a reference book. I explained my 'disability' and that I

needed to borrow it, to read in detail, so they helpfully found me a loan copy from another library. Once or twice my library has actually purchased a new loan copy of a book I've wanted.

- Ask about **book finding tools** For instance if you want to find out what books are in print on 'arthritis', you can find out from *British Books in Print*, indexed not only under author and title, but also under keywords like 'arthritis' too. It may be in bulky volumes or on microfiche; your librarian will probably be guarding it close to his or her bosom so you might need to coax them to let you use it!

Medical information

Apart from your doctor and healthcare team, a good guide to medical/health information sources is the College of Health's *Consumers' Guide to Health Information*. It tells you, for instance, what luck you're likely to have in finding and using medical libraries. One tip is that in addition to all public libraries, many academic and institutional libraries have obtained a Library Licence, which means that they have to agree to be 'open' to the public and not just to their own academic staff and students. So they're obliged to provide a reference service (though not lending service) to the general public.

The guide includes 'Where to find books in a medical library', 'Consumer health information services', 'Journals, newsletters and bulletins', 'Reference books'. It mentions too the British Library Medical Information Service. This can supply photocopies of specific medical journal articles for a small charge or do a 'search' for you (can be expensive) of some of the masses of computer medical and health databases. Contact the British Library number given in Appendix 2 for more details. See too Health Information Service (page 121), Help for Health (page 121), Medical Advisory Association (page 122) College of Health (page 119) and Patients' Association (page 122).

Self-help/patient support groups

One of my main reasons for joining ARC, Arthritis Care, and Young Arthritis Care was to get information, to find out all I could about arthritis and about how best to help myself. Since then I've joined other support groups too, for instance one concentrating on driving for disabled people, and another, the Association of Disabled Professionals, which focuses on employment. Self-help groups now exist for almost every condition under the sun!

Some people are put off joining a group. They may have a fearful vision of regular moan-ins, where everyone sits around swapping demoralising horror stories. Maybe some groups *are* like that, but fortunately I've managed to avoid them so far. You could always resign, or simply subscribe to the magazine. Other people question what benefits there can be in joining a group of people brought together by the very thing they would surely most like to forget? Fortunately, on the whole, the benefits far outweigh any drawbacks.

Groups vary considerably in what they do and how they do it. Some concentrate on fund-raising and research, or act as pressure groups to educate and change society. Others help with information, welfare, finance, counselling, and practical matters. For many people social contact through a group is important; it can break feelings of isolation and be a source of information and inspiration to 'keep going'. If shyness puts you off going try contacting the secretary asking to meet just one or two members first. Invite them in for coffee maybe, so you'll know someone before going along. If getting there's the main problem, see if the secretary can help.

People who already lead full social lives may choose to join because they value the information and ideas in the group's magazine, or because they feel they'd like to help other members in some way. Members have the advantage, over professionals, of firsthand experience. Good self-help groups can also give healthcare professionals and sufferers a special opportunity to learn from each other. The pros can learn more about the effects of treatment they recommend and a condition's social impact, and the non-pros can learn more about the illness than rushed surgery and hospital visits allow time for. Ideally, both sides can work together to educate society as a whole.

People like us with a chronic disorder may find different groups helpful at different times. Besides the specifically arthritic groups, we might at various times find helpful others focusing perhaps on parenthood, driving, coming off tranquillisers, employment, swimming and other leisure activities. To find out whether any specific group exists, consult reference books or, better still, the College of Health Self-Help Clearing House (send an SAE for information). Or, at the end of the phone: Help for Health (page 121).

The main self-help group for under 45s with arthritis is Young Arthritis Care. It most definitely does *not* go in for regular moan-ins! Nor do its members sit around passively, looking Grateful-with-a-capital-G, while they're given a pat on the head and a cup of tea. Instead, it's an active, lively group, sharing friendship, support, and fun. Members' lurgies include RA, AS, lupus, psoriatic arthritis. (Other self-help groups specialise, eg there's NASS for AS, Lupus UK, the Psoriasis Association, and others mentioned in chapter 3.)

Regardless of its mildness or severity, a younger person with arthritis can feel very isolated. Those of us going through bad patches can benefit tremendously from the support of other members who've been through the bad patches but who know the good times too, and who've seen light at the end of the tunnel. Having the opportunity to talk to and share feelings with fellow YPAs is a wonderful escape valve for something you can't discuss at length with other 'non-arthritic' people, however loving and concerned. Here are the comments of three members in their 20s, the first two are girls, the third a fellow:

"One of the worst things about being young is that one rarely meets anyone in a similar situation and one is therefore very isolated. I do not wish to meet other people like myself in order to sympathise with one another, rather to break the isolation and the feeling that one is somehow inferior to able-bodied friends and to be accepted as a person in my own right."

"The advantage of talking to another 'sufferer' besides sharing helpful tips and experience is you both know there is no need to explain anything and you can be perfectly natural."

"Of the 35 Group [now Young Arthritis Care] *it needs to be said, they are the best people I know. I have changed, just by joining them. Gone is the introverted shy man I once was. In his place strides, with head high, an extrovert, confident and without fears. Not scared to play the fool, if it makes someone else laugh. Not too scared to take responsibility, if it is given to him. Quite simply the 35 Group are fun to be with, they make me happy when I should be sad."*

For me the main benefits have been first, access to masses of information and ideas through the group's magazine *Young Arthritis News* and the newspaper *Arthritis News*, and second, making a special friend like Gwen. We found plenty to talk and laugh about besides RA – boyfriends, French, German, cooking, eating, travelling, etc, – and it was Gwen who inspired me to take up singing and came with me on hilarious singing courses. Gwen too who inspired me to think I might learn to drive one day.

There's more information about ARC, Arthritis Care, and Young Arthritis Care in the alphabetical list of organisations which follows, below. Other self-help/patient support groups are mentioned in chapter 3. Other chapters include yet more helpful organisations!

Selective guide to further sources of help and information
(in alphabetical order; for addresses see Appendix 2)

Access Committee for England
National focal point on access to the built environment. Ask about local groups. For local access guides, see RADAR, page 278.

Age Concern

Charity. Mainly for older people, but some of their information is helpful for anyone, eg *Know Your Medicines* (Pat Blair), *Gardening in Retirement, Heating Help in Retirement.*

Arthritis Care

Charity. Membership open to anyone with any type of arthritis. Doesn't give medical advice, concerned more with social and welfare aspects. Parent body of Young Arthritis Care (see page 123). Over 500 local branches, also specially adapted holiday centres and self-catering units, and a residential home. Has welfare department, the Wyeth phone helpline (page 112) and gives grants for equipment, holidays, etc. Publishes *Arthritis News*, excellent quarterly newspaper packed with information. See also the other publications mentioned on page 113. (One YPA commented: *"Arthritis Care are liberal with information, caring support and have given me a grant to install a gas fire."*)

Arthritis and Rheumatism Council (ARC)

Charity concerned mainly with research, also education. Nationwide network of groups raising funds for research. Membership open to anyone who has or is concerned with arthritis. Publishes *Arthritis Today*, £2 a year for three issues. Excellent buy, containing articles written specially for the layperson – general interest and news about research. Also excellent free handbooks, listed on page 113.

British Red Cross Society

Voluntary organisation, with branches nationwide. Can help solve practical problems, eg transport for housebound people, short-term loan of wheelchairs, commodes, short-term help for someone returning home after an illness or operation. Some branches also visit housebound people, eg to help with foot care, cooking, shopping, changing library books, posting letters, transport for hospital appointments, provision of escorts on journeys. (The St John Ambulance can sometimes help in similar ways, too.) Priced publications include *Home-Made Aids for Handicapped People*, and *People in Wheelchairs – Hints for Helpers.*

Care and Repair

National coordinating body of Home Improvement Agencies, projects which help elderly, disabled, or other low income households to repair, improve and adapt their homes. They employ people to visit and advise people in their own homes, arrange and supervise whatever building work is needed, and help to find and organise the money to pay for it.

Centre for Accessible Environments

Information service for the building professions, rather than the general public, but useful to know about if, say, you wanted to tell your office or local shop where to go for advice on improving access. Publishes journal, *Access by Design.*

Centre for Independent Living

Source of helpful information, run by disabled people. The Hampshire CIL publishes *Source Book Toward Independent Living*, to help people assess their needs for care support and then approach agencies for the money to pay for it. Another helpful body is the Community Service Volunteers' Independent Living Scheme, which provides volunteers to enable disabled people to live and study independently in their homes. See also *Recruiting a Personal Care Worker*, under Disablement Income Group, (page 121).

Citizens' Advice Bureau (CAB)

Voluntary organisation, with over 900 local branches. Long-established and very helpful.

No appointment needed. Most staff are volunteers, but all are trained. Can advise on benefits, housing problems, local voluntary organisations, legal or financial problems, etc. Can help you deal with difficult bureaucrats and phone calls, filling in forms, drafting important letters, and obtaining specialist advice. Can sometimes arrange home advisory visit if you're housebound.

College of Health

Non-profit-making body, set up in 1983 by Michael Young, founder of the Consumers' Association and Open University. Gives information on keeping healthy, on self-care in minor illness, on making the best use of the NHS, and sources of help outside the NHS, such as self-help groups and alternative medicine. Runs *Healthline*, confidential telephone information service (081 681 3311 between 4pm and 8pm any weekday) which gives detailed, *tape-recorded* information about medical and health problems, written by medical experts. An operator takes your call and plays the tape you want. The only charge is the cost of the call. A directory's available, listing all the topics, which include:

- *Arthritis: What it is and How it is Treated*
- *Hip-Replacement Operation*
- *Rheumatism: What it is and How it is Treated*
- *Rheumatoid Arthritis: What it is and How it is Treated*
- *Ankylosing Spondylitis*
- *Adaptations to Your Home for the Disabled*
- *Changing Your GP*
- *Sex and Contraception after Childbirth*
- *Masturbation*

There's also a helpline giving information on hospital waiting list lengths (see page 56). Write for a full list of the College's clearly written, low-cost publications, eg:

Guide to Alternative Medicine
Guide to Going into Hospital
Guide to Hip-Replacement Operation
Guide to Hospital Waiting Lists (England and Wales)
Consumers' Guide to Health Information

Community Health Council (CHC)

(Look in phone directory under 'Community' for the address of your local CHC, or get it from the Association of Community Health Councils for England and Wales)
Aims to be the consumer's voice in the NHS. Local CHCs consist of members of the public representing various voluntary and statutory bodies. They provide information on local health services, and advise patients on rights and complaints, etc.

Consumers' Association

Independent non-profit-making body, offering consumer advice and information to members. Publishes the newsy quarterly magazine *Which? Way to Health*, and the monthly *Which?* magazine – good for shopping around from your armchair (or public library chair): you can study information about products and services before buying. The CA also publishes clearly written treasure troves of information, eg:

- *Living with Stress*
- *The Which? Encyclopaedia of the Home*
- *Divorce: Legal Procedures and Financial Facts*
- *Earning Money at Home*
- *Starting your own Business*
- *Which Subject? Which Career?*
- *Making the Most of Higher Education*

Councillors
(Find out names and phone numbers from your local town hall, library or CAB)
Part-time, locally elected representatives on Parish/Community Councils, County or District or Borough Councils. If you're having problems with your local authority see if your councillor can help. They know how the council works and have useful contacts. Most councillors hold regular 'surgeries' where you can ask for a personal interview.

One YPA was elected as one of two Labour Councillors for a ward of Thanet District Council. She wrote in *In Contact*:

"How did I cope? Well my knees hurt like...much of the time, but our local pharmacist is a great guy and advised me on which pain killers I could take over a long period. Thanks to him I managed about four hours on the doorsteps every day, although the inflammation in the joints was almost constant...

"I hope to specialise in planning, and I have already made the Chief Executive – who I have known for some years because of my agent's work – look carefully at access for disabled people. He has now come to understand that disabled people should use the same doors as the rest of the public – not be pushed 'round the back'. He has been pushing wheelchairs and is coming to understand the problems."

Department of Health (DoH) and Department of Social Security (DSS)
(Look in your phone book under 'Health, Department of', or 'Social Security, Department of' for your local office, or under 'Health and Social Security, Department of'.)
Until 1988 these were both combined in the DHSS. The DoH now deals with the NHS, personal social services (including child care services), primary and community care, pharmaceutical issues, preventive health care, mental health, and hospital services.

The DSS deals with social security matters, state benefits, National Insurance contributions, occupational and personal pensions, and disability issues. There are free phone helplines giving general information on benefits: see page 127. For information on some DSS publications see page 128, and for more about benefits, see chapter 17. Look too at chapter 18 for tips on dealing with bureaucrats, and remember that people in your local CAB or DIAL can help you find your way through what can be a difficult system.

DIAL Groups (Disablement Information & Advice Lines)
(For your nearest DIAL Group, look in the phone book, or contact DIAL UK.)
Independent local advisory and information services run by people with direct experience of disability (eg former OT student and YPA Sue now works for her local DIAL). Free, impartial and confidential. Write, phone, or visit. Some groups offer counselling as well as practical and personal help. Questions covered include, for instance, local welfare services, access and mobility, education, aids and equipment, income and benefits, accommodation, personal care, personal relationships, sexual problems. They can also help you deal with officialdom, eg can help with form filling, accompany you to a tribunal.

Disability Alliance
Set up in 1974, national federation of over 90 organisations of and for people with disabilities. Campaigns for a comprehensive income scheme and aims to promote a wider understanding of the needs and views of people with disabilities, especially their living standards. Runs a welfare rights information service but has only two workers, so they ask you to use them only as a *last* resort (letter, with SAE, or by phone, afternoons only). Most questions are probably already covered by their excellent, regularly updated and low-cost *Disability Rights Handbook* (see page 127). Local CABs and Arthritis Care Contacts have copies.

Disabled Living Foundation (DLF) (see also page 144)
Registered charity. Information service for disabled people and professionals, and an 'aids for disabled living' centre. Will answer enquiries about specific problems (except anything purely medical). Can give up-to-date information about manufacturers, stockists and prices of many gadgets. Write, with stamp, for their list of really excellent information sheets and publications, which include those on page 171, and *Coping with Disability* by Peggy Jay, handbook of practical advice and information. Every library should have a copy.

As I write, there are plans to merge the DLF and RADAR, to form a new organisation that may be called the Royal Disability Association.

Disablement Income Group
Registered charity with local branches. Aims to improve the financial situation of disabled people. Runs an advisory service, does research and produces publications, which include *Compass: the Direction Finder for Disabled People* (money matters, aids, equipment and services, plus referral agencies covering everything from arts to writing, angling to wheelchair dancing), and *Recruiting a Personal Care Worker* (helpful advice on rates of pay, conditions of service, tax and national insurance, drawing up a job description, placing an advert, and interviewing applicants).

Family Planning Association
Don't be put off by the name – their books mail order catalogue *Healthwise* isn't just about family planning but a very good introduction to books on personal relations and physical and emotional health generally, as well as sex and sexuality.

Health Information Network
Publishes over 500 health booklets, for laypeople, written and edited by leading specialists and professors. Send an SAE for the list. Cost of each booklet in 1991: £2.95 inc p&p.

Health Information Service
Funded by Hertfordshire Library Service, North Herts NHS Trust, NWTRHA and charity. A local service but can also give information (phone, letter or personal enquiry) to people outside the area. Specialises in providing up-to-date and reliable health information for the layperson, in ordinary language.

Help for Health
Funded by the Wessex Regional Health Authority. Answers enquiries from health professionals and the public. Specialises in information on self-help groups (several thousand!). Also produces factsheets on different illnesses and disabilities and a series of bibliographies (including one on works of fiction and biography with a medical content).

Legal advice (See also Network for the Handicapped, on the next page)
Many Citizens' Advice Bureaux (page 118) have Honorary Legal Advisers – solicitors or barristers – who can give free advice. In larger cities *Law Centres* offer help with legal problems (addresses from local library, CAB, or Law Centres Federation). Staff are qualified lawyers, who can help you obtain legal aid (if you're not eligible for legal aid their services are free).

Legal Advice Centres give free legal advice. Usually run on a part-time basis by groups of lawyers, with restricted opening hours, and usually offer only limited assistance, eg writing letters, contacting other agencies, referring a case to a firm of solicitors.

Many *solicitors* operate the 'Fixed Fee Advice Scheme', where you can go to a solicitor's office and receive half-an-hour's legal advice for £5 maximum. The Law Society publishes a booklet called 'The Legal Aid Referral List' (LAR), which lists solicitors' names, addresses, and specialisations (eg family, accident) by area, or CABs have their own list of local solicitors.

Medical Advisory Service (MAS) (see also page 39)
Charity. Runs phone helpline, staffed by nurses, providing non-diagnostic medical advice.

MPs and voting
Our elected representatives in Parliament — there to work for us! You can write to your MP at the House of Commons. If you want to find out who s/he is, phone and ask for the Information Service. MPs have local 'surgeries' where constituents can see them about problems. As their time's limited, sort out what you want to say before writing or meeting your MP. Keep it short, to the point, and polite too, even if you're angry.

It's worth writing about anything you feel strongly about, especially health, arthritis, and disability issues — keep reminding MPs of *our* needs and existence. Write to the Prime Minister, too, at 10 Downing Street, London SW1. It all helps, and you usually get some sort of answer even if it's not the one you wanted.

There's an All Party Disablement Group, a group of MPs and peers who take a special interest in disability issues. Several MPs specialise in health and disability matters, eg Labour MPs Alf Morris, and Jo Richardson. Jo Richardson MP has had RA for nearly 30 years. In Michael Leitch's *Living with Arthritis* (Lennard/Collins) she talks about herself:

"My constituents know about my arthritis and they have always been sympathetic. Nobody has ever said, 'You shouldn't be doing this'. They just pile more work on me. Perhaps some people find it easier to relate to me because I have a disability. 'You've got your problems', they say, then pour out their own.

"My friends in the House of Commons give me help and support. They will pick up a bag for me without being asked, that kind of thing. There is one set of interview rooms in the House which has very difficult door handles: you have to twist them. I can't manage that so I have to ask someone to do it for me..."

Former Labour MP Jack Ashley did a considerable amount for disabled people. The impact of his acquired disability (total deafness) on himself, on his actions and on his family makes his autobiography particularly fascinating reading.

If you can't get out to vote, get a postal vote. Apply, at any time, to the electoral registration officer at your local town hall. The leaflet *Don't Lose Your Vote* (by post from the Home Office) explains what to do.

Network for the Handicapped
Formed in 1975, a free expert legal advice service for disabled people and their families, specialising in benefits, education and employment. Can help with tackling discrimination, for instance by an employer, and, with sufficient notice, free representation on tribunals. Does not cover divorce, conveyancing, criminal cases or large personal injury claims.

Patients' Association
Helps and advises patients, and publicises the patient's viewpoint. Publishes a newsletter *Patient Voice*, information leaflets, and a self-help directory. With the Consumers' Association they've published *A Patient's Guide to the National Health Service*.

PHAB (Physically Handicapped/Able Bodied)
(For the address of your nearest group, contact PHAB headquarters)
Aims for membership of equal numbers of physically handicapped and able bodied young people, for leisure activities and holidays.

Post Offices
Source of useful leaflets on DSS benefits, on free and 'season ticket' prescriptions, etc. Open a post office account for cash flow convenience when there's no bank nearby.

RADAR (Royal Association for Disability and Rehabilitation)
Important source of information on access, education, holidays, housing, mobility, employment, etc. Coordinating body of nearly 400 member organisations including Arthritis Care. Campaigns for the recognition of the needs and rights of disabled people.

Publishes a regular Bulletin (a few pounds a year) with news on legislation, employment, mobility, conferences, exhibitions, etc. Also free booklet for newly disabled people *If Only I'd Known That a Year Ago...* Send large SAE for publications list, full of enticing low-cost bits and bobs, eg access publications covering theatres, cinemas, nature reserves, London underground stations, public conveniences, cities and towns. (Many towns and cities also have their own Access Guide, available from the local Council office.)

As I write, there are plans to merge RADAR and the DLF, to form a new organisation that may be called the Royal Disability Association.

Religious bodies/churches
Many people find a lot of emotional, social and practical support through religion and from local churches.

Samaritans
(In your phone book under 'Samaritans', or phone Central London Branch, 071 734 2800)
The Samaritans' 24-hour telephone helpline is best known for providing a confidential ear for suicidal people, but they're also there to help *anyone* who's especially miserable, not only people who are suicidal. The Samaritans' international name explains their work best: 'Befrienders International'. In 1987 they answered 2¼ million calls.

Social Services: see page 143.

SPOD (Association to Aid the Sexual and Personal Relationships of People with a Disability) Gives factual help, information, leaflets to written enquiries, and there's a phone counsellor. SPOD can refer you for local advice and counselling too. (See page 225)

Young Arthritis Care (see also page 117)
Nationwide group (formerly the 35 Group) of young people (under 45) with arthritis and their friends. Parent body is Arthritis Care. Concerned mainly with social and welfare aspects (including holidays); doesn't give medical advice. Contacts (YPAs themselves) run local groups and are available just for a chat or if you need advice or help of some sort. Some work, others have families to look after. Some arrange get-togethers, eg with a speaker, or social evenings, or swimming sessions. Joining is an excellent way of finding out how to cope with arthritis, and can also help break feelings of isolation. Particularly helpful, too, are the Group's Personal Development Courses (open to non-members too), which include health and welfare advice, confidence skills, and educational, employment and careers development advice. Membership is cheap and entitles you to receive *Young Arthritis News* plus the quarterly newspaper *Arthritis News*, both splendid.

Other Voluntary Services
Women's Royal Voluntary Service (WRVS) has about 1500 branches nationwide, providing social help to elderly and disabled people (eg 'escort' services for disabled people, meals on wheels). Other groups who can help in various ways include the scout and guide movements, Voluntary Bureaux, Lions, Rotary Club, Round Table.

Chapter sixteen

AM I A DISABLED PERSON? – OR NOT?
Some thoughts and definitions

Some thoughts

Talking about disability may make some of you cringe and say 'that's not me'. Disability often conjures up the image of a severely disabled person, possibly in a wheelchair, and with a physically static condition, unlike many of us.

Sometimes we may feel, and be, very disabled; sometimes quite the opposite. Chronic arthritis is a see-saw experience, and many of us with largely invisible arthritis don't fit tidily in either the 'disabled-bods' camp' or the 'ablebods' camp'. If I'm having a 'good' day, or if my problems are invisible, then people with a very visible disability or a benefits assessment officer may deem me a fraud if I claim to be a disabled person. However, on a 'bad' day I'd be disbelieved if I claimed to be anything but! Sociologist Carolyn Wiener (see page 90) described the various ways we may deal with the dilemma.

Would that we were all regarded as being in one camp, a camp of human beings, but back to reality. Why shouldn't we, instead of considering it a dilemma, turn it to our advantage? The arthritis may sometimes dictate which camp's label is most appropriate at any particular time, but we can also to some extent choose which to wear when. Why shouldn't we choose whichever is most advantageous at a particular time? Even better, let's, at the same time, educate society into understanding that there is such a thing as 'partial disability', 'an intermittent disability', 'a variable disability'.

Let's also educate society into understanding another crucial characteristic of a chronic inflammatory arthritis, a difference often misunderstood, especially by officialdom, ie the handicap or disadvantage we may experience resulting from 'the interaction of different disabilities', clearly described in a WHO report (see page 194).

Back to existing labels. Why bother with the disabled label if you don't feel disabled? Well, for better or worse, it's a form of shorthand for 'someone with special needs', widely used by doctors, social workers, employers, etc, and from time to time, whether we like it or not, each of us will find the label applied. We do have special needs, eg functional problems, mobility, employment, finance problems to be overcome. It does at times help, when, for instance I ask for a special seat in the theatre, or apply for help with adaptations. There's also the 'stand-up-and-be-counted' advantage, when using the label means we can exert influence by the power of numbers.

Sometimes, swallowing an aversion to the disabled label can paradoxically even help to *lessen* a disability. – For instance, it's well worth looking at gadgets 'for disabled people', or special arrangements 'for disabled people' in holiday guides (eg ground floor bedroom in a hotel, or special arrangements at the airport). That 'disability' information may actually be all you need to make you 'non-disabled' again.

Problems come if the label's misused by other people, eg the *Does He Take Sugar?* attitude, for instance, where the disabled person is disregarded, a 'non-person', or when people talk about 'the disabled' as if we're all alike, and as if our most important characteristic is lack of ability, instead of all being very different people each with different talents and characteristics. Talking about 'the disabled' all too easily leads people into the trap of underestimating any disabled individual's capabilities, eg in education or employment, thus imposing artifical restrictions and additional handicaps where there need be none. For instance a Careers Adviser may assume that certain openings aren't worth mentioning to disabled clients (eg desktop publishing to someone like me with grotty-looking fingers), thus denying them financial, social and personal opportunities and benefits, with knock-on effects in other areas of life.

In *The Experience of Handicap* (Methuen) David Thomas says:

"To become disabled is to be given a new identity, to receive a passport indicating membership of a separate tribe. To be born handicapped is to have this identity assigned from the moment of discovery and diagnosis. Both involve a social learning process in which the nuances and meanings of the identity are assimilated. Those who become handicapped in adult life have to cope not only with the practical implications of impairment, but also with a host of behavioural-attitudinal adjustments."

Imposing language! But it's a crucial aspect of what chronic arthritis may mean. The practical implications of arthritis mean that in some ways I'm like a wooden doll, with disability caused by functional problems of reaching, bending, gripping, moving, walking, but the crucial difference between me and a wooden doll is that I'm a *living* doll, who experiences pain and aches, fatigue and stiffness, frustration and anger and depression, not only because of the arthritis itself, but also because of other people's misunderstandings, and reactions to it.

If you want to explore in more detail the sociology and psychology of disability, the DLF publishes a reading list. Susan Lonsdale's *Women and Disability* (Macmillan, 1990) examines the effect of physical disability on women in a social and political context. Other chapters of this book go into more detail about the emotional aspects of arthritis and disability and other people. Let's concentrate now on practical aspects.

Definitions

The words impairment, disability and handicap are generally used very loosely. The World Health Organisation has produced definitions which are slowly being adopted by professionals. To paraphrase these:
-   Impairment refers to having a body part or body function which doesn't work properly or is missing because of disease or injury.
-   Disability is the resulting lack of function.
-   Handicap refers to the limitations on daily activity that result from the disability.

All of us with arthritis have an impairment, but the extent to which it disables us varies considerably. Hip and foot problems most disable me; I'm not handicapped by them at home, where everything's the right height, etc, for me, but I can be considerably handicapped elsewhere, for instance if I'm in a room where all the seats are too low, or if I come across steps that are too high. Someone who needs glasses for reading has a disability too, but is only handicapped if s/he has no glasses.

Though someone with RA may not be noticeably disabled by it, they may often be handicapped by factors outside their control, for instance rigid working hours from 9 to 5 may prevent someone holding down a job, whereas flexitime might allow them to work at times when the RA is at its most manageable. The worst handicaps are caused by other people's attitudes and thoughtlessness, by non-disabled people parking in designated areas, by unthinking architects and planners, by inflexible rules and regulations. 'I have a disability, but they are my handicap.'

Registering as 'disabled'

There are two different registers, one kept by the local Social Services Department, and the other, the *Disabled Persons' Register,* kept by the government's national Employment Service. Registration on either (or both) is voluntary, though medical evidence of your eligibility is required.

1 The Social Services Department Register   The qualification for being put on the Register is a 'substantial and permanent disability'. Registration can be an advantage because you may get help and information about special provisions more easily. Though you don't *have* to be registered to get help, the Register is also an administrative tool which helps the local authority plan its budgeting and facilities for disabled people, so your registration benefits other disabled people too. Some authorities give you a registration card, others don't.

2 The Disabled Persons' Register   Kept by the Employment Service, the Register relates specifically to employment. This is the Register which gives you the famous 'green card'. Apply through your local jobcentre. (Ask for leaflet PWD 5, or send a second-class stamp to RADAR for one by post). To be put on the Register you have to be:

   "a person who, on account of injury, disease or congenital deformity is substantially handicapped in obtaining or keeping employment, or in undertaking work on his own account of a kind which apart from that injury, disease or deformity would be suited to his age, experience and qualification."

You have to be likely to remain disabled for at least 12 months, and be actively looking for and have some prospect of getting work, or already be in work. Registration (renewable) may be granted for any period from one year to 10 years or until retirement.

   Employers with more than 20 employees are supposed to have at least 3% registered disabled employees (the 'Quota', currently under review). Some special Employment Service help is reserved for people on the Register. More about employment generally in Chapter 31.

Chapter seventeen

FINANCE AND BENEFITS

Without committing yourself at all you can find out what's available by:

- phoning BEL, the free Benefits Enquiry Line on 0800 882200 (weekdays between 9am and 4.30pm), specially for people asking about disability-related allowances, including people seeking advice on filling out forms. You don't have to give your name, and the telephone adviser won't have access to your papers, but it's an excellent way of arming yourself with all the background information you need before going into specifics with your local social security office. For general, non-disabled information on benefits, phone free on 0800 666555 (0800 616757 in Northern Ireland).
- contacting your local Citizens' Advice Bureau (CAB, see page 118). A home visit can be arranged if you're housebound.
- contacting the Wyeth Helpline, at Arthritis Care, free on 0800 289170 (see page 112).
- sending by post for relevant Social Security leaflets (free from DSS Leaflets Unit). Two for starters are *Which Benefit? (FB2)* and *Sick or Disabled? (FB28)*.

Disability Alliance produces the low-cost *Disability Rights Handbook* (1992 £6.95, inc p&p), updated each year, a detailed guide to rights, benefits and services for all people with disabilities and their families. It tells you who to approach and how best to do it, takes you through all the benefits available, and explains the bewildering array of rules and procedures and exceptions applying to claims and appeals against decisions. It's good, but wordy, and does take some ploughing through! Advice workers, eg at the CAB, Arthritis Care, and other support groups have copies and can give you guidance on what it says, or you could get your own direct from the Disability Alliance.

Benefits and services are changing considerably as I write, and some of what I say may have altered by the time you read it. For up-to-date information see the latest update of the *Disability Rights Handbook* and/or contact the phone numbers and bodies I've mentioned.

General information and definitions

Some benefits are means-tested; some aren't. For means-tested benefits you have to give details of your income, circumstances, and any savings. Some benefits are available whether or not you've paid National Insurance contributions; others relate to any NI contributions you have made. You'd lose out on something like Invalidity Benefit, for instance, unless you'd paid sufficient NI contributions linked to paid employment with earnings over the 'lower earnings limit'. You's apply instead for SDA (see page 129).

Where to go

You apply for most benefits through your local office of the Social Security Benefits Agency (SSBA, formerly part of the Department of Social Security), where you can also make general benefits enquiries, and get SSBA/DSS leaflets. What your local office is called may be changing or may already have changed. For instance unemployment benefit offices are merging with jobcentres and will simply be called 'jobcentres', but with Claimant Advisers to advise on benefits. The best thing is to phone BEL, free, if you're not sure what office to contact. Here I'll use the abbreviation SSO (social security office), as a general term.

Don't delay, and get advice

Don't let apparently complicated forms or procedures put you off applying for a benefit. If you're not sure whether or not you qualify, apply anyway. Don't delay, because back-dated payments may not be allowed, or may be restricted by time limits. Bear in mind that for disabled people regulations which apply to non-disabled people may not be relevant, and exceptions may sometimes be made in your favour. Always keep a dated copy of any correspondence and a dated note of any phone call or meeting with an official. Look too at my notes in chapter 18 on dealing with bureaucracy.

Going about a claim in the right way can make all the difference. So does knowing how to appeal against a decision, and the time limits within which the appeal must be lodged. Get help from an independent and experienced adviser, eg social worker, CAB, Arthritis Care Officer, or Young Arthritis Care Contact. The *Disability Rights Handbook* is helpful too, and includes other sources of help (eg local law centres, Tribunal Assistance Units, Welfare Rights Officers). Many people are awarded a benefit after an appeal even though they were turned down when they first applied. If you're turned down once, don't let that put you off trying again if your circumstances change.

Assessments

For some benefits you may be asked to have a medical assessment. Most of us spend our lives putting a brave face on things, grimacing inwardly while telling the world that the pain's not too bad. You need to do the *opposite* when being assessed. Don't lie, but tell the truth, from the pessimist's, not the optimist's point of view. Stress how much it hurts and if pain starts right away, say so. Stress how much you *can't* do (but don't overdo it!). An optimist describes a glass as being 'half full'; a pessimist says it's 'half empty' – both statements are true, but benefits are decided on the evidence produced by the pessimist, not the optimist.

With a variable condition like RA, it sometimes helps, too, to keep a diary, from which your assessor can balance up the good spells and the bad, and come to a decision about your 'average' condition. Look too at my comments on page 194 on the problem of 'how to explain its oddities'. When preparing for an assessment, take advice from someone with experience of what's likely to happen, someone like a CAB Adviser, Arthritis Care officer, or Young Arthritis Care Contact. It may help, too, if you can provide for the assessor a statement about your disorder from your rheumatologist, since non-specialists so often misunderstand rheumatic disorders. See what your rheumatologist thinks.

Initial applications for the Disability Living Allowance (DLA), and the Disability Working Allowance (DWA), are now based on self-assessment, though you may still be able to choose to have a medical examination if you think that would be more in your favour. An adjudication officer decides your claim based on the self-assessment form which you complete, but the same principles apply as for a medical assessment: complete the form wearing your pessimist's rather than your optimist's hat, get advice from a CAB or self-help group adviser (eg Arthritis Care, NASS), and include a supporting letter from your GP or rheumatologist if s/he agrees.

See my notes on page 137 about completing forms. You can get help with the DLA form either from the helpline number given on the form, or from a CAB Adviser. Take care over drafting your answers, and be sure to read your draft(s) through pretending to be the adjudication officer (AO). – Does the completed form tell you, the AO, all you need to know? Does the claim convince the AO of the applicant's eligibility or raise doubts?

Going into hospital, studying, and doing paid work may all affect your benefits. You'll find more information on pages 57, 132, 133, and in the *Disability Rights Handbook*.

Proving incapacity for work

For some benefits the applicant's 'incapacity' for work may have to be assessed, by an adjudicating medical practitioner (AMP), eg for Invalidity Benefit or Severe Disablement Allowance. The *Disability Rights Handbook* goes into detail.

An intermittent disability like a rheumatic disorder can sometimes make proving 'incapacity' more difficult than a static disability. The assessment shouldn't just depend on your condition on the day or time of day you're examined. If your condition varies, the AMP should work out an average assessment taking into account your 'good' and 'bad' spells. Keeping a diary beforehand may help, and you could consider mentioning a Social Security Commissioners' ruling (R(S)9/79) on intermittent disability::

> *'A person who because of intermittent disablement, could perform the duties of a paid employment only on an average of, say, three days out of a five day working week...could rightly be held to be continuously incapable of work...'*

If you can't predict the days when you'd be fit for work, an employer might not want to risk taking you on – even for a part-time job. Part-time or full-time jobs

> *'that a claimant would be capable of doing only irregularly or unpredictably should be left out of account – CS/19/87.'* (Quoted in the 16th *Disability Rights Handbook*)

You might also be deemed 'incapable' of work, even though you're not, if:

- – you're under medical care for a disease or disability
- – and a doctor certifies that you shouldn't work *'for precautionary or convalescent reasons consequential on such disease or disablement'*
- – and you don't work.

However, even if you're deemed as 'incapable' of work, you might be allowed to do a little light work if your doctor considers it 'therapeutic' (see page 133) and of benefit to your health, *provided* you seek approval *beforehand* from your local social security office, and provided you earn less than a certain amount a week. If you do more work, even part-time, your benefit might be stopped on the grounds that you're considered fit for work.

Some of the basic benefits

Statutory Sick Pay (NI 244)
Most employed people (including women paying NI contributions at a reduced rate) receive SSP automatically from their employer for up to 28 weeks in a spell of sickness lasting more than four days in a row. If you don't get SSP you can claim Sickness Benefit. SSP relates to NI contributions and to your average weekly earnings.

Sickness Benefit (NI 16)
Payable for up to 28 weeks, after a spell of sickness lasting more than four days in a row, to people who are self-employed or unemployed, or employed but not receiving SSP. It's not payable to married women paying reduced NI contributions unless they're claiming because of an accident at work or an industrial disease. Relates to NI contributions. Not means-tested. Get a claim form from your employer (form SSP1) or form SC1 from your Social Security office or doctor.

Invalidity Benefit (IB) (NI 16A)
People who are still incapable of work after 28 weeks SSP or Sickness Benefit can claim, but only if they've made sufficient NI contributions. People in low-paid work may not have done so, and would therefore fail to qualify. See the section on page 128 about assessments and proving incapacity for work. If your incapacity starts before you reach 55 (women) or 60 (men) you can claim Invalidity Allowance as well. Not means-tested.

Severe Disablement Allowance (SDA) (NI 252)
People aged 16 or over and who are incapable of work for 28 weeks or more, but can't get Sickness Benefit or Invalidity Benefit because of too few NI contributions may be able to

claim SDA, depending on their age and extent of disability. You have to prove that you're at least 75% to 80% disabled and have been so for 28 weeks. If you receive DLA mobility and/or care component you'll be automatically 'passported' on to SDA provided you meet all other criteria. SDA's tax-free and not means-tested.

See my notes on page 128 on assessments and on proving incapacity for work.

Invalidity Care Allowance (ICA) (NI 212)
Payable to people of working age if they have to spend at least 35 hours a week looking after someone who gets the higher or middle rate DLA care component, but not the lowest. Doesn't relate to NI contributions, although for each week of ICA, the recipient gets an NI Class I credit, important if at any time s/he needs to claim another benefit. ICA is taxable. Claim the allowance through your SSO.

Disability Living Allowance (DLA) (NI 205)
From April 1992 this replaces the old Attendance Allowance and Mobility Allowance. (AA is still payable to people over 65.) DLA consists of a 'care component' payable at one of three different rates, and a 'mobility component' payable at one of two different rates. DLA's tax-free, and doesn't depend on NI contributions. Your first application for DLA is based on self-assessment rather than medical assessment (though you can choose a medical if you think that would be more in your favour). See my notes on self-assessment on page 128. Subsequent decisions are usually made by a special review procedure or Disability Appeal Tribunal, which must include at least one person with a disability.

Details and procedures for DLA are still being finalised as I write, so get the latest information from the sources I mention on page 127. Claim DLA through your SSO.

- *Care component* If you need considerable practical help from another person because of severe disability, you may be able to claim one of the two higher rates, even if there isn't anyone actually to give you that practical help; what counts is your *need* for such help, not whether there's anyone there to give it to you. Which rate you're eligible for depends on whether you need this help all day or all night, or both. The lowest rate may be claimed if because of your disability you (1) require, in connection with your bodily functions, attention from another person for a significant portion of the day (whether during a single period or for a number of periods – the *Disability Rights Handbook* 1991/92 (16th edition) reckoned that a 'significant portion' would be roughly 40 minutes or more), or (2) can't prepare a main meal for yourself even if you have the ingredients (or can't perform a similar task). If you're trying to claim this, you might find helpful the quotation on 'interaction of disabilities' on page 194.
- *Mobility component* Replaces the old Mobility Allowance, and is for people between 5 and 65, who are unable or virtually unable to walk. See page 187 for more details.

Income Support (IS) (SB 20 and SB 1)
Payable to help people aged 16 or over who don't have enough money to live on. It's means-tested. You can't normally get IS if you or your partner (married or unmarried) work more than 24 hours a week, or if you have savings of over a certain amount. The '24 + hours rule' might be disregarded if, because of your disability, your 'earning capacity' is cut to 75% or less of what you would, but for that disability, be reasonably expected to earn.

You might qualify even if you get other benefits, or earnings from part-time work. It's means-tested and relates to your age, but not to NI contributions. In addition to IS you may also qualify for one or more 'premium payments' if you have 'special needs' (eg because of disability, children). You may also qualify for Housing Benefit and certain other accommodation costs not met by Housing Benefit. If you receive IS you also qualify for free NHS prescriptions and NHS dental treatment.

Housing Benefit (HB) (RR 1)

People on low incomes can claim HB for help in paying rent and/or the community charge ('poll tax'). You may qualify whether or not you are working full- or part-time, and whether or not you receive Income Support. It's means-tested, and not payable to people with savings over a certain amount. Not linked to NI contributions.

Social Fund (SB 16)

This is to help people with exceptional expenses they can't meet from their ordinary income. Some payments are made as grants, which don't have to be paid back; others are interest-free loans, repayable over a period relating to your income and circumstances.

The first three payments listed below are at the discretion of Social Fund Officers (SFOs). SFOs have to keep all payments within the local office budget, so the success of your claim may depend as much on *when* you apply (eg early in the Financial Year) as on *why* you're applying. If you're refused a discretionary payment, you can ask for a review, but you have to do this in writing within 28 days of the date the decision was given or posted to you.

- *Community Care Grants* Not repayable, so preferable to a loan. They're to help people, usually already on IS, and in certain priority groups, eg elderly or disabled or chronically sick people, lead independent lives in the community. Grants may be made for items such as furniture, removal costs and house repairs. If you have savings over a certain amount (yours or your partner's) you must put those towards your needs. Claim through your SSO on form SF 300. If your application's refused, and you think you've got a good case, it's worth asking for a review. One YPA (writing in *Arthritis News*) received a very expensive estimate for crucial repairs/replacements in her bathroom, and was turned down at first for a grant. But she persisted, and eventually got not only the maximum permissible grant, but more!

- *Budgeting Loans* Repayable interest-free loans. If you've been getting Income Support for at least 26 weeks, this may help you spread a payment for essential exceptional expenses (eg for a cooker, other furniture, repairs). Any savings over a certain amount (yours or your partner's) are taken into account. In 1991 the smallest loan made was £30, the highest £1,000. Claim through your SSO on form SF 300.

- *Crisis Loans* Repayable interest-free loans. You don't have to be already getting a benefit such as IS to qualify. They're for people unable to meet short-term expenses in an emergency, or following a disaster, where there's serious risk to the health and safety of a family, and may be made for instance to cover living expenses for up to 14 days, or essential household equipment or travel costs. Apply through your SSO on form SF 400.

The following three payments are legal entitlements for people on low income:

- *Maternity Payments(FB 8)*
- *Funeral Payments(FB 29)*
- *Cold Weather Payments*.

Family Credit (NI 261)

Means-tested benefit for families on low wages who have children. You or your partner must normally be working for 24 or more hours a week, and mustn't have savings or capital of more than a certain amount. Claim through your SSO using form FC1.

Child Benefit (CH 1)

Tax-free benefit for each dependent child. Not means-tested.

The Independent Living Fund (ILF)

Charity set up by the Department of Social Security in cooperation with the Disablement Income Group to make payments from a government-funded trust fund. Due to close in 1993. Its purpose is to 'provide help to some severely disabled people who need domestic support if they are to live in their own homes. The aim [is] to prevent such people having to enter residential care if they cannot afford the support; and to enable people in residential care, who are capable of living independently, to do so'. Funds are limited, and the qualifying criteria strict, but to people who qualify, the ILF will normally help pay the actual weekly cost of domestic help/personal care, however much it is. For more information write to the Independent Living Fund. For more information on help with independent living generally see 'Centre for Independent Living' on page 118.

Maternity payments

See DSS leaflet *Babies and Benefits* (FB8). The Maternity Alliance can help with queries on benefits and practical support from the social services and health services. For rights at work during pregnancy, maternity pay and return to work after maternity leave, see *Employment Rights for the Expectant Mother* (PL710, free from jobcentres and some advice centres).

Help through your local social services department

Look at chapter 20 for help available, and for notes on other ways of getting special gadgets and equipment free or at reduced cost, including how to get VAT relief on certain items.

Studying and financial support

Whether or not benefits such as Income Support or Unemployment Benefit can be paid to you while you're on a course depends on your age, on whether the course is full or part-time, and if part-time, for how many hours; on your disability and its effect on your ability to work; and on whether you're required to sign on as available for work in order to qualify for benefit. Seek advice; it's complicated! *The Disability Rights Handbook* explains the various rules, including benefits and government training opportunities and allowances for adults.

Be careful; if you receive a benefit because of 'incapacity to work', taking a course might raise questions about your 'incapacity', so find out *beforehand* what your position is. Whether you're considered 'incapable' depends on all sorts of things (see my notes on pages 128/9). The *Disability Rights Handbook* gives helpful tips and the Social Security Commissioners' ruling about 'intermittent disability', quoted on page 129, is useful for someone with inflammatory arthritis to be aware of and perhaps quote, if necessary.

Over 19, although IS isn't usually paid to students, you might qualify as an exception if you're disabled. If you're 19 or older and required to sign on as available for work, you can usually do a part-time course without problems provided it doesn't last for more than 21 hours a week (excluding private study, lunch breaks and travelling), but do check first.

Some benefits relate to NI contributions. You pay contributions if you're working, but they can also be 'credited' in certain other circumstances. If you're studying, you might qualify for credited contributions, depending on the type and length of course. Don't miss out on being credited if you can help it; the credits may make a difference to entitlements later. Some courses count for automatic NI credits, for others you have to apply specially. Check with BEL (page 127), the Social Security Benefits Agency, CAB or other independent adviser. For more information about finance, grants, etc, relating to studying, look at chapter 30.

Employment and benefits

The Disablement Resettlement Officer (DRO) and other jobcentre staff can advise on employment services generally, and those specially for people with a disability. See chapter 31, eg page 258, for more information. How benefits, employment and disorders like RA affect one other is a horribly complicated area. For detailed up-to-date information, contact the bodies on page 127.

Some benefits (eg DLA mobility component) are payable whether you're in work or not, some are paid only if you're deemed 'incapable of work'. Other rules apply if your doctor says you'd normally not be able to work, but recommends a few hours for 'therapeutic' reasons. If you *can* work a little, but what you can earn is limited because of your rheumatic disorder, then you might be interested in the Disability Working Allowance (DWA), described below, or the Sheltered Placement Scheme (see page 253).

Take advice on how your benefits might be affected if you try to find work. You could lose Income Support, the right to free prescriptions, dental and optical treatment, help from the social fund, and help with fares to hospital. If your mortgage interest is met by IS you could lose that, and the Building Society might ask you to make full capital and interest payments. In some low-paid work you might not pay National Insurance contributions and would then have no entitlement to Invalidity Benefit if you were later off work ill for a long time. Seek expert advice, and weigh up all the pros and cons.

- *Disability Working Allowance* may be paid to people on low wages aged 16 or over who work at least 16 hours a week as employees or are self-employed, who have recently been getting a qualifying benefit, are considered to be at a 'disadvantage in getting a job', have limited savings, and who pass the DWA means test. The amount of benefit paid decreases the more you earn, and stops completely above a certain limit.

- *The 'therapeutic earnings rule'* applies to people who've been unemployed for a while because of ill-health, but who are thinking of trying some part-time work. With the *prior* approval of your doctor and your local DSS officer you can earn a small weekly amount, while still claiming sickness benefit. It's crucial you get approval from the DSS beforehand, though, and find out exactly how your other benefits might be affected. The *Disability Rights Handbook* (16th edition) warns:

  "The work must be clearly seen as 'therapy' (in a broad sense) for you. When working out your total earnings, certain work-related expenses can be deducted...If you are considering doing more substantial work (eg a few hours a week in an office) you should be aware that the Adjudication Officer may consider that you are fit for light work and stop your invalidity benefit altogether. The point is that invalidity benefit is not there to insure against a drop in your earning capacity; so if you are fit and capable enough to do an ordinary part-time job, you are considered to be fit for work. It is important to make sure your doctor agrees that you shouldn't take formal paid work, but that you can do odd jobs for therapeutic reasons. If the work can be organised flexibly or is arranged on a charitable or friendly basis, the AO might well agree that it is therapy for you."

- *Unemployment benefit* may be paid rather than sickness-related benefits if you're out of work, but still considered 'capable of and available for paid work'. It relates to NI contributions. You claim through your local Unemployment Benefit Office (soon to be part of your local jobcentre), using form UB461. You'll also be asked to fill in form UB671, a questionnaire about your availability for work. You might find parts of this difficult to complete. *The Disability Rights Handbook* explains in detail how to tackle UB671 bearing in mind your state of health. You're allowed to take the form away from the UB Office for up to three working days, so you could ask an adviser, eg CAB officer, for help. Keep a photocopy or exact note of your completed UB671.

- *Income Support and work* If you're unemployed and don't get UB, you may be eligible for Income Support. To receive IS, you're normally required to 'sign on as available for work' but you might qualify for exemption if you're disabled or submitting evidence of incapacity for work in support of a claim for sickness or invalidity benefit, or SDA.

I repeat − the whole area of employment/benefits/rheumatic disorder can be highly complicated, so seek advice, and cross-check it if possible.

Other sources of finance

Throughout the book, I've included other information to help you financially. Take advantage of any concessions and benefits for which you qualify; please don't be too proud. Why be poorer or more handicapped than you need? Isn't there some truth in the saying 'to each according to their needs, from each according to their ability'?

It's always worth asking around to see if help can be given, even if you've no idea who might help or how. Try your local social services department, your doctor, the local CAB, DIAL, church, local and national charities. Some businesses and commercial organisations have charity funds for certain purposes. Find out about local charities through your local library or church; the library should have the following:

−   *The Charities Digest* (Family Welfare Association)
−   *The Directory of Grant-Making Trusts* (Charities Aid Foundation)
−   *A Guide to Grants for Individuals in Need* (Directory of Social Change)

Keep your eyes skinned for books and leaflets giving tips on money management. Bulk purchases bought alone are expensive, but could you perhaps share the cost with friends, to save money? Visit jumble sales, Oxfam and other charity shops, and car boot sales. Some second-hand goods and equipment are real bargains, provided you avoid rip-offs. See too my note on page 161 about the Furniture Recycling Network, and Care and Repair on page 118.

Fuel costs are a high cost item. Ask your local British Gas showroom or Electricity Board about different payment methods, eg regular monthly budget payments, or 'fuel stamps', etc. Make sure your home's as efficiently insulated as possible. Cash help's available under the Home Insulation Act 1978 and some local authority housing departments give grants for loft insulation, hot water tank jackets and cold water tank and pipe lagging. More is refunded if you're getting Disability Living Allowance plus Income Support and/or Housing Benefit. Send for free leaflets *Help with Winter Heating* (Energy Management and Information Unit), and *Help with Heating Costs* (SB17 from DSS). Two other helpful free leaflets are available from the Building Research Establishment: *Homeowners' Guide to Affordable Heating* and *A Tenant's Guide to Affordable Heating*.

Economise on telephone costs by using the cheap after 6pm rate for personal calls, or save them for the weekend. Keep the most expensive time, 9am − 1pm, for emergencies only, and from 1pm to 6pm make only unavoidable business calls.

Check whether you qualify for free prescriptions and dental treatment. If you normally have to pay for your prescriptions, don't forget that you can save money by getting a 'Prepayment Certificate' (see page 43).

Budgeting on a fixed income isn't easy. If debts mount up, try not to panic, but contact your CAB or consumer advice centre for help in working out what to do. The booklet *Debt, A Survival Guide* (Office of Fair Trading), gives an action plan, personal budget chart, etc. There's a national phone helpline giving free confidential advice on housing debt: Housing Debtline, on 021 359 8501/2/3, Mondays and Thursdays between 10am and 4pm, and Tuesdays and Wednesdays from 2pm − 7pm. Housing Debtline also produces helpful leaflets: *Rent, Rates and Water Rates Arrears, Mortgage, Rates and Water Rates Arrears*, and *Dealing with Your Debts*.

Chapter eighteen

DEALING WITH BUREAUCRACY

"Quite often the obvious sources of help seem to be programmed to 'fend off' and 'fob off' so that at the moment when the individual is most in need of help and at his/her most vulnerable – he/she comes up against the horrors of bureaucracy and the result can often be DESPAIR!" (YPA)

First contacts with an impersonal bureaucracy like the DSS or social services can be alarming. So it helps to know something about how they and 'the System' operate. Remind yourself, too, that caring officials *do* exist. Some try hard to interpret rules and regulations in the most humane way possible:

"Once past the impudent switchboard operator and the apathetic Duty Officer – the Occupational Therapist, Home Care department and the Social Worker have all been perceptive and helpful. My Social Worker makes me laugh too – which is a terrific bonus!" (the same YPA)

If you're unlucky enough not to winkle out any humane officials, do remember there are plenty of caring and informed 'allies' around who can help (eg CABs, Arthritis Care Welfare Officer or Young Arthritis Care Contact, NASS for people with AS, Lupus UK, Raynaud's and Scleroderma Association, Law Centre or Network advisers).

Telephoning tips

It's easier and quicker to pick up a phone than to compose a letter. Straightforward queries might get a quicker answer on the phone. A call can be followed up in writing, to ensure important facts like names, dates and other facts have been correctly understood. For tips on overcoming physical difficulties in phoning, see page 147.

Before phoning get clear in your mind what you want to ask and, if possible, whom you need to speak to. Jot down some notes to help. What happens when you get through? Bureaucracies have big switchboards. No one seems to answer your endless ringing. This may just mean there's a stacking system, where your call (represented by a light on a switchboard/computer screen) has been put into a queue. So let it keep ringing and keep your place in the queue. If instead the number's engaged, put the phone down and try again, without pausing. Again and again, so that your call leaps into the queue as soon as a line's freed, and before any other call sneaks in (a last number redial button makes this easier).

Be sure you're phoning the right place and asking for the right service or person. You'll discover for instance that for information on DLA mobility component you might as well phone Blackpool direct, rather than your local DSS office, and for advice on special equipment at work, you need the jobcentre DRO, not social services. A quick phone call or visit to your local library can identify appropriate bodies, in reference books like the *Social Services Yearbook*, the *Hospitals and Health Services Yearbook*. Ask a switchboard operator for 'general enquiries' if you've no idea who to speak to!

Don't waste your breath going into detail to the switchboard operator. Keep it brief, eg 'I'm phoning to ask about Home Help services'. Homework beforehand helps, for instance if the switchboard operator at the College of Further Education's flummoxed when you say 'I want to ask about access to courses', instead you'd know to ask for the Student Services Officer/College Counsellor, or the adviser for students with special needs.

You might be confused by having to speak to several different people. The first person you speak to may not be the one who actually ends up dealing with your query. At the social services department, for instance, you'll find yourself speaking first to a Duty Officer/Intake Person. They'll refer your query to a specialist section or officer (eg Home Help organiser maybe, or the Children's Resources Team for information on child-minders, or to the Mental and Physical Health Team for queries on disability aids, community OT or chiropodist). You may end up being referred to several sections/ officials!

Keep costs down by phoning after 1 pm. Ask if they can call you back if the answer's not readily available. Make sure you know the name of the person you speak to (write it down) in case they don't call back or if you need to call again.

Don't assume a particular official knows everything! Or will tell you everything! For instance, no one told one mum (writing *In Contact*) that the 'limited hours of study ruling' didn't apply to her son. Because she discovered a particular clause in the DHSS rules herself, her son (with AS) was able to study full-time *and* still get his benefits.

Your homework can also uncover lesser-known wonders *outside* the statutory services like, for instance, the British Red Cross escort scheme, where someone will accompany a disabled person on a journey, or drive them to a hospital appointment.

When talking to officials, keep to the point (jotted down beforehand). Don't assume they can read your mind or see what's invisible and needs explaining (so often the case with inflammatory arthritis). Be firm and gently persistent if necessary but avoid being rude: it only antagonises and as likely as not s/he hasn't made the rules and regulations. Speak to officials as if you *expect* them to behave as civilised human beings and, hopefully, that's how they'll react. Keep a note somewhere (eg in your Infokit, see page 112) of the day you phoned, who you spoke to, and what was said.

If the first official you speak to is unreasonably unhelpful, find out who's next in the hierarchy. In benefits offices, for instance, your first contact will probably be the Counter Clerk. If you're not happy with what s/he says, ask to speak to the senior Adjudication Officer (AO) or Supervisor, who has a wider knowledge of the law and policy and may be the person who has made the decision. If you still feel your claim's been handled badly, write to the Manager (keep a copy), and seek advice on whether or not to appeal to the Social Security Appeal Tribunal. Remember you can get help from outside 'allies' like the CAB, a disability organisation, your MP. Sometimes you just have to keep at it.

Letter-writing

Sending a letter has several advantages. You have time to think about what you want to say and how best to say it. No one can butt in while you're speaking. It gives the recipient time to give you a more considered and more informative answer than if you'd phoned. Letters can be kept as evidence if there are misunderstandings or if things go wrong, and they can be copied to other people for information. Copied to the boss or local councillor or MP, they can be a powerful way of speeding up inaction!

For tips on overcoming physical difficulties in writing, see page 148. Spend time and effort composing your letter.

● Who's the right person/body to deal with your query? Get name, title, and address.
● Make a rough list of all your points/questions. Leave it for a while. Look at it again, cross out anything unnecessary, then arrange the points in order of importance.
● Think about the person you're writing to. What facts might s/he need from you? What questions will s/he ask when dealing with your letter? For instance 'Has Ms X written to us before?' (Quote their earlier reference, so they can quickly find previous papers.) 'Has Ms X already tried anywhere else for a grant?' 'How old is Ms X?' 'From what date has Ms X not been able to use public transport?'
● Compose a rough letter first. Keep it short and to the point. Be clear about what you say

and don't obscure the main point. Avoid ambiguity. Number points if there are a lot of them. Avoid rudeness, which achieves nothing. Finish with a summary of what you would like done. Put the rough draft away for a while. Look at it again later, this time pretending to be the recipient. Can it be made clearer or improved in some way?

- Make the final version legible, especially your name and address! If you or a friend can type it, so much the better. Date the letter, and keep a copy. Consider whether to send a copy to anyone else, eg the recipient's boss, or to an 'ally'. You could let the recipient know you're doing this by writing 'cc Mr X' at the bottom of the letter.

Filling in forms

- Write your anwers out in rough first, on a blank photocopy of the form if possible, and in pencil. That way you can work out first whether they'll fit the space available.
- Get help/advice beforehand, from someone knowledgeable and experienced, eg CAB/social worker/professional friend.
- Write legibly, in black ballpoint (it photocopies better than blue), and in capital letters (unless you're asked not to).
- Are some of the spaces too small? Against the relevant item number, eg '16', write 'see attached sheet'. On the attached sheet (staple it to the form) write the number '16' and the full details.
- If you're not sure whether to send full details at this stage (eg about your disorder/disability) give a brief response and add 'Further details available on request'.
- If the form's questions don't bring out something important that you think should be taken into consideration, write it legibly on a separate piece of paper (cross-referring to it on the main form). I needed to do this with my Mobility Allowance application – it was so difficult otherwise to explain what my problems were.
- Keep a copy in your Medikit or Infokit so you know what you wrote (essential, this!).
- Check that you've included all the information requested. Do you need to enclose any documents? Send copies, not originals, if so, unless originals are asked for.

Complaining

Christopher Ward wrote a whole book on the subject! *How to Complain* (Martin Secker and Warburg). Here's just one helpful extract:

"Cock-ups are often the result of a simple human or mechanical error. A clerk forgets to make a note in the order book. A secretary takes a week's sick leave to go on holiday with her boyfriend, leaving a memo about your lawn mower in her Kleenex drawer. A pleasant telephone call or letter to the right man will often sort out the problem in minutes. No need for threats, angry letters, telegrams to the managing director."

If that doesn't produce results, however, you have to escalate the complaint.

"Write to A's immediate boss (B) asking him to sort out your problem. Mention A's incompetence, by all means, but don't let it become more important than your original object – getting your lawnmower back – or you'll get a letter back apologising for A's sloth, but making no mention of your mower."

If you still don't get anywhere then you have no alternative but to take it to the top.

"The bloke who employs all these cretins might hold the title of Managing Director, General Manager, President, or Chairman. Find his name and title from someone on the switchboard and also his business address if there is a head office.

"When you write or phone, be scrupulously polite and reasonable. He will already be looking for someone to blame, and if you come over as yet another aggressive difficult and unreasonable customer, his sympathies will be with his incompetent staff and not you."

The basic rule with complaints is that the method you use should reflect its nature or severity, while being dealt with as near to the point of origin as possible. The remedy may be simple. By keeping calm and firmly polite, you're more likely to get the problem sorted out right away, rather than being condemned to *'return to the bottom of someone's in-tray because they don't like the tone of your voice'* (Christopher Ward). Annoying, but true! Send in any written evidence in support of your complaint. Here's where keeping copies of letters and forms comes in useful. Quote references, dates of letters and phone calls.

Your local Community Health Council will advise you how to register a complaint about the NHS, or your GP. The system's complicated. If you've a complaint about a local authority service complain first to the department responsible for organising that service. If that fails to produce results, complain to your local councillor or MP, and/or write to the local newspaper.

Allies

'The System' is frightening and many people give up before getting anywhere. Try not to give up. Remember the 'allies', who can help us work our way through the impenetrable jungle. Allies like CAB, Network, Skill (on educational questions), the Disability Alliance, the Association of Disabled Professionals (on questions of employment), NASS, Arthritis Care or other patient support group, or a DRO, a social worker, GP, local DIAL office, the Patients' Association, MP, local councillor. Find out too how other people have coped.

Confidence can reach a low ebb when you're out of sorts and in pain and the bureaucrats who should be lifting the burden are adding to it. But remind yourself that you have the right to be treated as an intelligent, capable and equal human being, by anyone – stoney-faced bureaucrat/highly qualified doctor/whoever, and that you have the right to ask, politely but firmly, for what you want even though you may still not get it.

Further Reading

- *Working the System*, by Tony Roberts (BBC Education Booklet, 1987)
- *How to Complain*, by Christopher Ward, (Martin Secker and Warburg, 1974)
- *Business Letters* (Elliot Right Way books)

Chapter nineteen

INSURANCE

When you apply for insurance cover, whether for car, holiday, mortgage protection or life insurance, you normally have to declare any medical condition or disability. If you don't, then any claim you make later may not be met, so it's important to be truthful. However your declaration may mean the premiums are loaded, and may be unreasonably high. It pays to read the small print and to shop around for better deals. Check that any company you deal with is a member of the Insurance Ombudsman Bureau. If you have a dispute with the company, then the Ombudsman can (sometimes) help settle it.

Car insurance
The sort of car you get can make a big difference to the amount you pay in car insurance, even before any medical condition's taken into account, so find out about insurance ratings before deciding which car to buy.

You're required by law to tell your insurance company about any disability. RADAR, the Disabled Drivers' Association, the Disabled Drivers' Motor Club, and the Mobility Information Service (see page 187) can all provide information on car insurers with experience in dealing with disabled people, and there's a helpful chapter in Ann Darnborough and Derek Kinrade's *Motoring and Mobility for Disabled People* (RADAR) (page 180), which includes specialist brokers who say that premiums won't be loaded on account of disability. Included, too, are insurers for manual and powered wheelchairs. Two motor insurers which particularly cater for people with a disability are M J Fish and Co, and Leslie and Godwin.

Any driver or would-be driver who has a disability or medical condition requiring more than three months' treatment must by law also inform the Driver and Vehicle Licensing Agency (DVLA) in Swansea (MVLA in Northern Ireland). DVLA has its own medical panel of specialists who will ask to see your medical files if necessary and liaise with your GP or hospital specialist. They may also ask you to undergo an independent medical examination. If DVLA is satisfied and grants a licence then there should really be no need for an insurance company to insist on a separate note from your doctor, though some do.

Shop around. Always seek a number of quotations before signing on the dotted line for car insurance and consider whether the cover's adequate. Check too whether the policy covers personal accident. Some insurers delete this cover for disabled drivers. If you think you're being ripped off by an insurance company because of your disability, try the Insurance Ombudsman, and/or take your business elsewhere. Write too to your MP and the Transport Under-Secretary at the House of Commons. He's responsible for transport for people with disabilities.

Some organisations run special priority car breakdown services for car drivers and passengers with a disability. Some are limited to Orange Badge holders. Services and costs vary, including for instance roadside help, and help getting car, driver and passengers home or to their destination after a breakdown. More information from AA RADAR Group, Autohome Disabled Travellers' Motoring Club, National Breakdown, RAC Response.

Holiday insurance
Read the small print before taking out holiday insurance. See what it says about 'pre-

existing medical conditions or defects'. You may not be covered if problems arise, which could result in horrific expense somewhere like the USA, for instance. Get RADAR's very helpful Holiday Fact Sheet listing insurance brokers who offer policies which don't exclude 'pre-existing medical conditions'. Insurance information's included too in RADAR's publications mentioned on page 278.

The Holiday Care Service, in association with the Home and Overseas Insurance Company, has a travel insurance policy for people with disabilities (send SAE for leaflet).

Household insurance

Arthritis Care has joined forces with insurance brokers Leslie and Godwin to devise a special home insurance policy called Arthritis Homecare. It provides standard cover, with special additions, eg wheelchairs and stairlifts.

Endowment mortgage, mortgage protection policy, life insurance, etc

If you want to take out an endowment mortgage, mortgage protection policy, or life insurance, you'll probably be asked to declare any medical condition or disability, and the insurance company may ask for a medical report on you. Since January 1989 you have a right to see a copy of any medical report.

When a company writes to a GP asking for a report they also have to write to the patient explaining that s/he has 21 days to obtain a copy if s/he wishes. Take this opportunity to check that it's accurate and to query anything you disagree with. If you and your GP disagree, you can include a note giving your views.

Sometimes you may have no problem getting the cover you want. After all, most rheumatic disorders don't reduce life expectancy. But some insurance companies won't, as a matter of principle, take on anyone with what they call 'impaired' or 'substandard lives', or they may make the premiums horrifically expensive. Again, it pays to shop around. One company which specialises in various types of insurance cover for disabled people is M J Fish and Co Ltd.

The National Ankylosing Spondylitis Society (NASS) has found that because many life insurance companies don't fully understand AS, they're apt to put a loading factor on a policy. NASS advises people to shop around if this happens, and if that fails, then NASS can give further advice. Over the last few years NASS has intervened with many companies on behalf of its members and got them to reverse their decision.

Chapter twenty

SANITY-SAVERS
Gadgets, adaptations and alternative methods: general information

How can we outwit the arthritis in a practical way, in our everyday activities, from washing and dressing, or coping with cooking and housework, to getting out and about or coping with work? The world simply isn't designed for people like us with weak grip, stiff joints, and limited strength – frustrating enough before you even begin to add the aches and pains that multiply the misery. All too easy to feel very handicapped and disabled, however able-bodied we may look.

Fortunately there are plenty of ways of getting over practical problems, to maximise abilities and retrieve some sanity! 'Tools for living' is the jargon phrase to replace the old 'aids' (for disabled people). ADL is used sometimes, too, meaning 'aids for daily living'. Why not gadgets?

The right gadget or piece of equipment or adaptation can make a dramatic difference to keeping yourself as independent and sweet-tempered as possible, *and* can help you protect your joints and conserve energy. It doesn't have to be expensive, or even 'specially for disabled people'. A piece of wire, bent the right way, has served me as a boot zip puller-up in the past. Spending a few pounds on an extension plug (the sort with curly-wurly leads, found in hardware or DIY shops) can temporarily 'raise' an unreachable electric socket. Often the simplest and cheapest solution is the best, or maybe just a new way of doing something. – Or even, as one YPA put it 'some things I just leave'!

Some of us are too embarrassed to use special gadgets or adaptations; we feel we're making ourselves look 'odd' or 'different'. I'm still cross with myself for having delayed so long using an 'easyreach/helping hand' gadget at work, through embarrassment. It makes life *so* much easier. Using it is now so automatic that my embarrassment is long forgotten, and because I'm not embarrassed, other people too accept it as just a part of me, and forget about it. Any comments I get tend to be expressions of genuine interest or envy – even 'where can I get one?' If a gadget helps, use it! After all, people who wear glasses are using special 'aids', aren't they, and they're accepted as perfectly normal.

Using special gadgets doesn't mean you're 'giving in'. – Is it *really* better to carry on moaning (outwardly or inwardly) about problems which *could* be solved, or nagging other people to do things for you which a gadget would enable *you* to do instead? Why let the arthritis give you more problems than there need be? Defy it! – If a gadget helps, use it!

Special gadgets *aren't* only for severely disabled people. Look at all the 'aids' used by cooks, gardeners, car drivers, housewives, who aren't even mildly disabled. What's a computer or a drill or a food mixer if not an 'aid'? It's just that they're called gadgets or tools or labour-saving devices. So what if it's a gadget 'for disabled people'? – Magically, by using it, you're actually making yourself *more* capable and *less* disabled.

Moreover, one of the most important reasons why someone with inflammatory arthritis *should* use gadgets or adaptations (provided they're used the right way) is to *avoid* becoming severely disabled, to help *avoid* joint damage or deformity, and to conserve energy for more essential or enjoyable activities. Maybe you *can* struggle to open a tin manually, but at what cost to your joints? An electric can-opener (the right sort) could save time, energy, pain, *and* help avoid further joint distortion.

So do take joint-saving and sanity-saving devices and tricks seriously. They're as essential a part of your treatment as going to the doctor or taking the tablets.

Your doctor may give you some advice, but where can you find out more? Occupational therapists (also known as 'Disabled Living Advisers') are the experts. More about OTs on page 38 and in chapter 6. For referral to a community OT, it's usual to ask your doctor, though *not* essential. Ask for referral as early as possible: it's never too early, and there's a shortage of OTs in some areas, so you may have to wait anyway. If there's a very long delay try asking your doctor if s/he can help hurry things up for you.

Babette, a newcomer to RA, found just one visit from the OT solved several 'small' problems which added together had been getting her down. Lorraine Rogers' life was transformed by a bedsit extension with shower and toilet, built on to her family's home. A young housewife and her family got totally frustrated by her inability to do anything, especially in the kitchen, and her husband even gave up work to try to help. Someone suggested they contact the social services OT.

In the kitchen, the OT arranged for cupboards and surfaces to be lowered so they could be reached sitting down. A trolley helped with moving things around the kitchen, and a washing machine-tumble drier meant heavy wet washing no longer had to be lugged around. Cupboards were replaced by large storage drawers to avoid having to reach into awkward corners. Other aids provided by the OT included an automatic bath lift, a helping hand and a spring-loaded chair. The husband was able to return to work, and the whole family felt much happier generally.

Books and leaflets can give you ideas, too. I can't tell you here about *all* the gadgets and tricks available, but can tell you where to start looking. Other chapters will also help, and you'll pick up tips from other people with similar problems. Seek your OT's advice as much as possible, before buying things, especially anything expensive when you can, alas, all too easily 'be taken for a ride'. Find out all you can beforehand about different options and 'try before you buy'. Disabled Living Centres (page 143) or NAIDEX exhibitions (page 144) are good places to see what's available. And window-shop from your armchair by sending for the catalogues of commercial suppliers mentioned on page 144. Other helpful reading:

- Heather Unsworth's *Coping with Rheumatoid Arthritis* (Chambers). Excellent paperback, with lots of emphasis on joint care, and helping yourself.
- Peggy Jay's *Coping with Disability* (Disabled Living Foundation). Good, but covers all sorts of disability, not just arthritis, so not all relevant. Borrow it from the library.
- Publications from Arthritis Care, ARC and the DLF (eg see pages 113 and 144).
- Michael Leitch's *Living with Arthritis* (Lennard/Collins) is inspiringly full of tips from a variety of people who themselves have a rheumatic disorder.
- Your OT probably has some of the superb *Equipment for Disabled People* range of books. Copies (medium-price) are available to anyone, by post, from the Disability Information Trust. Each is illustrated and crammed full of ideas including useful everyday 'non-disabled' gadgets and 'make-it-yourself' aids too. The excellent *Arthritis − An Equipment Guide* has selected items and advice taken from the 13 other books in the range, and was sponsored by the Arthritis and Rheumatism Council. Others include *Personal Care, Parents with Disabilities, Clothing and Dressing, Housing and Furniture, Home Management, Outdoor Transport, Gardening.*
- *Equipment and Services for Disabled People* (free, from Health Publications Unit).

Look out all the time for ideas that could help. 'Disabled' literature can give you ideas, but don't overlook all the gadgets and labour-saving devices and tricks around for non-disabled people too. Look in magazines (including the small ads), and shop-by-post leaflets and catalogues like those on pages 177 onwards.

Train yourself (family and friends too) to look at the oddest things with the question 'could that somehow make life easier for me?' Try DIY shops, pet shops, even sports, camping and cycle shops. In an art shop I found just the right long-handled paint-brush for applying moisture cream to my dry, rapidly ageing neck! In a shop selling climbing or sailing gear you'll find carabina clips, used for clipping ropes together. They remain firmly closed in use but are opened easily by pressing down lightly on one bar. Attached to dog-lead clips they proved ideal for one YPA for attaching her baby's walking reins or safety harness. Simple plastic bags or long-handled dustpans become nifty devices for getting things out of the fridge or off shelves.

Let your brain ease the strain, and help conserve energy. Work out shortcuts or new ways of doing things, at home, at work, at leisure. Boil potatoes in their skins or cook jacket potatoes instead of peeling them. Use convenience foods. Plan the week's menus ahead. For non-perishables shop around from your armchair (see page 176 onwards). Make your home (even just a part of it) the one place where you feel as little handicapped as possible. List the obstacles to be overcome and set about finding the solutions.

Where to find out more

Social services departments
(In the phone book under the name of your local authority/county council)
For information about home care service, child care, meals on wheels, advice on housing, finance, education, aids and adaptations. Some run day centres, some have kitchen/bedroom/bathroom facilities where you can try out sanity-saving gadgets and adaptations. Social services alsowho administer the Orange Badge scheme which allows parking in certain restricted areas (see page 185).

By law, a local authority, through its social services department, is required to assess the needs of a disabled person for any of the following, if asked to do so by that person or by a carer: help in the home, recreational facilities in or outside the home, assistance with transport to such activities, aids and adaptations, holidays, meals, telephones.

They're entitled to charge for some services though can't refuse to provide the service if the disabled person can't pay. However what happens in practice varies a lot. Contact Arthritis Care or RADAR or other support group for advice if you have problems. Departments are also required to inform disabled people of any other possibly relevant service they're aware of.

You can ask to be put on the social services' *Register of Disabled People* (see page 125). You don't have to be registered though it may help with getting some services. You can request a social worker's visit if 'in need or at risk'. Social services also employ some physios, OTs and chiropodists. It's usual to ask your GP for referral, though possible to request their help directly. They can also liaise for you with other departments or organisations. If you can't get out to see them because of disability, ask for a home visit.

Some social services employ people part-time to visit disabled people regularly in their homes, eg to help with shopping or fetching prescriptions, or may be able to put you in touch with organisations like Home Start, which in some areas provide volunteer 'family friends'. See page 158 for the immense help one YPA got from her social services.

See the latest annual *Social Services Year Book* (Longman) in your local library for more background information.

Disabled living centres (DLCs)
Each centre (DLC) displays useful aids and has a professional, well-informed staff (mainly OTs and physios) to advise you, though the centre doesn't actually supply aids itself. Referral from a doctor isn't essential, though wise, as it helps the staff help you more effectively. They can recommend equipment, and supply leaflets, costings, and details of where gadgets may be bought privately or through the NHS or social services. Phone first to make an appointment and to check whether what you're interested in is available to see. For details of your nearest centre contact the DLF (details below).

The Disabled Living Foundation (DLF)
This is *the* national disabled living and information centre (based in London) on all non-medical aspects of coping with disability. By prior appointment, aids can be seen, demonstrated and tried out. You'll get information on costs and suppliers, though can't actually buy any gadgets there. Displays include wheelchairs, hoists, aids for kitchen, bathroom, bedroom, toilet, living room, aids for reading, writing, eating, mobility.

Also useful, if you can't get to London, or to a local DLC, is the DLF's *Information Service*, a telephone/letter enquiry service (SAE essential, as DLF's a charity). It operates five days a week, answering queries on aids and equipment, services, benefits, etc. DLF also publishes an incredible variety of low-priced, very informative leaflets, for instance *Advice Notes for People with Arthritis*. Leaflets include suppliers' addresses. Send an SAE for the publications list.

NAIDEX (National Aids for the Disabled Exhibition)
Held every spring and autumn, alternately in London and somewhere else in the UK. An excellent opportunity to find out and try out before you buy. Contact NAIDEX Conventions Ltd to find out when and where the next one's being held.

Arthritis Care, ARC, the British Red Cross
All good sources of information on gadgets. In conjunction with Keep Able (see below), Arthritis Care has produced a *Designed for Living* catalogue of useful gadgets. Buying through Arthritis Care means your purchase benefits the charity as well as you.

Commercial suppliers of gadgets and equipment for people with disabilities
I've room here to tell you about only a few (addresses are in Appendix 2). Find out about others through DLF leaflets/information service, through your OT or DIAL, or from the books on page 142. You'll find local suppliers in *Yellow Pages* or *Thomson Directory*. The Disability Information Trust's *Arthritis* also has an extensive list of suppliers.
–   *Keep Able* is Britain's largest commercial centre where you can try and buy over 2000 different products. They also stock second-hand wheelchairs. There's a car park, the centre's fully accessible, and on site are two OTs, two physios, an incontinence adviser, a chiropodist, and even a coffee bar. The manager was formerly at the DLF.
Some commercial suppliers produce free catalogues you can browse through at home, and order from by post. Why not send off for one for ideas not just for you, but for labour-saving presents for other people, too? Frankly, I think it's worth getting all the catalogues!
–   *Arthritis Care's Designed for Living* catalogue (see above).
–   *Keep-Able* (see above) also produce an excellent mail-order catalogue, available from their Northampton address.
–   *Homecraft Supplies*. They now also own *Chester-Care*. From the Chester-Care catalogue I've bought things like a folding walking stick, stick ferrules, folding easyreach gadget (ideal for travelling, hospital appointments, office drawer), harpoon weeder, one-handed tray, eye mask, etc. There are masses of nifty gadgets, for kitchen, garden, house, reading/writing, mobility, bathing, and a portable, wonderfully discreet (*not* bulky like a bedpan) female 'urine bottle' (Warwick SASCo Ltd's 'Cygnet') usable standing, sitting, or lying down (useful in the car, or if visiting friends with no downstairs loo). One for men, too. Also a tiny portable male/female chair/car loo. Homecraft also produce a larger catalogue, for health-care professionals.
–   Other catalogues you could try include those from *Nottingham Rehab Ltd*, *Medici Rehab*, *Coopers*, and *Llewellyn-SML Health Care Services*.
  Boots the Chemist produce a well-illustrated free *Healthcare in the Home* catalogue, packed with sanity-savers. Larger branches stock some items and all can order

catalogue items for you. Ask Boots Customer Services (address in Appendix 2) for the catalogue.

General Points

Beware doorstep salesmen

Arthritis News (summer 1987) quite rightly warned us to be wary:

- *"Think before you sign. Doorstep salesmen can be very persuasive, especially when they are offering you hope of relief from pain. Some suppliers of medical and massage equipment and special furnishings employ such salesmen. Whilst this practice is within the law, members are advised to be most careful before committing themselves to any form of direct purchase or hire purchase agreement under these circumstances. In the case of medical apparatus you should always consult your medical adviser. If in doubt, write to Head Office [of Arthritis Care] for advice.*
- *Do not sign any form unless you are quite convinced of the suitability of the equipment that is being offered.*
- *Ask the salesman to show you some form of authority for selling the company's goods.*
- *Do not pay over any money until you are quite sure that the equipment that you are buying is suitable and reasonably priced.*
- *If you pay a deposit, make sure that you obtain a proper receipt, stating the name of the company from whom the equipment is purchased, the amount paid and the whole clearly signed by the salesman."*

Payment for gadgets and equipment

Some gadgets are provided free on loan by the NHS or social services. For others you may be asked to contribute some or all of the cost. Don't let that put you off. If you can't pay, explain you have a problem. Special equipment for work can be organised through Disablement Resettlement Officers − see page 258 onwards. For studying, see page 251.

You may be able to get financial help from a voluntary or charitable organisation, eg Arthritis Care, or a local charity. Ask your local DIAL or CAB or library for advice. Books in your local library may give you ideas, eg:

- *Directory of Grant-Making Trusts* (Charities Aid Foundation)
- *Charities Digest* (Family Welfare Association)
- *King's Fund Directory for Patients and Disabled People*, by Kathy Sayer (King's Fund)
- *Directory for Disabled People*, by Ann Darnborough and Derek Kinrade (Woodhead-Faulkner)

Don't forget fairy godmothers and Father Christmas too. My notebook has a section 'Presents I would like', where I jot down not only idle luxuries but all the useful gadgets and labour-saving devices I covet. As soon as Father Christmas (or his helper) appears, sighing with lack of inspiration *'What* do you want for Christmas this year?' − sigh − yawn − sigh − out comes my notebook, brimful of solutions to *both* our problems.

Value Added Tax and 'aids for disabled people'

VAT relief is allowed by HM Customs and Excise on certain aids for personal or domestic use by a disabled person, eg wheelchair, long reacher gadgets, key-turners, stocking aids, stair rails. The order for the aid must be accompanied by a statement signed by you or on your behalf, confirming that you are a chronically sick/disabled person and that the goods are being supplied for your personal use. Most commercial suppliers of aids provide a ready-made declaration which you just need to sign and date, eg:

"I am chronically sick or disabled, and I am receiving from [name of firm] the goods on this order form, which are being supplied for my personal use. I claim that the supply of

these goods is eligible for relief from VAT under group 14 of the Zero Rate Schedule to the Value Added Tax Act 1983. [signature and date]"
Full details in VAT leaflet no. 701/7/86 *Aids for Handicapped Persons*, available from your local VAT office (look under 'Customs and Excise' in the phone book). Sometimes repairs, adaptations or services may qualify for VAT relief too – ask your VAT office.

Borrowing aids
Some of us need only occasional use of something like a wheelchair or commode – on holiday, for instance, or visiting friends with no downstairs loo, or when we're temporarily less active than usual. Useful to know that the Red Cross or St John Ambulance can loan some equipment on a short-term basis for home use.

Some firms hire out wheelchairs on a weekly or monthly basis (DLF has details). More and more places like the National Trust and some shopping complexes are providing wheelchairs for temporary use by visitors. Phone first to check. Don't forget hire shops, too, and 'Radio Rentals' for occasional use of labour-saving devices, even possibly as 'try at home before you buy' sources of household equipment (eg washing machines).

Buying second-hand
Be careful. Again, seek professional advice and 'find out and try before you buy'. Second-hand availability is very limited; your local DIAL might be able to suggest local sources. The DLF keeps lists of second-hand goods for sale, eg manual wheelchairs, pavement scooters, stair-lifts and electrically operated baths and beds. RADAR newsletters also carry adverts and *Exchange and Mart* magazine has a special section. See too my note on page 161 about the Furniture Recycling Network.

One-off or tailor-made aids
Maybe you've scanned all the booklets and seen gadgets galore but still have an unsolved practical problem? Write explaining the problem (with SAE) to the DLF; their vast records (of over 10,000 items!) may contain just the solution. Other possibilities:
–   Hospital or community OT may be able to get something made specially for you.
–   Your local DIAL may know of a local college or voluntary group who might like a challenge.
–   Try taxing the brains and talents of DIY friends and relatives. They'll enjoy using their skills to provide solutions.
–   Maybe 'Technical Equipment for Disabled People' (formerly REMAP) can help? It's a voluntary organisation with groups nationwide, who'll design, make, or adapt aids/equipment, free, for local disabled people. Volunteers include engineers, carpenters, machinists, handymen, DIYers, OTs, physios, nurses, social workers, doctors. Something already on the market might do, alone or modified, or something special might need to be designed.
Creations include a driving seat for a very short person, help for someone with RA in opening a car door and lifting the handbrake, a special chair for a hairdresser who couldn't stand for long periods, a bath hoist modification so a woman with severe arthritis could operate it herself, a dressing frame for someone with poor shoulder movement (based on upturned clothes hanger and two plastic balls), modifications to control knobs to make them more 'graspable', a variable height trolley so a heavy casserole from the cooker could slide across to the trolley at one height, and be lowered to work-top height at the other end of the kitchen, and a gas-fire control device for someone with bending problems.

Electronic and technical equipment
Roger Jefcoate is an electronic equipment adviser to many organisations including Arthritis Care, the OU, and the Employment Service. He can advise disabled people at

school, home or work, on computers, communication aids, and electronic reading and writing aids, ie on the practical application of electronic technology to increase independence. There's no charge to disabled people for the advice, and he can sometimes assist in getting financial help towards the cost of equipment. The Electronic Equipment Loan Service can arrange free loans of used electronic aids like typewriters, page turners, communicators and computers.

The British Computer Society has a specialist group for disabled people and can provide information for employers and potential employees.

Special assessment centres

Hopefully most of us won't need to go far for the help we need. But in case there's anyone reading this who's like Theresa Dinsdale (with severe RA), I'll mention the Mary Marlborough Lodge at the Nuffield Orthopaedic Hospital, Oxford, which specialises in assessing severely disabled people.

In her autobiography, *The World Walks By* (Collins, 1986), Lady Sue Masham (paraplegic following a riding accident) recalled how she met Theresa and suggested that she should go to the Rehabilitation Centre, Mary Marlborough Lodge. Theresa's GP had never heard of it, but arranged for her to go there. She had several operations, and to her delight was given an electric typewriter and an electric wheelchair, and was later re-housed with the persistent help of the staff. (She had been living in a terraced house up three large steps.)

Sanity-savers for overcoming particular difficulties
Phoning – writing and gripping – reading – eating and drinking

Telephones

How *would* we manage without the phone? In our frailest moments it keeps us in touch with the outside world, lets us chat to friends, do mail-order shopping, even talk on radio phone-ins. A phone means you can work from home and even, by using a computer fitted with a modem, talk to other computers many miles away.

Some people are nervous about using the phone, especially at work, or for talking to officials. Overcoming any fears is well worthwhile. The phone can 'do your walking' for you, and help you gain 'access' to physically or bureaucratically inaccessible buildings. (See chapter 18 for tips on phoning technique.) Invisibility on the phone is valuable: make the most of it. No matter how weak and frail you look, you can sound authoritative and get responses which might be difficult face-to-face. Or you can 'put a smile' in your voice, when talking to friends or business contacts, no matter how immobile or painstruck you really look and feel.

BT are keen to help people with disabilities overcome practical problems. Dial 150 for your local BT office, and ask for the free *Guide to Equipment and Services for Disabled Customers*, well-illustrated, with masses of variations of phone types and useful addresses. (Or write to BT Action for Disabled Customers.)

Always try before you buy if you've got special problems. Local BT sales officers can tell you about centres where you can do this. If you're housebound, they might be able to arrange a home visit. Some ways of making phoning easier:

● Sockets can be fixed at waist height, to save bending.
● Plug-in sockets for new phones can be fixed in more than one room, so you can move the phone about the house with you. (DIY kits are available.)
● Hands-free phones (eg Binatone's Speakerphones) turn the phone into a sort of intercom, with inbuilt loudspeaker and microphone. (One disadvantage: other people in the room can listen in!)
● Another device allows the receiver to be removed from the telephone and permanently

clipped to a stand adjustable to different heights and angles.

- One YPA who couldn't raise the phone to his ear extended the handle by fixing a stick or ruler to it with sticky tape. The 'extension' could be left permanently in place.
- On-hook dialling saves having to lift the handset until the call's connected.
- 'Last-number redial' saves fingers by automatically redialling the last one you called.
- Memory facilities store frequently used numbers. You just press one or two buttons for automatic dialling.
- Push-button sizes vary. Specially large pushbuttons may help. Handsets differ a lot too: some are easier to grip than others.
- With old-fashioned phone dials insert a pencil for easier dialling.
- Stop your phone slipping about by using a slip-resistant pad like Dycem, or go for a wall-mounted phone.
- Cordless phones can be carried with you anywhere, inside and out, provided you don't move more than 100 metres from the base unit. – Handy while you're in the garden or the bath or cooking the meal, or just resting. Real luxury. The base unit is electrically powered and connects to the phone socket and the electricity supply. The handset's powered by batteries which recharge automatically from the base unit. You'd need another ordinary phone in the house too, to rely on if the electricity supply fails, or the battery runs down. 'Cordless Door Entryphones' (address in Appendix 2) combine remote control of telephone and door entryphone.
- If you live alone and can't afford to pay for your phone apply to your social services department: you may or may not be lucky. Or try the other sources, under 'Paying for aids and equipment', on page 145.
- Keep bills down by making only emergency calls between 9am and 1pm (when it's most expensive), 'business calls' only between 1pm and 6pm (standard rate), and save all personal calls until after 6pm or any time at weekends (cheap rate).
- Directory Enquiries: Weighty phone-books are unwieldy for arthriticky hands. The Directory Enquiries service is, alas, no longer free. However, as a condition of its operating licence BT has to ensure that people whose disability means they can't use directories continue to have the service free, or are compensated for any charges. Phone 0800 919 195 (free) for details. Directory enquiries calls from phone boxes are still free.

Writing and gripping difficulties

Weak grip, and stiff and painful fingers are a warning to treat your joints with care. So do avoid straining them by trying to grip pens and pencils that are too thin, and avoid having to press down hard to write. Instead:

- Use felt-tip pens and soft lead pencils which need less pressure.
- Overcome gripping problems – enlarge the diameter of a pen/pencil by wrapping foam rubber around and fixing it with sticking plaster, or buy special plastic foam tubing, which comes in different diameters and lengths, or ready-made enlarging pen grips and finger yokes ((from mail-order suppliers listed on page 144). They look neater though may not fit every pen/pencil. Or you could mould your own 'grip': for instance 'Gripkit' from Homecraft Supplies uses two plastics you mould together, like plast-icine, but which sets solid. Or try inserting the pen/pencil through a 'holey' practice golf ball or foam rubber ball.
- You can buy magnetic writing boards which hold paper firmly in place as you write.
- Try a typewriter (especially an electric or electronic version) or word processor!
- If you're planning to write something lengthy like a bestseller, think about dictating into a cassette recorder, microwriter or work straight on to a word processor.
- Send tapes instead of letters.

Typewriters and word processors

Using these can be a godsend: quicker, easier on the joints, and on the reader! Taking up typing launched Marie Joseph on her successful writing career just before her 40th birthday: *'As my swollen hands skimmed over the keys, I felt a moment of sheer elation. This was something I* could *do. This was me...'* Pamela LaFane, whose hands became *very* crippled with RA, worked out a way of typing using a stick, and embarked on a correspondence course in journalism. One result was her moving autobiography *It's a Lovely Day, Outside* (Gollancz).

On an electronic typewriter or word processor you don't need to press hard, and the finished result is always even, however unevenly you press the keys. Automatic correction's often built in, so you can kid the world you *never* make mistakes. They're expensive, but don't despair. If you need one for work, ask the Disablement Resettlement Officer for help (page 259). See page 145 and 251 for other finance sources. Roger Jefcoate (page 146) is a wonderful source of free advice on electronic reading and writing devices, including computers, word processors and typewriters. I'd bought my electronic typewriter before I met him, but he told me some manufacturers do discounts for disabled people.

Try out as many as you can, and find out as much as you can before buying. Seek advice too from *Which?* reports (eg in your local library), and other users. I was horrified when I discovered the cost of the non-reusable ribbons on my electronic typewriter – not all are as costly. Some typewriter supply shops might even let you hire one first, on trial, so ask.

Reading

Put a book on a table or book rest to spare weak hands and finger joints. Some book rests, like those used for cookery books, stand on a table. Others look like music stands or fix with a clamp on to a table or are like those used by typists and computer operators (eg from Thousand and One Lamps or business suppliers). Or you can get special tables – some have castors, and others are cantilevered so that the base slides under a chair or bed. Some of the catalogues on page 144 have book rests; contact the DLF for other suppliers. A rubber thimble may help with turning pages, if that's a problem. See also 'Reading for Pleasure' in chapter 35, for information about books on tape – another solution to book holding problems. 'Prism glasses' are expensive but a nifty device. Worn like spectacles they allow you to watch TV or read a book while lying flat on your back. Could help avoid neck strain. Your eyes look up at the ceiling, but what you actually see is anything at an angle of 90 degrees to your eyes! (From various suppliers on page 144, eg Chester-Care.)

Eating and drinking

Increase the diameter of cutlery handles to make gripping easier and as good joint care practice to put less strain on finger joints. Page 148 gives some ideas for enlarging handles. Several different styles of ready-made cutlery with large, easy-to-grip handles are available commercially too. The Disability Information Trust's *Arthritis* book (see page 142) includes illustrations and suppliers of these and different-shaped plates and lightweight cleverly designed mugs and cups too. You'll also find pictures in commercial suppliers' free catalogues (page 144). A slip-resistant mat under a plate can help stop it slipping about while you're cutting up food.

Booklist

Helpful books and leaflets are scattered throughout this chapter: see especially pages 142 and 145, and list of commercial suppliers and catalogues on page 144.

Chapter twenty-one

PERSONAL CARE:
Keeping clean – clothes – shoes

Keeping yourself 'nice to know' can be difficult and exhausting if you've got a rheumatic disorder. Fortunately there are lots of gadgets and tricks to help. Please don't be too stubborn to take advantage of them. You'll also work out your own pet ways of getting things done.

Get the advice of an OT, and thoroughly look into what's available before investing in any gadgets or adaptations. Look back at chapter 20 for where to find out more, page 144 for a list of gadget suppliers, and Appendix 2 for suppliers' addresses. Contact the DLF for more information and addresses. Don't, too, forget all those nifty devices around for non-disabled people like a non-slip bath mat or long-handled back brush (useful for feet).

Keeping clean

The bathroom

Make sure it's warm. If other people use it, bully them into leaving it just as they find it. Train them to clean the bath and loo themselves after use and to put things back in the right place for *you*.

A bath doesn't just keep you clean. A long luxuriating bath can do wonders for the morale and for relaxing weary bones and muscles. So don't give up too quickly if bathing becomes a chore. Sometimes the solution's surprisingly simple. YPA Chris Wood was overjoyed to find that taking her exercises seriously and regularly actually meant she could manage bending and kneeling again, and, despite some difficulty, she could at last use the bath she hadn't been able to use for over six years!

Bath rails can help, positioned with an OT's advice, and fixed by someone skilled at the job, who knows which walls can take the strain. Also, as Peggy Jay rightly points out:

"...placing the feet correctly before moving, and timing the thrust which is needed from the feet at a particular moment, is every bit as important as the help given by a rail..."
(In *Coping with Disability*, DLF)

A bath board or bath seat solves the getting in/out problem for some people. Whatever you use, beware of slipping. Slip-resistant rubber mats are cheap and widely available. Other solutions are more complicated. Ask your OT about different types of bath and adaptations to existing baths. You can get high baths and low baths, walk-in baths and adjustable reclining baths, or you can get bath inserts to fit in or over existing baths. Bath hoists help some people, though aren't always easy for someone with arthritis to operate alone. My OT has loaned me a wonderful bath seat (Mountway's Aquajac; Mangar do one too) which rises up and down in the bath at the touch of a button, and operates on a rechargeable battery. However, very stiff hips, bent knees or difficulty lifting your legs over the side of the bath might make cause difficulties. I found I needed a grip bar on the wall to help, too.

Maybe taking a shower is easier than struggling to have a bath? Again, do get an OT's advice. Be sure you can get in/out safely, operate the taps, and cope safely with washing movements. Some showers have flat, walk-in access with no steps. Properly fitted grab rails may help – some fold up against the wall. You could sit on a special washable stool, some are adjustable in height. You'll also need shelves/hooks for soap and gadgets, and a non-slip mat. You might avoid the palaver of a shower-cap simply by working out exactly where the spray goes and keeping your head out of the way! Inexpensive adaptations might do rather than fitting a complete new shower unit. The DLF leaflet *Showers and Shower Equipment for Disabled People* gives lots more general information.

Lever style taps are usually easiest to manage and put less strain on wrist, thumb and fingers. Portable lightweight plastic levers are available which you can use on existing taps and when away from home, or you could have yours changed permanently to lever style. Only certain types are permitted for domestic use, so get your OT's advice. Some water authorities may be willing to modify your taps, changing not only the taps, but the position too, if necessary.

Bottom-washing's difficult if you can't get in the bath or shower. You could try a long-handled sponge, or flannel mitt over the end of a long handle (eg bath brush used wrong way round). Or how about a portable or fixed bidet?

Away from home, if you're not too handicapped to think about using a strange bath/shower, remember to take any easily portable gadgets with you, eg non-slip bath mat, long-handled brush, portable tap turner (or increase your grip using a damp cloth). Keep a note (in your Medikit, page 33) of what you'll need to take if you go away, so you don't forget.

Wherever you are, home or away, *before* you attempt to bath or shower, do first think through every movement from start to finish. Can you really manage everything, and safely? I well remember a wonderful bath (away from home) from which I had idiotically not pre-planned my exit. Eventually I solved the problem by soaking a towel completely (to stop it slipping), and only *just* struggled out by contorting myself on to it, over the side. My hostess was extremely puzzled by the sodden state of the towel!

Washing tips
You might prefer a sponge to a flannel as it lathers and squeezes out more easily. Or perhaps a homemade or bought flannel mitten; in France mittens are more usual than square flannels. Instead of a slippery tablet of soap you could try liquid or aqueous cream 'soap' (pharmacists sell big cheap pots), or get someone to make you a 'soap on a rope' to hang round your neck, or use soap in a home-made foam envelope. Sew two pieces of foam sponge together, inserting left-over soap pieces before you close up the edge completely.

Like me you might need a long-handled bath brush to reach feet and legs, and maybe your neck too. A long-handled dish mop might come in helpful! You can also buy special long-handled lambswool pads and sponges, and long oblong pieces of flannel with loops at each end for doing your back.

Try 'baby buds' for cleaning ears and/or give them (the ears) a regular good soak in the bath. Use lateral thinking for other difficulties, for instance if you can't easily take the nailbrush to your nails, take your nails instead to a fixed nailbrush.

Drying
Large or small towel? A large towel wrapped around you saves the bother of rubbing dry, but a small towel may be easier to manage. A towelling robe or cape helps some people. If you can't reach to dry your toes, try wriggling them in the towel to dry them, possibly using the other foot to help. Or shuffle them on the bath mat, and sprinkle talc into your slippers from aloft before stepping into them. A powder puff on a stick's another possibility.

Using the loo
Wear clothing (eg 'open-crotch' tights: page 155; trouser device: page 154) that makes moving/removing easier. Through your OT borrow a plastic 'seat raise' to overcome low loo seat problems and avoid straining bad knee and hip joints. Get OT advice on other adaptations, eg grab rails. Disability Information Trust's *Arthritis* lists ways of over-coming toileting problems, including loo-flushing (eg broadened cistern lever or foot-

operated flusher). Why not borrow a commode for bad times or if stairs are a problem, at night? Some disguise their purpose well. For temporary use, perhaps while staying with friends, a commode can be hired from the Red Cross. Or take a discreet plastic jug or portable 'urinal' (I do! – see page 144). Special bottom wipers are available, eg from suppliers on page 144 or Rehabilitation Engineering. They vary in price and effectiveness.

Some top to toe personal care tips

Hopefully, some of these will help increase your independence, conserve energy and cut down on pain and stiffness problems. Look back at page 148, under 'writing', for basic tips on enlarging handles to overcome gripping problems and improve finger joint care.

Difficulty	*Possible solution*
Hair care	● Use long-handled brush/comb, or attach comb to a ruler or other long stick with sticky tape. Wash hair while having a shower. Apply shampoo with long-handled bathbrush, instead of hand. Ask if a local hairdresser does 'home visits'. Try sitting near a small wall-mounted convector or fan heater, but don't touch it and make sure no water can drip on to it. Use hair mousse or gel to make shape more interesting without having to blow-dry or use rollers. Apply by dipping comb/brush in the mousse if easier.
Teeth	● Rubber band wound round toothbrush handle increases grip. Or enlarge handle using suggestions on page 148. Try an electric toothbrush, lighter and cheaper than you'd think; more efficient than weak hands. Too house-bound to get to your dentist? Talk to your GP and/or contact the dental officer employed by your district health authority.
Skin care	● Instead of soap try low-cost scent-free aqueous cream (from the chemist). Use a soft long-handled artist's paintbrush to apply moisturiser to parts (like neck) which you can't reach. People with psoriasis or lupus may need special advice on skin care, and can get tips from the Psoriasis Association and Lupus UK or the British Red Cross.
Make-up	● Looking good will help you feel good too. Make-up brushes make applying eye shadow and rouge easier. Before you buy, test containers in the shop for ease of opening. A felt-tipped nail-polish pen is easier than the normal bottle and brush method. See page 178 for make-up and skin-care product buying by mail-order.
Shaving (men)	● Check weight and ease of use of electric/battery shavers before you buy Lightweight disposables may help on bad days. Rehabilitation Engineering do a long-handled wall-mounted electric razor holder, or try a homemade long handle for a disposable razor. For a wet shave try aerosol foam lather. Or grow a beard! A cordless electric beard-trimmer (eg Braun's) will keep it smart.
Depilation	● Sitting in the bath or shower apply cream or aerosol foam to legs using wrong end of long-handled bath-brush. Rinse off (thoroughly) using carefully directed shower spray or mugs of water. Or get it done professionally or ask a friend.
Foot care	● Chiropodists don't just cut nails. Their skills (see page 38) can ease many existing painful foot problems, and help prevent others. Footbaths are soothing; try a handful of bath salts in warm water.

Clothing

Taking trouble over the way you look boosts self-confidence, and focuses other people's attention on your best features. Stiff joints and dressing don't go easily together, but by choosing styles with care, using a gadget here, or a nifty trick there, you can work wonders. Tried and tested styles can be updated by bright and zany accessories. No need to go for specially designed clothing though it's available if necessary. If you or a friend can manage simple adaptations yourself, so much the better. Nellie Thornton's *Fashion for Disabled People* (Batsford) or Rosemary Rushton's *Dressing for Disabled People* (DLF), give tips. Have a go at learning to sew (see page 283). Worth remembering too that dry cleaning shops will do some alterations, eg fitting zips, shortening clothes.

Get helpful tips from other YPAs, OTs, and look out in *Arthritis News* for fashion and personal care articles. Celia Hart, who used to write these, now runs a small mail-order company, Easy-on Designs, which produces really warm easycare acrylic/polyester/mohair blend bedjackets, woolly bedsocks, and pretty step-in or easy fasten nighties. The DLF has a special Clothing Advisory Service (write with an SAE), and DLF's *Clothing* leaflet gives tips for men and women on overcoming difficulties, plus suppliers' addresses.

Choose loose-fitting rather than tight garments, clothes with roomy armholes and reachable, manageable fastenings. Go for front openings rather than back. Slippery, lined garments are easier too. Try dressing sitting down rather than standing. Opt for light-weight rather than heavy clothes. Several lighter layers are warmer than one heavy layer. Pockets save wear and tear on hands and feet, so include pockets in any clothes you make.

Jogging suits are comfortable and easy to get on, but choose them with ankle openings that aren't too tight. Girls: look in men's departments for bigger, looser clothes, easier to fit over swollen joints, eg gloves and socks and jumpers. Try sports departments for tracksuits/warm clothes for skiers/weatherproof gear for fishermen, etc. *The Special Collection* mail-order catalogue (from J D Williams) specialises in easy-fastening clothes, shoes, lingerie and nightwear for women *and* men.

Armchair shopping saves wear-and-tear on nerves and joints. You can sit and take your time 'window-shopping', buy on credit, and many firms now take phone orders. Many have special offers and sales from time to time. You do however need to be able to post 'returns' back. Avoid firms that expect you to run an agency unless you really do want to buy in a big way. Much more about mail-order shopping on pages 177 to 179. Many of the firms listed there, including some of the charity catalogues, have bright, easy fit T-shirts, sweatshirts and leisurewear.

One YPA wheelchair-user, Kay Jones, wrote a jolly article 'Fashion Frolics' in *In Contact*. She found a personal dress designer/maker, an expensive but ideal solution! Like Kay, some people with JCA are on the small side. Children's and teenage departments are worth looking at, for instance Etam's Tammy range. Stores with small or petite fitting ranges include Top Shop, Marks and Spencer, C & A, Dorothy Perkins, Hammells, Principles, Wallis, and Debenham's Anne Brooks collection. Richer (see page 179) does a mail-order range for women of 5'2" and under.

Dress agencies (look in your *Yellow Pages* or *Thomson Directory*) are a source of good quality cheap clothes. So are charity shops, favourites with Kay:

"Once you have a system you can pick up a bargain or several. I usually have in mind what sort of thing I'm after, then I look at the labels to either find a brand I know I like, or to give an idea of the quality of the garment. Anything with holes, stains or threadbare patches I don't buy. The material itself is something to consider. Is it a natural fibre (nicer to wear I think) or a strong well wearing material that keeps its shape, like denim or corduroy? I can often come out of a charity shop with a three piece outfit that's only cost around £6.00! One of my best bargains yet has been a fashionably baggy (honestly, it wasn't just stretched) lambswool jumper for £2.00 and it is so warm!

My sister managed to get a Next skirt once for a few pounds...The charity shop in a quite well off area will usually have clothes donated by those who can afford to refit their wardrobes every month or so! For example, in one shop I go in, regular donations come from a lady who only ever wears things once!"

Gadgets
- Lots illustrated in the catalogues on page 144. Dressing hooks are nifty devices, variations on the theme of a coathanger (with centre hook removed) plus hook end/rubber thimble. Gutter aids, flexible plastic devices with long tapes or rigid plastic handles, help you pull on socks/stockings/tights without bending down. Reaching aids (easyreach/ lend-a-hand/claw reachers) come in useful too. Tape loops stitched to the top of socks, pants, skirts and trousers may help pull them up more easily. Medici Rehab make the 'Coat On' device, which fixes on a door frame, to help people with limited shoulder movement get a coat on and off.

Buttons
- Big buttons and buttonholes are easier than small. You can replace buttonhole fastenings with easier-to-manage Velcro, disguised by sewing the button back on top (eg on collar or cuffs). Make no-need-to-unfasten cuff-links by joining two buttons together with elastic, or sew a piece of elastic between the cuffs which will stretch to let your hand through. Button-hooks can help with unavoidable buttons. Hugh Steeper Ltd do a telescopic dressing aid for buttons and zips, handy for pocket or handbag.

Zips
- Thread tape or cord through the tab hole for an easier grip. You can get special zip puller-up devices from haberdashery departments, or make your own with a big safety-pin/nappy pin plus length of string/cord. Someone with sewing know-how can adapt a top that's too tight to go over the head by cutting straight down the front (careful!), binding the two cut edges in a toning or contrasting binding, then putting a zip in. Or into side seams of garments for easier opening. Ease a stiff metal zip by running a soft lead pencil up and down it while closed.

Velcro ®
- Easy to use 'touch and close' fastening device, available in many colours and widths from shops or by post from Notts Rehab. Write to Selectus Ltd, for a leaflet showing what's available. Best used in small bits rather than long lengths. Put the two faces together when washing to avoid catching on other garments.

Hems
- For easier sewing of hems try iron-on hemming web. For quick repairs use double-sided sticky tape (but remove it before washing).

Rainwear
- A 'slinger' brolly keeps hands free till needed, though weak hands make coping with an open brolly difficult. Rain-hats can be squashed in a bag till needed and keep hair dry and hands free in the rain (except in high winds). Damart do rain-hats by post; so do the Three Jay & Co, who also sell sou'westers, waterproof capes and ponchos. Liberty's sell rainhats in glamorous fabrics and styles.

Coats
- Try lightweight quilted coats/jackets. Damart do a mail-order range. Some people prefer capes, not always easy to find in shops. Capes in various shades and weights are available by mail-order from Brenda Redmile. Other suppliers are in the DLF *Clothing* leaflet.

Trousers
- Trousers with waist pleats rather than darts may be easier. See DLF leaflet for useful trouser info, eg washable men's trousers with elasticated waist and fly/false fly/velcro fastening fly/other variations, also for a trouser 'pull-on', piece of flexible plastic which clips to the waistband with tapes attached so you can lower and pull up trousers without bending. Spencers Trousers do mail-order and made-to-measure trousers

	for all sizes.
Ties	● Tamar Neckwear Ltd do clip-on neckties.
Underwear	● Front-opening bras may help (eg by post from Woods of Morecambe), or fasten a back-opening bra at the front then swivel it round to the back. Loose-fitting knickers are easier than bikini briefs. Vests and long-johns/ passion killers are essential for keeping warm, and much more glamorous and colourful than they used to be! (By post from Damart or Woods.)
Natural fibres	● People with sensitive skin may need to keep to natural fibres (eg by post from Cotton on, Natural Fibres, Mail to Male Ltd).
Socks, underwear for men	● Finding comfortable socks can be a problem for men with arthritis. Clayton Socks and H J Hall sell socks without elastic in the tops, by post. Socks with linked (not sewn) seams across the toes are available from Cox, Moore & Co Ltd. Mail to Male Ltd sell men's underwear, socks, shirts, etc, by post; Damart too.
Tights/ stockings	● It may take practice to put on open-crotch tights or single-leg tights with a 'puller-on'/gutter aid, but they can be more comfortable and make going to the loo easier. By post from Buyona. DLF has details of natural fibre hosiery suppliers.
Jewellery	● Necklaces long enough to throw over the head avoid problems with tricky fastenings. For a choker effect get a really long string of beads and throw it around twice. If fastening real chokers is difficult, make your own from beads threaded on to round cord elastic. Once made, get it over your head with, say, a longreach gadget. Similar elastic (black) will do, too, instead of a chain, for avoiding fastening problems with a locket or pendant.
Keeping warm	● Several thin layers of clothing rather than one thick layer are warmer. Vests and long-johns/'thermal' underwear are available by post from Damart. Lots of body heat escapes through the head, so wear warm headgear and a scarf. Wear gloves – work out what suits you best – mittens or gloves or fingerless mittens with a flap over the finger ends (try Raynaud's Association). Large wool or sheepskin gloves are warmer than man-made fibres, and men's sizes allow more room for swollen joints. You can get 'furry' lined shoes/inner soles (from Damart or Clifford James), or line footwear with foil. A shawl or bed-jacket (eg from Easy-on Designs, see page 153) is comforting.
	Low-voltage electrically heated gloves/mittens/socks (by Healthaction Ltd or Camp Ltd) are available for people extra-sensitive to cold; the Raynaud's Association can supply information (send SAE) on these and other heating aids, many available by post through them, eg magical tiny portable handwarmers/bodywarmers (by Mycoal or Thermogel), activated by touch and some reusable again and again. Look in sports shops and camping shops too (skiers, anglers and polar explorers are clever at keeping warm).
Woollens	● If you prefer jumpers and sweaters to easier cardigans, go for shawl collars (turned up or down) or yoke or turtle necks (*not* polo). They're easier to get on over the head. Man-made fibres are lightweight, but wool and wool-blends are warmer – and some, like mohair, lightweight. Peter Nightingale has some useful tips for dressing with stiff shoulders:

"To get jumpers and T-shirts on and off use a long stick. I use a walking stick, or sometimes a folding snooker cue. [Or a dressing hook or longreach gadget]. Put your arms in the sleeves of the jumper first and then with the stick up the front of the jumper (with the end resting at just below the neck) push it over your head. To get a jumper off: put one end

of the stick up the back of the jumper and rest it near the top at the back of the neck. Rest the other end of the stick against the corner of a wall, or in a recess (eg hollow grip of a chest of drawers) at about neck height or just below. Walk backwards. The jumper will come over the top of your head. Release the stick and pull the jumper off from the front."

Shoes

For problem feet, get professional advice from doctor/physio/OT/chiropodist (who can be very helpful in choosing or adapting footwear). DLF's Footwear Advisory Service low-cost leaflets include one on footwear for swollen feet, and another on *Footwear and Hosiery: Hints on Dressing When You Cannot Reach Your Feet.* Glamorous high heels aren't really a good idea, alas. Choose styles that give your feet good support and are easy to get on and off. Some people find that trainers, with velcro fastenings, are best. OT Heather Unsworth (in *Coping with Rheumatoid Arthritis,* Chambers) gives helpful general guidelines:

"Shoes held on by lacing, bars or ankle straps are generally best as they stop the foot from sliding forward and so cramping the toes. Some slip-on styles are not good, if they are only kept on because of compression between the toe and the heel. Mules are similarly not recommended as you are reliant on the toe bar to keep them in place.

"Choose a shoe with a supple and soft upper, preferably without seams that will cause pressure on the toes. This upper may or may not be leather.

"Choose shoes that are well-cushioned, flexible and non-slip. Thin inflexible plastic soles will not be comfortable, neither will leather. Similarly, a thin rubber sole glued to a leather sole will not improve the comfort at all, although it will make it non-slip. For soles, synthetic materials win every time!"

If your consultant recommends surgical shoes, take heart from Jacqueline S:

"Another traumatic experience was being reduced to wearing surgical shoes! The tears started...but after getting my first pair I found them so comfortable and the styles are quite acceptable. Now I have three pairs in different colours and two different styles. Since I started wearing them I find I can walk a good mile if I take my time."

My solution to the shoes problem came when I found a theatrical shoemakers who produce reasonably priced leather Twenties-style shoes, with a bar strap. Not exactly high fashion, but not too dowdy either, and oh what comfort! They're just right for my size 8 monstrosities after I've got extra heel pieces fitted one side (one leg's slightly shorter than the other), and replaced the button fastening with elastic so although the shoe still looks the same I can slip it on and off still fastened. Leather soles are lethally slippery so I roughen them with a cheese grater. YPA Kay Jones, writing in *In Contact*

"...invested a hefty sum in 'Adams and Jones' who are a Glastonbury set-up that hand make shoes and will make them for people with feet problems. Admittedly the cost is high for the first pair but once your shoe last is made (the model for your particular feet), the cost of future shoes is less. Also due to the difficulty of dealing with problem feet you may have to send the shoes back a few times until the fit is as you want it...This is a mail-order service so you don't have to hike up to Glastonbury!"

Adams and Jones do shoes, moccasins, sandals, boots, in assorted colours – also a fun multi-coloured 'tropical' range. If you want to investigate a specialist shoemaker independently, you could also try to find one in your area. However they *are* expensive and you need to be sure you're getting value for money. The DLF Footwear Advisory Service produces an annually updated Footwear List with names and addresses, and the British Footwear Manufacturers' Federation's booklet *Footwear for Special Needs* lists firms with specialist services including made-to-measure shoes. There are some 'foot hospitals' (eg London Foot Hospital) which give advice, and can fit shoes too.

Chapter twenty-two

'HOME, SWEET HOME?'

Do you ever feel your home's a nightmare, where housework and furniture and electric sockets and unthinking family all seem to conspire against you? Or maybe you wouldn't put it quite so strongly? Nonetheless, even a few minor changes can work unexpected miracles. Home really should be the one place you feel you have some control over life with the arthritis, an 'enabling', not a disabling place. Above all, somewhere you feel physically and emotionally comfortable, a haven, *not* a prison.

Get cracking now on making it a haven. Finding solutions to problems of stiffness, weak grip, reaching, access, and mobility will cut down on aches and pains, and cut down too on frustration, stress and other bugbears. Aim for as much feeling of independence and 'being in control' as possible, even if it's only in a small corner of your house, or only a maddeningly tiny part of your life compared with your pre-arthritis days.

Solutions may be simple or complicated, may involve getting gadgets or labour-saving devices, may mean retraining the family, or simply just finding a new way of doing things. Often the cheapest and simplest solution is the best. For general advice, look back at chapter 20, if you haven't already read it, before looking at this chapter.

Top priority: your own special corner

Make at least one room, or corner of the house, exclusively yours; a place where you can relax, where everything's in reach, and where you can be quiet or do your own thing. Make sure anyone else who lives with you understands, and drum into them never, ever, to move anything in your corner unless you ask! Here's what makes my two special corners just right for me:

Bedroom   Bed at right height (on blocks). Firm mattress. Light but warm duvet. Electric blanket or hot-water bottle. Reachable light switch and well-positioned light. Bedside table for books, radio, drink/vacuum flask, alarm clock. Phone accessible from bed. Longreach gadget hanging by bed. Though the TV's not directly in view, I can actually watch and work it by remote control by bouncing the control's rays off a carefully-angled mirror!

Living room   Carefully chosen seat: right height (with 'raisers'), firm base and arms (from which hang plastic bags of goodies for the current activity (eg letter-writing, sewing, armchair shopping). Seat is next to a high table topped with magazines, typewriter, etc. 'Clutter' is what some people call it; I prefer 'sanity-savers'! Within reach are phone, radio, TV remote control, foot stool, well-positioned light, longreach gadget, and electric socket on a curly-wurly lead. Seat faces a window so I can enjoy the view.

Priority no.2: making the rest of the house, and housework, easier

Sit down and think about how you need to use the house, and what problems the arthritis creates. What might make things easier? Be systematic, making notes so you don't forget. There'll be blank spaces here at this stage, but you'll gradually fill them in. Go through the house mentally, from top to bottom, and through your week, from the Monday morning alarm call through to the weekend's activities and unwindings. Get family and friends to feed in their ideas too. Follow the 'Replanning exercise', below.

Look back at chapter 20 for the basics on how and where to start looking for solutions. Combine them with other ideas in this chapter. Study too those cunning books produced to make *any* houseperson's life easier (some in the list on page 171). For 28 year old BS, with husband and two children the social services were the starting-point. She swore she wasn't 'on commission from them'!

> *"They are absolutely marvellous. It took a little while to get started, but since then, things have run very smoothly. They came to the house to see what aids I needed. They supplied a high backed armchair, a high stool for working in the kitchen, raised toilet seat, hand rails both sides of stairs, amd also appliances to help me in and out of the bath. After that I received a helping hand, foot stool, and something to help put tights on. Then they raised our bed and now I have a shower in the bedroom which is marvellous. This was done through a grant."* (She may get a stair-lift now, too.)

Just as important, (cheap too) develop 'Planning ahead' and 'Using your brain to ease the strain' habits, like Sue, on page 97.

The replanning exercise

Good planning is as important in running yourself and your home as it is in running a business effectively, and something you can do however bad your arthritis. Aim for a good balance of rest and activity. List the tasks you feel need doing, tasks like housework and preparing meals and cooking and washing up and shopping and washing and shoe cleaning and car care and gardening and DIY. For each task ask yourself three key questions:

● can you *eliminate* it (simply not do it)?
● can you *facilitate* it (make it easier in some way and less of a strain on your joints)?
● can you *delegate* it (get someone else to do all or part of it instead?)

The art of good management lies in *eliminating* unnecessary or wasteful use of resources (ie your limited energy and physical abilities), budgeting the limited resources you have for essentials only and in the most efficient way possible (ie in the *easiest*, least painful way possible, least likely to damage weak joints).

It means prioritising too, listing tasks in order of importance, so if time/energy/good days are limited, you can get important tasks out of the way first and it doesn't matter if those lower down the list don't get done. Last but not least, good managers learn to *delegate*, how best to get other people to do the work for them. – Not forgetting however to keep everyone motivated and happy, too, and that includes you, the manager!

If you live on your own, you still need to do the replanning exercise. Restyle your home life to make the most of limited resources. Though being on your own has its drawbacks, especially not having someone close at hand to 'help', you do have the distinct advantage of also having no one around to 'hinder', however unintentionally!

A closer look at the key questions

1 Can you *eliminate the task* (simply not do it)? Do away with the non-essentials, like cleaning and dusting everything every week. Stick to the *real* essentials like preparing meals. Be ruthless. Prioritise what's left. Now's the time to give up any perfectionist habits. Striving for perfection's a bad habit if it strains you and your joints and leaves you no time for things that really matter like happy family relationships.

Can you *eliminate parts* of the task, eg ironing? Stop ironing things that aren't visible like bedlinen and underclothes. Use crease-resistant materials, and hang things to dry so they avoid creasing. Can essentials be done less frequently? Why not wash the bedlinen every other week instead of every week?

Don't worry about 'what other people think' if you and your house aren't perfectly spick and span. They're probably too busy thinking about themselves anyway. Are their opinions really more important than your family's (and your) health and happiness? If necessary, hand them a duster and let them get on with it themselves! People who care about you won't be critical, especially if you explain how it's part of your plan of self-help, eg beam happily and nonchalantly 'I've decided visitors will just have to take me as they find me, dust, clutter and all!'.

2 Can you *facilitate* the task (make it easier on you and your joints)?
Get all the gadgets/labour-saving devices you (or your fairy godmother/godfather) can afford to make life easier (some come cheap or free through OT or social services). Use easier recipes and cooking methods too – books and magazines will give you ideas, and there are some on pages 168 and 172.

Rethink housework, for instance dry clothes inside instead of traipsing in and out and fighting with a difficult washing line. Train other members of the household to clean up after themselves. Train them at least not to *hinder*, even if they don't always *help*. Use techniques like doing only half a task instead of a whole one (eg vacuum one room instead of doing the whole house), and doing bits at a time, in advance (eg when preparing meals).

Use lists: for shopping, for the day's meals and tasks, and for the week's. Do your thinking and planning from your chair, not while you're on the move wasting limited energy rations.

3 Can you *delegate* all or part of the task? For instance make the most of family, friends, outsiders, especially if they actually *offer* help of some sort. Don't say 'no', but instead 'thank you for offering', while you work out how best to make use of the offer, eg could they change the duvet cover for you, pick up x, y and z for you at the shops, move the rubbish bin outside, empty the vacuum cleaner, get things out of a low cupboard for you? People like to feel needed, so in a way you're actually helping *them!* Many need to feel they can do something to ease your burdens. Looking on helplessly can itself be a burden.

Can you make tasks involving other people DIY affairs? For instance make breakfast a DIY and clear-away-after-you affair, or visitors coming for coffee or tea? Why not?

Break essential household tasks down into light and heavy work. Work out between you and the family who's going to do what and when, during the week. Write it all down, and pin it up, so no one can make bad memory excuses!

For regular jobs you could have a rota (get the children to design a colourful chart which can be ticked, or use gold stars or whatever) for things like doing the vegetables, laying and clearing the table, washing up, shoe cleaning. For irregular jobs have a 'watch-this-space noticeboard', or use fridge magnets, where you can put notes saying what needs doing (helps overcome the problem of getting a rude retort for asking at the wrong time).

Delegating, especially to the family, calls for great psychological tactics. Keep people motivated and happy! Minimise nagging and instead maximise 'rewards' for volunteers/victims. Avoid asking at the wrong time, avoid criticising the way something's done, avoid saying 'I could have done it better'. Instead, give praise and thanks in abundance, especially to the children, however tired you get of hearing yourself saying thank you.

Children enjoy feeling they're being useful, and spouses too, so even when they buy the exact opposite of what you wanted, try making a joke of it rather than scolding. Train yourself to criticise only inwardly. If you must criticise outwardly, turn it into a joke, or save it up for a 'how about' comment *next* time the job needs doing, eg 'how about saving time by putting the saucepan on to boil *before* you start peeling the potatoes?'.

Maybe your family's got into the habit of leaving almost everything to you to do. Re-educate them! Explain, with your doctor's help if necessary, that you need their help in replanning what needs to be done. You need their understanding, too, so they don't feel you're shirking when you're resting or looking on from the sidelines. Get everyone to contribute their ideas in the replanning exercise so they each feel involved and responsible.

Worth pinning up somewhere, a quotation from Don Aslett's *Who Says It's a Woman's Job to Clean?* (Exley), compulsory reading for all those uneducated in modern day homecare truths:

"I once heard a non-housecleaning husband say to his wife on Mother's Day, 'Dear, is there any way that I can help you with the housework?' Her reply was: 'Dear, if you just clean up all your own things there won't BE any housework.'

"Picking up and cleaning after yourself are the most useful things you can do. There's nothing wrong with making a mess, that's often progress in the works; it's leaving it that is wrong. So...

- *If you open it, close it.*
- *If you turn it on, turn it off.*
- *If you unlock it, lock it.*
- *If you break it, fix it.*
- *If you can't fix it, throw it away and buy another.*
- *If you borrow it, return it.*
- *If you make a mess, clear it up.*
- *If you've finished with it, put it back.*
- *If you don't know where it goes – ASK!"*

By the way – delegating doeesn't mean you, the manager, sit back and opt out of *everything*. Sorry! Except when the arthritis is at its worst, don't shift *everything* off on the rest of the household. Bad for them and for you too. It could lead to resentment, or it could lead them to over-protect you, seeing you as a disabled invalid rather than someone with abilities. Not good. You'll feel better if you feel needed and a person of abilities first and foremost.

Heather Unsworth explains how one family tackles things:

"Your biggest ally could be your husband. I am lucky enough to have an understanding and domesticated husband who cheerfully undertook all the heavy chores in the early days, such as hoovering, shopping and ironing. After a full day's work he would come in and make a cup of tea and give me a short spell with my feet up, recuperating from the demands of the children, and this I found invaluable and it enabled me to continue with the supper, etc afterwards. If this is not possible then you must *at least train both your husband and the rest of the family not to hinder. This sounds odd, but you will be so grateful for the energy spared when you have taught them to put everything away as they use it, collect their dirty washing and put it in the right place, not to leave tools, toys, etc all over the floor where you can trip and do yourself an injury.*

"My maxim has become 'If you cannot help, then please do not hinder.' Other children must be taught to do the same and encouraged to help as much as possible. In the darkest days my nine-year old would give me half-an-hour after school each day for any special tasks I needed done. He became very good at chopping vegetables and tasks that I found dificult. He was also very good at fetching and carrying for the baby and entertaining him for a short while so that I could sit down or put my feet up for ten minutes if things got on top of me. You can supervise just as well sitting down!" (In *Coping with Rheumatoid Arthritis*, Chambers)

Practical ideas to help
throughout the house

Look back at chapter 20 for all the help available from the social services, OTs, Arthritis Care, the DLF, commercial suppliers, etc. Look too through the leaflets and books mentioned on page 171. Don't forget that some gadgets/equipment can be borrowed, loaned, or bought second-hand thus saving money. Remember, anything that makes life easier for you will probably benefit the rest of the family as well.

Lots of labour-saving items can be bought in ordinary high street stores, but have a chat first with your OT. S/he can supply some gadgets direct, and help you avoid expensive mistakes buying others. *Which?* magazine reports (try your library if you're not a subscriber) help you judge 'best buys'. *Good Housekeeping* magazine has useful factsheets and runs a telephone information service on a range of subjects like *Choosing....a freezer/ iron/microwave/washing machine* etc. Use things like the *Argos* catalogue or the *Comet* newspaper, too, for window-shopping from your armchair. Where possible go for light-weight devices, eg for campers and travellers, like a travelling iron. Above all, *think* before you buy, and *try* before you buy. Make sure you can operate it *before* you sign the cheque!

Local newspaper second-hand columns are useful hunting grounds for expensive things like automatic washing machines (provided you're extra careful). People in wealthy areas often advertise machines for sale not because they're faulty, but because they want a newer and fancier model. I bought a third-hand automatic machine for £25.00 which did good work for four years. Don't forget boot fairs too. The Furniture Recycling Network volunteers will collect any unwanted usable second-hand furniture and electrical appliances, repair them, then pass them on to needy people (referred through the social services) either free or for a small charge.

Names and addresses of suppliers I'll include only the names of a few lesser-known suppliers here (for addresses see Appendix 2) – most things you'll find available from the suppliers on page 144. Others are listed in DLF's leaflet *Household Equipment* and in the Disability Information Trust's *Arthritis – An Equipment Guide*. In case of difficulty, contact the DLF's Information Service for the name of a supplier. Remember the DLF and some disabled living centres (see page 143) have displays where you can actually see and discuss what's available.

General reaching up and down, and storage Get longreach aids (also called Helping Hands, grabbers, Easyreach gadgets). Save journeys by having several, hanging in the most important places, eg bedroom, kitchen, by chair in living room. Plan storage so most frequently used, fragile or heavy things are at or near waist level. Fix shelves, work surfaces and hooks within your 'reaching zone' too. At higher levels store non-fragile things which can be edged down or dropped (using a reaching aid) on to lower surfaces for retrieval. To reach things stored at lower levels, use longreachers or edge them into plastic bags or on to a clean long-handled dustpan you can then lift up. See also DLF's leaflets on page 171.

Rethink storage generally. If everything has a home, then the family's got less excuse for not putting things away. ('A place for everything and everything in its place'.)

Think 'safety first'. Avoid having slippery or uneven floors. Avoid loose mats and deep pile carpets. Avoid clutter by making sure there's sufficient storage and drill into everyone 'if you get something out, put it back' and 'tidy up as you go along'. For a fun solution to the problem of constant floor clutter, one mother strung a hammock (from a camping shop) across her children's bedroom into which they happily flung all their toys. Do away with trailing flexes. Think before you act – will your weak wrists really let you carry that heavy kettle? – Why not leave the kettle where it is and fill it from a plastic jug or carafe, for instance? Keep a special fire-smothering blanket handy (eg from Tutor Safety Products).

Carrying things Use a trolley (doubles as a walking aid), or a basket on wheels. Or apron with big pockets. Or a long handled bag/basket slung over your shoulder (lightweight things only), eg from cycle shops (called musettes), or the sort used by newspaper delivery boys and girls.

Security and doors   Do take precautions, especially if you're on your own. The Crime Prevention Officer at your local police station will give you free advice on request. Fit a door spyhole, and consider getting an entryphone. Instead of a fiddly door chain, some people might find easier something like the Chainlock door lock ((Wadsworth Security Products), or Yale's 'Checklock', which engage a safety chain automatically every time the door is opened from the inside. Flicking a lever on the lock releases the chain. These and others are available from hardware shops. 'Password' (Friedland) is one of several lower-priced door intercoms. One unit, fits outside the door, the other inside the house within 30 metres of the front door. Cordless Door Entryphones make a combined remote controlled entryphone and telephone for people who can't get to the door or phone easily, plus other security devices. OT and DLF can advise on special alarm call systems if needed.

Keep door lock and hinges well-oiled. Replace round door knobs with lever handles. Modify small-headed Yale-type keys for easier grip with special 'key turners' or build up the head with mouldable 'Gripkit' (eg from Homecraft) – also good for cupboard door handles, kitchen appliances, etc. Try metal skewer/knitting needle to turn keys with large holes in the top. Soft rubber 'knob turners' help turn Yale-type latches. Fit a shelf by the front door to rest shopping or bag while you open the door. Wire basket below letter-box saves bending. Fix a milk bottle holder to the wall or get one on a long handle.

Windows   Sliding windows may be easier than sash. Fixing long levers may help you, eg on a fanlight window. A long piece of wood, with a hook fitted in one end can be used for a window with ring fitted in the framework, or fit a remote opener (eg by Easiaids). Use helpinghand/easyreach to draw curtains or fit a pulley cord or even ask DLF about electrically controlled systems.

Steps/stairs   Consult OT about fitting hand-rails both sides, and other aids. Make sure the stairs are non-slip. Going down backwards or sideways needs extra care but may put less strain on knees. Cut down on up-and-down journeys by fitting a downstairs loo (OT might assist), or use a commode or even a discreet urinal (see page 144). Plan needs, like BS:

> "When my husband comes of an evening he takes the ironing which I do late afternoon (sitting on my high-backed stool of course!) and anything which I put on the stairs. Our stairs are usually filled with things to go upstairs. I have all underwear kept downstairs for the children. I also have a downstairs toilet."

If you're considering having a ramp anywhere, talk to your OT and try one out first – shallow steps suit some people better. If stairs are proving permanently impossible, ask your OT about getting a stair-lift (eg Stannah stair-lift).

Electricity   For a temporary solution to low power points try portable sockets (plug one end, socket at other), perched on a reachable shelf, but beware of overloading them and beware of trailing flexes. A 'Handisocket' or 'Extend-a-Plug' are neater devices for converting a low socket to a higher position without rewiring. For permanent new sockets, consult a properly qualified electrician; the local Electricity Board will have a list. While you're having sockets raised, get any single sockets replaced with double sockets.

Plugs can be made easier to pull from the socket by using 'Handiplugs' or 'Pullplugs' which have in-built handles. Try elbow action instead of fingers for difficult light switches. Rocker switches (eg Crabtree Electrical's Corinthian) need less pressure than flick switches. Two-way light switches, eg one by the bedroom door and one by the bed, might help. Think about fitting time switches, eg on room heaters, kitchen appliances, to save constant getting up and down. Get *Making Life Easier for Disabled People* from your local electricity showroom, the Electricity Association, or RADAR.

Gas   Get the booklet *Getting the Best from Gas: Advice for Disabled People* from your local British Gas showroom, the British Gas Home Services Department, or RADAR. Your local Home Service Adviser can tell you about gas appliances, aids, specially adapted controls, handles and knobs, and will make a home visit (free), if necessary. A gas meter that's in an awkward position can be moved to a better one. A special extended handle can be provided (free) if you can't operate the coin mechanism of a pre-payment meter.

Heating   Heat at least one room well, and wrap up well too. Time switches on convector heaters (eg in the bedroom) save having to get up and down, though may be fiddly for your fingers to set. Berry Magicoal Ltd manufacture a remote controlled electric fire. See also page 155 for tips on keeping warm. Ask your local gas or electricity board for advice on economising on fuel and fuel costs (and see page 134).

Chairs   Essential to have at least one which is your very own, but don't rush into buying one that may be unsuitable. Consult your OT and get ARC's leaflet *Are You Sitting Comfortably?* (free, send SAE). Avoid low chairs and soft chairs. HSL Ltd make a range of firm, comfortable chairs up to 20" high. Avoid chairs you have to flop into; you'll jar your poor joints too much. A chair should be high enough for you to get on and off with least possible joint stress. Chair leg extenders can raise the height. Hardboard under the cushion might make a firmer base. The arms should be well forward to support you. Avoid sitting with your legs crossed: that encourages joint deformity. Change your position frequently to avoid joint stiffness.

You'll need good back support and should be able to rest your feet on the floor (or footstool). Something called a 'gout stool' can be found in some antique shops. It's angled, and can rock backwards and forwards, allowing gentle movement in foot, knee and calf muscles.

When you get out of a chair, wriggle forward first, place the flat of your hand over the padded end of your chair to help you push and spread the strain through your forearms and over as many joints as possible. Don't push up with bent fingers as that strains delicate finger joints. Try a rocking movement, so that the weight of your head (about 9lbs) helps move you forward, using the principle of swinging a weight to make it lighter. Avoid twisting as you rise. Special riser chairs seats might tempt you. They can be helpful, but *do* try some out first. Some are a bit *too* energetic or stiff!

Plan the area round your chair so everything's at hand, eg table, phone, light, radio, remote control for TV, longreach gadget. A book rest on the table might help spare your hands. Some people find a baby's pillow or a butterfly pillow eases neck strain. You can buy butterfly pillows, or make one by tying a long strip of material firmly around the middle of an ordinary pillow. Around the house, keep a bar stool or two, eg in the kitchen, by the telephone, for shorter periods of sitting or perching (more about stools on page 165).

Bathroom   See chapter 21.

Bed   Low, sagging beds strain weak joints, and increase pain. A firm bed may take some getting used to, but will make all the difference in the long run, especially for people with AS, hip and back problems. That *doesn't* mean investing in an exorbitantly priced so-called 'orthopaedic' bed, unless your doctor recommends it. Such beds *may* have a stronger spring system than an ordinary bed, but have no special medical properties. An ordinary but firm bed may be just as good. Mine's blissfully firm and perfectly ordinary, bought in a sale and carefully tried for firmness *in* the shop. I prefer a pine bed to a divan type, because it has individual legs which fit on bed-blocks to raise the height, and the wooden slats under the mattress give it a firm base. And it's perfectly stable, even with two occupants!

Having the bed the height of an ordinary dining room chair suits many people, and avoids strain on hips and knees. If you're raising the height with bed-blocks, *don't* use them on beds with fitted castors; ask your OT about alternatives. Some people have difficulty lifting their legs into a raised bed. Ask your OT for tips. A special 'bed hopper' device or a stirrup-like gadget on a long strap might help. An electrically operated inflatable air bag device is available, but expensive (eg Centromed Leg Lifter). Portable bed-boards may help you be sure of a firm bed away from home.

Aim to keep your hips and knees straight – don't ease aches with cushions under your knees or hips, as that can distort joints. Do use any leg cylinders or night-resting splints you've been prescribed. They may take some getting used to, but they help prevent deformity by keeping your joints in a good position while you rest.

Go for lightweight, easy-care bedlinen (eg polyester/cotton mix), and a light, foam filled pillow. Avoid using more than one pillow as otherwise your head will be pushed forward too much. A small pillow may suit your neck (eg butterfly pillow). Duvets are light, warm and minimise bedmaking, especially if someone else (spouse? home help? good friend?) can change the cover for you. If you prefer blankets, go for lightweight cellular ones. Keep unnecessary weight off your feet – a bed cradle might help, or hang the bed-clothes over a dining or bedroom chair at the end of the bed.

Tucking-in sheets (if you must !) may be easier if you create a slight gap by fitting small blocks between the mattress and bedlinen. If you like fitted sheets but find the bedmaking awkward, try slitting one corner and fastening it with tapes instead. If you have handles on your mattress devise an 'anchoring system', sewing tapes to sheets which then tie round the mattress handles.

Instead of a hot-water bottle, weak hands might prefer an electric heating pad or a sort-of 'hot-water' bottle that's permanently sealed and contains something like wax (eg the Snuggler, by Innovations International, by post from the Raynaud's Association – send SAE for details). Be wary of leaks or splits. Or a special hot-water bottle holder helps hold a bottle steady while you fill it. A light electric overblanket suits some people.

Have accessible storage near your bed for books, water, thermos flask, radio, and a light switch nearby too. Some people like over-bed adjustable tables, but be sure you can still get in and out easily.

Wardrobe   Get the hanging-rail lowered if necessary. Shelves with pull-out baskets may be easier than drawers.

In the kitchen

Oh for a purpose-built kitchen, with every latest gadget and design feature! Unlikely to happen for most of us, so it's a matter of making the most of what we've got and adapting or adding to it as necessary. Discuss difficulties with your OT. Try before you buy for reachability and operability, and think about cleanability. Check weight and knobs/handles. Look for things that overcome weak grip problems, and help avoid joint strain and damage.

OT departments in larger hospitals, and the DLF and some other disabled living centres (see page 143) have kitchen displays. If finance is a problem, ask your OT or social worker whether you might qualify for a grant (and see page 161). There's useful advice in the *Disability Rights Handbook* (mentioned on page 127).

Radio Rentals now hire out not just TV sets and video equipment, but washing machines, tumble driers, dishwashers, microwaves, etc, one way of 'trying before you buy' expensive appliances. Contact one of their superstores in Bath, Blackburn, Sheffield or Southend for information. Ask local hire shops whether they run a similar service.

Storage and layout   Good storage arrangements are crucial. Aim to reduce too much walking about and stretching and bending and lifting. Aim to avoid straining your joints, or using them in a bad position. Try to have an unbroken continuous working surface between the food preparation area, sink and cooker, with a heat-proof working surface one side of the cooker. Slide, rather than lift, heavy things. Keep out at reachable level heavy, awkward things like food processor/mixer, electric can-opener, kettle, even saucepans if necessary, and things you use frequently, like salt and sugar and cooking oil and coffee and tea. Plan 'activity centres', eg keep everything you need to make tea and coffee together by the kettle at a socket near the sink; other centres could be for baking or vegetable preparation.

Lots of reachable open shelves may be easier than cupboards with awkward doors, though shelves get dustier. 'D' handles on cupboard doors and drawers may be easier to use than knobs. Tape looped through cupboard door handles might help with opening. Fit hooks everywhere for hanging tools and gadgets, not forgetting one for a longreach gadget. Check and adapt electric sockets, cooker and appliance control knobs, taps, all handles, and windows for reachability and operability.

Ann Macfarlane uses a special gadget − a stick with a cup hook screwed in one end and a rubber thimble over the other (often sold as a 'dressing stick'):

"I use the hook for opening doors, for lifting cups by the handle and all sorts of other things. If I drop something on the floor − which I often do − I can sometimes pick it up by pushing the thimble end of the stick inside the object and levering it into the air; if that doesn't work I always have plenty of plastic bags available; I then push the object inside the bag and use my stick to lift the bag." (From Michael Leitch's *Living with Arthritis*, Lennard/Collins)

Fix baskets and shelves as reachable back-of-door storage. How about a vegetable rack on castors? Maybe another if there's room, for gadgets and utensils?

Vertically divided deep drawers might make reaching easier. In corners and on work surfaces carousels/turntables swing out-of-reach things towards you. Pull-out racks or shelves in base units make access easier, and can sometimes be fitted in existing units. Pull-out worktops fitted below existing working surfaces make extra surfaces.

Get a high stool to sit on. Try a bar stool with a foot rest (some are easier to slide on and off than others) or a special high perching stool with a sloping seat (details from DLF and/or the commercial suppliers on page 144).

A non-slip surface (eg a 'Dycem' mat) saves straining fingers gripping a mixing bowl. Other tricks are to wedge the bowl (or whatever) in an open drawer at waist-height, or to stand it on a damp cloth, or rest it on your lap.

Cooker   Try before you buy. Can you reach everything and operate the controls without straining? Is the grill convenient? Ask at the local Electricity/Gas Board (or write to the manufacturer) about special switch and tap handle adaptations for people with weak hands. Avoid ceramic hobs if you can't lift saucepans − they scratch easily. Self-cleaning ovens and automatic timing devices make life easier. A split level oven may overcome bending difficulties. A drop-down rather than sideways opening oven door can be used for resting things on briefly, but may make reaching inside and oven cleaning difficult.

Some people prefer an all-in-one oldfashioned cooker raised on a plinth. I use a cheaper but smaller alternative, a Tricity Coronet mounted at waist-height on a strong purpose-built trolley, handy for one person or a couple. Some models are plug-in but you can use only one ring when the oven's on. The wired-in model lets you use both rings plus the oven at once. You could also have a separate plug-in table-top hob unit. Other makes of table-top cooker include Baby Belling, Berry Magicoal Minorcook, Tefal Compact Cooker, Rowenta FB11 petite, Moulinex, Vival, Sona, British Gas's Flavel Vanessa. (Ask *Good Housekeeping*.)

Microwave ovens are a boon and save working with heavy saucepans and dishes. Dishes are easier to clean, and special lightweight plastic cookware is available, eg by post from Lakeland Plastics or Studio Cards (you can't use metal containers). Some (the cheaper semi-disposable plastic) become too hot to handle without oven gloves. *Which?* magazine (December 1987) found two types made of pricier, durable plastic (TPX, polysulfone) which didn't become too hot to handle without oven gloves.

You can cook vegetables in less water than on a hob so they have a better flavour and retain more vitamins and minerals and you can cook fish or eggs with less fat. Food can be cooked and served in the same dish, saving on washing-up. There are some disadvantages: small capacity; large odd-shaped foods such as a chicken may cook and defrost unevenly; judging correct cooking times can be difficult; overcooking may cause food to catch fire. Good microwave cooking doesn't come automatically, it's a skill you need to learn. General information's available from the Microwave Association. A wall-mounted microwave may save space though getting things out could be difficult.

Other useful alternatives to ovens can be placed on a work surface, making for easier cooking without extensive adaptations: electric table-top hob or portable grill or slow cooker or 'multi-cooker pan' (electric tabletop pan for frying, baking, casseroles).

Sink and taps   Tips on bathroom taps on page 151 apply equally to kitchen taps. Lever-taps needing only a quarter turn from off to full on are ideal. Move taps or detachable tap-turners with your palm, to save your finger joints. A swivel spout (or small hose fitted to the spout) means you can fill a saucepan beside the sink without lifting, and it helps with the washing up.

Washing up tips   Pour water into a food-encrusted saucepan the moment you've emptied it: it'll clean much easier later on. Leave dishes to soak before washing them. If rubber gloves are a problem, try a larger size, or try wearing just one, on your strongest hand and keeping the other out of the water. Dusting talc inside makes them easier to slip on and off. Just drain dishes, don't waste limited energy rations drying up (see Pamela's tips on page 170). Using a brush (enlarge the grip if necessary) is less strain than a dish cloth, but if you prefer a dish cloth, wring it out by wrapping it round the tap top then twisting it. Some people find a shallower than usual sink easier or raise the washing up bowl to save bending. Leaving cupboard doors open under the sink may mean you can sit closer and avoid bending. Best of all get someone else to wash up or ask your fairy godmother for a dishwasher, but before she writes the cheque make sure you can load and unload it!

Fridge   Planned fridge use saves on shopping journeys and allows advance preparation. A small one can hang on the wall or stand on a table-top. A larger one could be mounted on a plinth for easier reaching. Difficult-to-reach non-breakable items on shelves can be edged out on to a clean long-handled dustpan kept specially for the purpose, or into a plastic bag.

Freezer   Useful if you've a large family, but needs careful planning and organisation, not just for what you put in, but *how* you put it in and how you'll get it out. Loading and unloading and defrosting difficulties need to be thought through before you buy. A small table-top freezer might give you less bother while still allowing you the advantages of having some ready-cook frozen food.

Trolleys   One with a heat-proof tray at oven height avoids heavy lifting and carrying. Specially designed walking aid trolleys are higher than normal trolleys. A pull-out mobile trolley which lives under a worktop when not in use is handy if you've got room. Social services might provide a trolley if essential and if you can't get one yourself.

Kettle   Get one with an automatic cut-out device. Fill with water using hose on tap spout, or using light plastic jug or carafe. Save lifting by fitting kettle on a tilter base – useful for a teapot too (though tea-bags in mugs are even easier, or try a teaspoon-sized tea infuser – available from hardware and cookery departments/shops). Jug kettles are lightweight, and can be filled through the spout, though the height might cause difficulty. A Jug Kettle Tipper is now available (eg from Medici Rehab) to avoid lifting and tipping problems. A filled vacuum flask can keep you going through the day, and a small one can be carried in a bag even if you're using two sticks. An 'elephant flask' with a spout doesn't have to be lifted for pouring. Or avoid lifting and pouring problems altogether by fitting a wall-hung electric water boiler (eg Creda Corvette) near the sink. Or get an individual electric beaker-heater element (eg Pifco Mini Boiler).

Opening tins   The old fashioned key type tin-opener strains joints. Get an electric tin-opener, instead, with a magnet to hold the lid. Some are more stable than others. Beware of hand-held electric openers which may be too heavy to hold.

Jars and bottles   As a general rule, if you can't avoid using your own hands, open with your stronger hand and close with the weaker one as this will stop you closing them too tightly. Better to use a gadget to take strain off the joints, eg by holding the jar or bottle firmly so you can use both hands to twist. Or use the long lever type of opener like the Strongboy. Besides using a non-slip mat (eg Dycem) to hold the jar steady there are also devices to stabilise jars and bottles leaving both hands free. Try a rolling pin (moved with palm or forearm) to roll out the last remains from tubes of tomato paste, etc. If ketchup refuses to come out of the bottle, insert a drinking straw to let air in, then remove it. The ketchup should start to flow.

Opening plastic packets   The 'Slitapac' is a useful gadget, fixed to any smooth, grease-free surface by adhesive pads. The edge of a plastic packet is slid along the guide bar and pressed against the blade. Some electric can-openers have a special blade for slitting packets. Look for lightweight scissors with large finger holes, or try special scissors with no finger holes but instead a special looped spring-action handle design.

Saucepans   Stainless steel, though more expensive, last longer and are easier to clean than aluminium. Enlarge long pan handles (see page 148) if necessary. Non-stick pans save on cleaning problems. Lift one-handled saucepan handles with one hand, while using your other forearm to support the handle, or try double-handled pans. Preferably avoid lifting altogether, and instead slide pans across work surfaces, provided they're heat-proof. Keeping the lid on a pan when simmering reduces cooking time and saves on fuel.

My favourite saucepan is an old-fashioned steamer, a double-handled pan with a holey bottom, which sits on top of a saucepan of boiling water. It's economical on fuel (potatoes cook in the bottom while veg steam in the top), retains healthy vitamins, and steamed veg are much tastier not soggified by boiling water. I've also worked out a way of doing quick-cook individual steamed puddings, using little dariole moulds topped with aluminium foil!

Kitchen tools   Top priority is a really sharp knife (used with care). Blunt knives need too much pressure. Enlarge handles if necessary (see page 148). A special design may help, eg the 'Rocker' knife, circular with a central wooden handle, which can be held in different ways and cuts by rocking from side to side. Other people prefer 'angled' knives and kitchen tools (roughly L-shaped). Get plenty of plastic bowls and containers – ideal for food preparation and fridge storage, and can be kept at low or high levels with no danger of breakage.

Some optional extras   Food processor: has its advantages, eg for mixing pastry and chopping things, though is fiddly to set up and fiddly to wash. Heavy too. Check operability before you buy and check too you can dismantle it for cleaning. Keep it where you can just slide it towards you when needed. *Electric mixer:* go for a cheaper, lighter one. Before you buy, try it for weight and grip, try out the beater release button, the on/off switch, try for ease of fixing and releasing from a stand. *Kitchen timer:* saves frequent treks to see how the cooking's doing; the sort you hang round your neck are good. *Electric knives* might be useful though the blades are fiddly to put in and take out. *Cookrest/ bookstand* keeps the cookbook open for you. *Egg separator* is a handy gadget for separating yolks from whites.

Waste bins   Separate waste bins for 'dry rubbish' and 'wet or potentially smelly rubbish' mean you don't have to empty the former quite so frequently. Swing top waste bins are easier than pedal bins. Polythene bags put inside a bin save cleaning it out. In smaller bins plastic bags with handles on, saved from shopping trips, make handling easier. Bin carriers are available if you have to take rubbish outside yourself (eg from Ease-E-Load Trolleys). Some local authorities will let you off having to move a wheelie-bin to the gate if you provide a doctor's or OT's certificate explaining that you can't.

Cooking tips

Sit and *think through* all the steps first. Read the recipe all the way through and picture how best to tackle each stage. Next collect together everything you'll need from start to finish, then sit down again to get on with the actual preparation and cooking.

Change your cooking methods   Switch from making hot and heavy casseroles to oven-top stewing, pot roasting, grilling and steaming, or use table-top appliances like the slow cooker, portable grill, or microwave.

Use more convenience foods, eg canned, frozen, packet, ready-made. The nutrition and healthy eating guides listed on page 69 will help you judge the nutritional value of differently processed and packaged foods.

Go for sliced bread, soft easy-spread margarine, etc. Keep a good stock of tinned meat and poultry, tuna and sardines (forget the key – use an electric can opener), packets and tubs of dried vegetables and flaked onions to see you through days you can't get out. Even a small freezer compartment in a fridge can be used for stocks of frozen cod steaks, beefburgers, chickenburgers, as good 'basics'.

Mix convenience with inspiration, eg get sweet or savoury pie fillings and add extra veg or personal toppings. Enliven grilled sausages and other meats with packet sauces (eg Crosse and Blackwell 'Bonne Cuisine' – simply add water and stir) or with instant garnishes like garlicky soft herb cheese or red currant jelly (good on lamb chops). Tins of soup or packets are an easy way to make stews and casseroles tastier, or can be adapted (using less liquid than for soup) for use as a sauce (eg half a packet of make-in-a-cup chicken soup makes a lovely sauce for grilled chicken pieces). Adapt stir-fry techniques for healthier, less fuel-consuming dishes. More time has to be spent on cutting up and preparing the food (which some people may find difficult) but food prepared in advance can be stored for a few hours in plastic bags in the fridge. Use all-in-one recipes, eg for cakes.

Vegetables   Simplify traditional ways of peeling/serving veg, eg runner beans don't really need slicing and taste juicier if simply broken into bite-sized chunks, and steamed, preferably. Boil or bake potatoes in their cleaned jackets for eating as they are or for DIY peeling by everyone at the table. Or plunge them into cold water after boiling, then peel. Or use instant spuds. Or serve rice or pasta instead (a little oil in the cooking water stops it all sticking together).

If you can't avoid peeling veg, try a spiked board to hold the veg still and choose from the variety of peelers available – I use a swivel type (eg Skyline speed peeler), which can be used towards or, as I prefer, away from me. Enlarge the handle if necessary. Other people prefer a wide-grip peeler, with a handle you can slip your fingers through, and which needs little wrist movement. Or reverse the process and rub the potato against a stationary grater/peeler device.

Avoid lifting heavy panfuls of hot water to strain veg by cooking veg in a lift-out wire-mesh basket, eg a chip basket: some fold. Or lift the veg out with a large perforated straining spoon. Or rest the pan on the sink edge and tip it out over a strainer/colander. Or try my favourite double-decker steamer instead.

Pastry Use frozen ready-made, or use the food-processor to mix your own. Make more than you need and store some. Shortcrust pastry mixture, before water's added, keeps for several days in a jar or plastic bag in a fridge. With sugar added it's a handy quick crumble mixture. Use a pastry brush dipped in cooking oil to grease pastry dishes and cake tins, or use Bakewell parchment non-stick lining paper.

Pastry substitutes for savoury dishes Top thick stew-type tinned fillings with instant mash, flavoured with butter or cheese. Or use scone dough topping (*cobbler*) – lighter and easier to roll than ordinary pastry. Or buttered crumbs, freshly made in a food processor, or crushed crisps (crush in a plastic bag using rolling pin). Or try a *moussaka* topping: – blend two well-beaten eggs with two rounded tablespoonfuls of flour, beat in a carton of natural yoghurt. Pour over the filling and bake in a medium oven for 25 – 35 minutes till set and golden. Or use a *charlotte* topping: – cut the crusts off sliced bread, butter well, arrange in slices or triangles over cooked dish, and bake for 15 – 20 minutes in a medium oven till crisp.

Line a greased pie dish with **instant mash** made up with half the usual quantity of water plus an ounce of melted butter. Press out and line a pie-plate using your fingers. Fill for example with sliced tomatoes, and pour over 1/4 pint single cream or top of the milk mixed with cheese. Bake for 15 – 20 minutes in a hot oven until golden brown. Or line a pie dish with overlapping slices of buttered bread, or crushed cheesey biscuits. Or use scone dough as a pizza base. Or, even easier, cut **rounds out of bread** slices with a biscuit cutter, spread with a little melted butter, fit each one gently into a tartlet tin, put a small piece of foil in the centre of each held in place with dried beans and bake in the centre of a hot oven for 10 minutes or less till crisp and golden. Take out and add filling (eg cooked anchovies/tomato paste/onions/egg).

Pastry substitutes for sweet dishes Adapt cobbler, charlotte, crumble topping or bread slice rounds for sweet dishes by adding sugar and using tinned fruit fillings. Or top with marshmallows arranged over a cooked filling and grilled till lightly browned.

Make a base for sweet flans with crushed digestive biscuits, 4 oz mixed with 2 oz melted butter, crushed in a food processor or broken into a plastic bag and bashed with a rolling pin. Or use Rice Crispies or cornflakes: – melt together 2 tablespoonfuls of syrup, and 1 oz butter to 3 oz Rice Crispies. Toss well to coat, then press into the flan tin and chill. Fill with Angel Delight or icecream or fruit and jelly. Slices of swiss roll held together with jelly also make a good base for a sweet dish.

Look at the recipe books listed at the end of this chapter for more ideas on making cooking easier, without cutting down on interest and variety.

Homecare

First, some tips from Pamela Waterhouse:

"The main thing is to do only a little at a time and to do only what is strictly necessary.

The good thing about having arthritis is that people do not criticise when they see a layer of dust! Invest in a good lightweight Hoover and slosh disinfectant on various surfaces and it's surprising how clean the house seems! I wear rubber gloves when doing dishes to protect the joints from exposure to extremes of temperature. Ron has mounted a large drainer on the wall for me. I keep all the everyday dishes on this so I never have to dry dishes. I also have a tube which I push on the tap so that I can rinse the dishes on the rack without having to hold them. Better still is when my husband does the dishes – which is most nights, luckily!

"I usually dry clothes indoors because it saves all the bending and stretching and the running out when it rains. I arrange the clothes really carefully and ease out any creases. It's surprising how this cuts down on the ironing."

If you can't manage heavier housework yourself it may be worth paying someone to do it for you, or ask if the social services can help. You may or may not have to pay something. Have a planned routine for each visit, to make the most of the limited time available.

If you do it yourself, don't try to do everything at once. 'Think before you act'. Spread it over the whole week. Balance activity with rest. Wear working splints if prescribed. Avoid concentrating strain on one or two joints; spread it over as many joints as possible, eg use both hands to carry objects or use a trolley. If you live with other people *do* stop them *creating* unnecessary work for you and *do* make them do at least their share (eg get the men to iron their own shirts, make everyone swop careless TTJA habits ('throwing-things-just-anywhere') for PETA ('putting-each-thing-away') habits.

Cleaning A long-handled dustpan and brush saves bending. Pad handles for an easier grip. Go for an upright lightweight (and cheaper) vacuum cleaner, or a lightweight electric carpet sweeper. Make sure you can empty it OK. The Sunflower Vac handle fits on most upright vacuum cleaners, carpet sweepers, etc, so you can use both hands (Notts Rehab).

Clean floors with a long-handled squeegee type sponge mop, one of those with a special hinge on the handle for squeezing dry. A similar, smaller version with a telescopic handle exists for window cleaning. Use a long-handled feather duster for dusting. A clean long-handled artist's paintbrush helps get dust out of awkward cracks – try a dab of furniture polish on it. Cottonwool 'buds' are useful too, eg for getting behind taps. For cleaning the bath use a long-handled sponge or a cloth/sponge gripped in your longreach. Better still, keep a long-handled brush and washing up liquid permanently by the bath and train bath users to clean up after themselves.

When using aerosol cans, push down with the palm of your hand, instead of thumb or finger tip. You can also get special aerosol handles (eg from Medipost) to make aerosol cans easier to use or the OT department might make you one.

Laundry Try spreading it through the week. Some town dwellers might find taking it to a launderette for a service wash easier than doing it at home. Someone from a local voluntary organisation might help fetch and carry it.

For washing at home, a combined automatic washer-tumble drier is best. I find a front-loader easier than a top-loader, as I can load it with my longreach gadget and unload it using gravity to help pull things out into a basket below the door. A low machine could be raised on a plinth. Washing machines are expensive, so wait till the sales are on or consider buying second-hand (see page 161), but do make sure it works safely, and that you can operate it OK before buying.

A folding laundry basket (eg Chester-Care's 'Laundry Maid') holds a machine-load of washing at waist height. For outdoor drying try a rotary drier fixed at lower than normal height. Some have a winding handle so clothes can be loaded at a convenient height and then raised by turning the handle (*do* try before you buy in case it's too difficult). Or go for a clothes line with a pulley system to allow loading from one position. Try hangers on the line to drape blouses, shirts, trousers, skirts, for quicker drying in better shape.

Or dry inside over the bath to avoid rushing in and out when it rains. Look in hardware and department stores at the variety of washing lines and airers available before buying.

Ironing Cut down on ironing by folding wet clothes carefully to avoid creasing while they dry. Eliminate any unnecessary ironing, eg of bedlinen, of underclothes. For unavoidable ironing try a lightweight travel iron. Sit down to iron. A wall-mounted folding board without legs might make this easier, eg from Relax Housewares or Panilet Tables. Or do occasional ironing on a very well-padded kitchen table. Consider paying someone else to do it for you if there are no eager volunteers around.

Further information

Low-cost starter information

- *Your Home and Your Rheumatism*, by Barbara Ansell MD FRCP and Sheila Lawton MBA OT, free booklet produced by ARC (send large SAE). Includes lots of photos showing joint care and housework dos and don'ts.
- Also from ARC *Are You Sitting Comfortably?*, guide to choosing easy chairs.
- *Ideas to Assist Those with Arthritis, Aids and Ideas to Help Those who Cannot Bend*, and *Household Equipment* (the most detailed), three low-cost leaflets produced by DLF, packed with information and suppliers' addresses.
- Alas, no longer in print, but so good I mention it so you can agitate for a reprint!: *Rheumatoid Arthritis: Helping Yourself*, 30 page booklet, packed with brightly written and illustrated self-help guidelines, produced by the Occupational Therapy Department and Department of Health Education, Doncaster Health Authority.
- The catalogues of the specialist suppliers listed on page 144 are free, packed with ideas and usually have helpful illustrations. Send for all of them!

Other useful books

- *Arthritis – An Equipment Guide*, and *Home Management*, both in the Disability Information Trusts's *Equipment for Disabled People* series. Really excellent, well-illustrated guides full of up-to-date ideas and suppliers' addresses for ordinary as well as disabled equipment, plus DIY ideas too. Even if you don't get your own copy, do see if your library or OT can let you see one.
- *The Arthritis Helpbook* by Kate Lorig and James F Fries (Souvenir Press) has two well-illustrated chapters 'Protecting your joints' and 'Self-helpers: 100 hints and aids'
- *Coping with Disability*, Peggy Jay (DLF, 1991)
- *Kitchen Sense for Disabled People*, edited by Gwen Conacher (DLF, 1986)

'Non-arthritic' books

- Shirley Conran's original *Superwoman* was commissioned by a male editor who wanted a book which would teach him housework. Since then there's been a spate of books (including a revised edition of *Superwoman*) aimed at making life easier for housepersons, bachelor men and working wives, many of them the sort of tips a clever grandmother passes on. Scour them for tips to make life easier.
- *Tips and Wrinkles* (a treasury of ways to save time, energy and money around the home), collected and edited by Mary Sansbury and Anne Fowler (Pan).
- *Household Hints* by Hilary Davies (Fontana), full of ingenious tips on dealing with day to day problems and chores.
- *Supertips 1* and *Supertips 2* by Moyra Bremner (Hodder and Stoughton Coronet) – masses of useful tips, how to look after home, stomach (food and drink, buying and

storing), yourself (clothes and shoes, laundering and stains, gloss and glamour, possets and potions) and pets, etc, at least cost and with greatest ease

And three books specially aimed at educating men who claim they don't know the first thing about the skills (and benefits) of housework:

- Don Aslett's *Who Says It's A Woman's Job To Clean?* and *Is There Life after Housework?* (Exley Publications) and
- Sonya Mills *Bachelor's Buttons* (Corgi), written to educate the sort of fellow who tried to reheat a plastic bowl of pudding in the oven and found it welded to the metal shelf. Aimed at bachelors on their own, but helpful tips for anyone.

Healthy eating

You need to be sure that your diet is healthy and well-balanced, even if mobility and other problems limit what shopping and cooking you can do. Two booklets will help: *Eating Well on a Budget* (Age Concern), and *Guide to Healthy Eating* (free from the Health Education Authority), which includes a guide to further reading. There's also a fascinating, low-cost book *Manual of Nutrition* (HMSO), packed with information about all the important nutrients, including vitamins and minerals, the foods that provide them, and how they're affected by different methods of cooking and processing, etc.

Recipe books

Once you've got one or two good basic cookery books (eg by *Good Housekeeping* and/or Delia Smith), go for a few 'theme' hardbacks or paperbacks, too, especially if cookery's a hobby, as it is for me. By theme books I mean work out what sort of cooking suits you best, and borrow or buy books specialising in those areas.

For instance I go for 'quick cook' books full of shortcut tips and ways of making convenience food more interesting. I also go for 'cook ahead' books, 'ices and frozen dessert' books, and books that teach me the basic principles of these specialities so I can then devise my own variations. Other themes you might go for are microwave cookery, steamed foods, stir fry, deep freeze cookery, or books which include interesting sauces to dress up plain grilled or roasted meat. If you find a particular product you like to use (eg tuna, sardines, Angel Delight, canned fruit) why not write to the manufacturer to see if they produce any free recipe leaflets to give you further ideas?

Here's a handful of recipe books (mostly paperbacks) to be going on with:

- *Are You Cooking Comfortably?* by Ann McFarlane (sponsored by British Gas for Arthritis Care, 1986). Imaginative practical ideas and shortcuts, culled from Ann's personal experience of having RA since she was four.
- *Quick Cook* (recipes in under thirty minutes) by Beryl Downing (Penguin). Includes chapters on low cholesterol and slimmers' recipes.
- *Easy Cooking for One or Two* by Louise Davies (Penguin). Written with the over-60s in mind, but ideal for anyone who wants to cook interesting, nourishing food with as little as possible elbow grease!
- Shirley Goode's books, eg *Goode for One* and *The Shirley Goode Kitchen* (BBC Books) are cheap, chattily written, and packed with excellent hints and recipes.
- *Microwave Cookery for One* by Cecilia Norman (Grafton)
- *Microwave Cookery for One* by Annette Yates (Elliot Rightway Books)
- Good Housekeeping's *Family Microwave Cookery*. The whole Good Housekeeping range is worth finding out about. Write for a publications list to Ebury Press.
- *Ices Galore* by Helge Rubinstein and Sheila Bush (Hodder and Stoughton Coronet)
- *Making Ice-Cream and Cold Sweets* by Bee Nilson (Mayflower)
- *The Yoghurt Book* by Arto der Haroutunian (Penguin)
- *Steaming Cookbook* by Hilary Walden (Collins)

Chapter twenty-three

SHOPPING

How you manage your shopping depends on so many things – where you live, how near and accessible your shops are, whether or not you can drive, what help friends, relatives, or other people can give, what your finances are like. It depends too on what problems the arthritis lumbers you with at any particular time. Shopping around and impulse buying, once taken for granted, may have to give way to a carefully thought-out plan of campaign. This chapter looks at ideas from which to pick and choose to suit your needs.

Plan ahead

As always! Use the brain to ease the strain. Keep a spiral-bound notebook in the hall, in the kitchen, in your bag. Jot down what you'll need as supplies run out. That way you'll avoid forgetting things and having to use your limited energy rations to go back for them.

Bulk buy if feasible and affordable, and if you can solve carrying and storage problems. Would one or more neighbours go halves with you on special bulk buy offers? Consider bulk buying small non-food items as well as large (eg before the bad winter weather sets in, stock up on 'toiletries' – shampoo, soaps, face cream, toothpaste, sanitary tampons, etc) and 'stationery' – envelopes, paper, stamps, greetings cards, etc).

Stocking up on freezer food and other convenience foods helps cut down on shopping trips and ensures you've food in stock for any housebound periods. Make use of any local delivery services, especially for heavy goods. Milkmen, for instance, often deliver a range of goods besides milk, eg fruit juices, potatoes, bread, chickens, eggs. Home deliveries from food shops are less frequent than they used to be, but it's always worth enquiring.

Lots of shopping, and 'window shopping', can be done from your armchair. More about that in a moment. For any unavoidable 'shopping around', make your phone work for you. Find out about prices, store access, etc, by phone before you leave the house. Phone when you know the shop won't be too busy.

Where to shop?

Local shops may be nearer and more accessible, though sometimes more expensive. However, friendly staff who know your needs are a bonus, and some local shops do still make home deliveries. Town centre shops may pose problems with parking and walking. Getting an orange disc may help. If ramped pavement kerbs would be a help but aren't where you (and probably other people too) need them, write to the local council asking if they can do something and/or contact your local DIAL and Access Group too.

Some shops without public lifts have a staff or goods lift you can use on request, for instance in Boots, Marks and Spencer, C & A, and Littlewoods. Some shops perversely have only one escalator, going *up*. However, when I asked in one such shop if there was any way of coming down other than the steep stairs, they said 'yes'. – All I had to do was ask, and the escalator would be stopped, and put into reverse action. Wonderful! So it's always worth asking.

Superstores, with everything under one roof, have certain advantages, though can sometimes prove *too* large if you have walking problems. Writing a list beforehand avoids wasting time and energy (and cuts down impulse buying), especially if you can write the list in the order you're likely to come across the goods.

Superstores get horribly crowded, so avoid peak times if possible, especially Friday and

Saturday. Phone to ask when the quiet times are. If you shop alone and need help loading and unloading a trolley, or reaching up and down, phone in advance to see if an assistant could come round with you: at quiet times this can sometimes be arranged. In February 1987, *Good Housekeeping* published a survey of seven superstores. Those which specifically said staff assistance was available for disabled shoppers were Co-op superstores, Presto, Safeway, Sainsbury's, Tesco, Waitrose. When her local Gateway supermarket ran out of special trolleys for disabled people, one shopper with arthritis was given the services of a member of staff to go round with her to pick items from inaccessible shelves. The manager said the service was available to anyone who asked.

My little electric scoota is ideal for whizzing round superstores. However I still need someone with me to load and unload it from the car, it can't carry much, and I still need to overcome the reaching up and down from shelves problem... The great advantage is that I can see just what's available, instead of having to guess from my seat at home. An occasional refresher trip helps keep me up to date for when I'm writing the list for my gallant friend who normally does the shopping.

Carrying shopping
Avoid carrying heavy bags or handbags: they'll strain and damage your joints. Use shoulder bags and shopping trolleys on wheels. Cycle shops sell good-sized shoulder bags. Always keep with you a spare plastic bag or two 'just in case' – those with big handles so you can slip them over your forearm instead of having to grip them. Some shopping trolleys have built-in seats, so you can take a rest now and again (eg from suppliers on page 144). Some shopping trolleys have two wheels, others four. Some are better pushed, some better pulled. Handle designs vary a lot, so look at different types before buying. If necessary enlarge the handle (see page 148) to improve your grip.

Stopping to rest
Try a shopping trolley with a seat, or a folding stool/stick seat (see page 182). Try asking for a seat if you need one. Persuade shops to join the 'We Care with a Chair' campaign, which encourages shopkeepers to provide a chair for elderly or disabled people and display a sticker showing a shopkeeper offering a chair. (Details from Age Concern.)

Paying
Avoid purses with a tight catch and press fastening. A children's long flexible pencil case was my solution, the sort that opens with a zip. Ask the cashier to count the change into your purse (while you watch carefully) rather than into your uncooperative hand. Or ask "Can I take the change from *your* hand, please?". Or use Switch or credit cards, or cheques which can be machine-completed in the shop.

Loos and getting caught short
Needing a loo can be a nightmare when you can move only slowly and with difficulty. Watch what you drink before going out. Avoid drinks like coffee or tea or cola drinks which are 'diuretics'. By definition they make you need to pass urine more frequently!

Many superstores now have loos. Larger chain stores like Marks and Spencer will let disabled people use a staff loo on request. If you look fairly healthy (as many of us deceptively do) you might need to explain briefly "Could I possibly use the staff loo/ toilet? I've got rheumatoid arthritis and have problems walking far..". If you're shy about asking see if your doctor would write a short note for you to produce when needed.

Public loos aren't always accessible. The National Key Scheme for toilets for disabled people provides you with a key to unlock some special loos. Ask your local social services for one (there may be a small charge), or apply to RADAR (small cost), who also publish a national list of these special loos, handy if you're going on a long journey.

For some people getting caught short becomes such a problem it stops them going out. Why not think about wearing a discreet yet efficient incontinence garment or using a discreet urinal (eg in the car)? Some can be bought by mail order. Try Attends Advisory Service, Procter & Gamble, or write or talk to the DLF's sympathetic, well informed Incontinence Adviser, or start by looking at what's available in commercial catalogues listed on page 144, and see my note on the same page about portable urine bottles.

Help from other people
Many of us have to rely on friends and relatives to shop for us. My wonderful friend loathes shopping, but armed with my list, whizzes round Safeways for me every fortnight or so. I manage on my own to get to a smaller, local shop, now and again.

Some friends really enjoy the chance to help, and the chance to spend someone else's money for them! Those of us who go out to work may find workmates willing to pick up odds and ends in the lunch-hour. One regular visitor to the local fruit and veg market knows I'll go halves with her on any particularly good special offer she comes across. Train your friends (subtly) to let you know which shops they're off to so you can place an order. Keep it within reason though – don't go asking for stamps when they're doing their darndest to avoid wasting precious lunchtime minutes on post office queues.

Ask people to tell you about special offers they come across, and to bring back any free leaflets. To help when you're compiling a shopping list keep yourself informed of what's in season, and therefore cheaper. Some local free papers have a weekly good buys column, and many cook books contain 'what's in season when' guides.

Some local authority Home Care schemes will do some shopping for you if you're badly disabled and there's no one else to help. Ask the Home Care Supervisor. Or members of local voluntary organisations (eg youth groups, good neighbour schemes, WRVS or British Red Cross) may be able to help. Find out through your social worker or OT, your Citizens' Advice Bureau, your local council for voluntary service, or DIAL.

Communicate your needs
Help yourself (and others too – other YPAs, mothers with prams, elderly people) by writing in with suggestions for improvements. Join your local Access Group if there is one. RADAR publishes a factsheet on how they work and how to contact a local group. Write to big stores about seats, creches, heavy doors, access problems; to the local council about access and mobility problems, eg ramped pavements, parking facilities, road crossings, public loos. Copy your letters to the local MP/councillor. Comment on any reported planning proposals – does the proposed new shopping centre have loos, rest areas, mother-and-baby facilities, level access? Keep your letters polite. Avoid being aggressive. Keep the reader on your side. Many omissions or hazards aren't intentional, but due to a lack of awareness.

Special schemes
Various schemes now exist to help people with mobility problems shop, though some are limited in the hours and days available. In some areas there are excellent shopmobility schemes, providing manual or powered wheelchairs. For details send an SAE to the National Federation of Shopmobility, or find out what's available locally from an access guide, DIAL or local tourist information office. Some Dial-a-Ride schemes have regular shopping trips to specific superstores or high streets. Some shops arrange special opening hours for disabled people, especially just before Christmas. You'll hear through the local newspaper or radio, or perhaps if you're on the social services register of disabled people.

Futuristic shopping schemes
Some people are already shopping by computer. Some libraries and community centres, eg

in Gateshead, have special arrangements so disabled people can transmit shopping orders to a telephone centre and have the goods delivered to their home. Chris Curry, former head of Acorn, has been working on a special shopping-by-computer system, called Keyline. The plan is to give the computer away free, and that it will let armchair shoppers buy goods or services from Littlewoods, Mothercare, Gateway, Asda, Ladbroke, William Hill, Freemans, Grattan, NatWest and Midland Banks.

Armchair shopping

You can get practically anything by post except daily food supplies. As shops get unbearably overcrowded even for the fittest of the fit, more and more mail order opportunities are springing up. I certainly don't know how I'd manage without! Here are just some of the things I've bought by mail order over the years – clothes, shoes, garden equipment/seeds/plants, all sorts of presents, toys, stationery, toiletries, cosmetics, exotic herbs and spices, books, handcraft materials, kitchen gadgets and equipment, disability gadgets, furniture, wines, buttons, catering-size packs of Clingfilm and aluminium foil, dress fabrics and patterns, theatre tickets, maps, etc, etc!

Set up your own home shopping centre, using an old shopping bag or a cardboard box. Into it throw any promising leaflets or catalogues or small ads or newspaper/magazine items you and friends and family come across. Let everyone know you're a leaflet addict! Keep handy a stock of cheap envelopes, writing paper, and stamps. A stock of those tiny ready-stick labels with your address already printed saves finger wear-and-tear – (from Able-Label, Steepleprint Ltd). My cardboard box now houses a vast collection of leaflets through which I take a very enjoyable armchair shopping trip whenever I want. Even doing the Christmas present shopping is now a positive pleasure.

There are some pitfalls to be wary of, however. Some of the traditional mail order houses produce bulky catalogues, very awkward for arthriticky fingers. They pester you to become an agent, which can be complicated and involves you, in turn, having to pester people to buy from you, and to pay up when the goods arrive. You're responsible for all payments, and for sending back any unsatisfactory goods. These I avoid.

Admittedly I do know of one YPA in a residential home who actually enjoys being an agent as a hobby. If you wanted access to the vast choice in one of those catalogues *without* the hassle of becoming an agent yourself, you could ask for the address of an agent nearby, but stress very firmly that *you* don't want to become an agent, and keep a copy of your letter as evidence.

I keep instead to the smaller leaflets and catalogues for the personal shopper, some of them produced by charities and high street stores, plus anything else that catches my eye in magazines and newspapers. Examples of just a few follow. Don't hesitate too to write to or telephone a manufacturer if you've seen an ad for something that takes your fancy but needs to be hunted out on unwilling feet. By writing instead of foot-slogging I managed to get a special bra for myself from one manufacturer and from another, the address of a cordless beard trimmer supplier for my boyfriend's Christmas present.

Before you do any mail order shopping, check on your legal rights by getting the free leaflet *Buying By Post* from the Office of Fair Trading. Follow these guidelines, too:

● Keep to reputable firms.
● Think carefully before you order, to be sure you get just what you want; if it isn't, you'll need to find someone willing to take the return parcel to the post office for you.
● Always keep a dated copy of your order in case of problems.
● Always write your name and address in block capitals (or use ready-printed sticky labels)
● Some firms now accept telephone orders. – Before you phone, write down exactly what you want, with any reference numbers (double-checked), so you don't waste costly

telephone time. Note too the price of the article, any delivery charges, measurements, sizes and colours. You might have to speak to a telephone answering machine, so be prepared!

● If the goods are unsuitable, make sure you send them back in immaculate condition within the time stated – usually 14 days from the delivery date. If the goods are actually faulty, you can claim the cost of the return postage. If you need to complain and don't get any result by writing direct to the company, contact the Mail Order Traders' Association. If the goods were advertised in a newspaper or magazine, complain too to the advertising manager.

● To avoid having to send large sums of money in advance, try the cash-on-delivery (COD) system. It costs a bit extra, but is sensible with a firm you know nothing about

● If the flood of mail gets out of hand and you want to stop it – or, alternatively, if you want more (on specific subjects) – write to the Mailing Preference Service.

Some mail order firms
Inclusion in this book does not necessarily imply recommendation.
Always check prices, availability, and suitability before parting with any money.

Details of other firms are scattered around the book, for instance:
–   books by post – see pages 114 and 281 (including J Barnicoat for paperbacks)
–   special gadgets for overcoming disabilities – see specific chapters, including chapter 20 and page 144
–   craft supplies, including DIY jewellery making – see pages 283/284
–   some clothing items (including men's) – see page 154 onwards
–   gardening goodies – see page 287
–   maternity wear and accessories, children's toys, etc – see page 236

Full addresses are in Appendix 2. Send a stamp, or large SAE for charity catalogues. Many charities now sell a colourful range of items not just at Christmas, but all year round. You'll find all sorts of useful items tucked away in the most unexpected leaflets, for instance in *Stockingfillas* toy leaflet (see page 287) you'll find an inflatable neck pillow.

Some charity catalogues
–   *ARC Cards Ltd* (part of *The Arthritis and Rheumatism Council* – cards, gifts, useful kitchen, gardening, household gadgets, etc
–   *OXFAM* Trading – wide variety of colourful goods from around the world, eg clothes, jewellery, bags, household items, cane and rattan items, toys, stationery, etc.
–   *Traidcraft* – similarly fascinating array of mainly third-world products includes colourful clothes and jewellery, recycled paper and cards, teas, coffees, dried fruit
–   *Unravel Mills* – small selection of products made by mentally ill people in Preston, includes economical dining seat cushions and practical folding wooden side tables
–   *World Wide Fund for Nature* – unusual and fun fashions (eg animal sweatshirts, T shirts), gifts, gadgets, books, etc
–   *Save the Children Fund* – packed with bright goodies and gifts

Two particularly good sources of an amazing variety of useful gadgets and knick-knacks
–   *Studio Cards* – nearly 300 pages, well worth getting. Not just cards and stationery, but also gifts and gadgets galore for kitchen, house, garden car and DIY, toys, toiletries, jewellery, fashion accessories. Discounts.
–   *Lakeland Plastics* – everything for home cooking, fridge, freezer, microwave, etc. Enormous range of labour-saving and space-saving ideas, eg plastic pudding basins with lids, catering packs of foil and clingfilm, storage containers, cake tin liners.

A miscellany

- *Marks & Spencer* – furniture, household goodies
- *Index* – all items found in Littlewoods' index shops. Home delivery is possible, free for some items, and at a small charge for others
- *Foam for Comfort Ltd* – will cut foam and latex to any shape or size, useful for specially firm cushions or wedges
- *The Country Garden* – kitchen, garden and household essentials and nifty gadgets
- *St Saviour's Nurseries* – lovely carnations and freesias by post, from the Channel Islands. Friendly and efficient service, cheaper than traditional ways of sending flowers long-distance. Will take written or phoned (credit card) orders
- *Gardeners' Royal Benevolent Society* – tiny leaflet, but particularly good for huge attractive lightweight PVC coated shopping bags
- *Nature's Best* – vitamins and minerals, evening primrose oil, fish oils and toiletries
- *Fox's Spices Ltd* – exotic spices by mail-order (see Culpeper, too)
- *Curry Club* – 'curryphernalia for the curryholic': spices, curry powders, pastes, utensils, pickles and chutneys, poppadums, coconut milk, rose water, recipe books
- *A E Rodda & Son* – for the occasional treat of clotted cream by post!
- *Ashdown Smokers* – vast range, eg smoked salmon, haddock, kippers, cheeses, prawns, game – nice for unusual presents or occasional self-indulgence
- *HMV (UK) Ltd* – records and cassettes by post
- *Video Club* – mail-order club: you make a commitment to order two introductory videos plus at least a further three during your first year of membership. *Britannia Home Videos* is another club.
- *Past Times* – unusual and attractive gifts, jewellery (good earrings), fashion accessories, etc, inspired by Britain's heritage, eg Celtic, Medieval, Tudor, Victorian, art nouveau, art deco
- *National Trust (Enterprises) Ltd* – attractive range of gifts, table linen, books, toiletries, practical gadgets (eg useful walking/folding stool)
- *V & A Enterprises Ltd* – unusual gifts, toys, jewellery, etc
- *Natural History Museum Collection* – includes rubber shark bicycle hooter, dragonfly earrings, sweatshirts, kingfisher teapot
- *Nature Company Catalogue* – all sorts from inflatable penguins to grasshopper glove puppets, from jewellery and toys to a rainforest jacket
- *Factory Shop Guides* – not exactly mail order, but cheap information-packed books on how, when and wear you can buy direct from a manufacturer, and save money. Includes wheelchair-accessibility and cup-of-tea availability.
- *The Poster Shop* – posters
- *Mandolin Puzzles* – special jigsaw puzzles by post, (500 to 1500 pieces)
- *Jigrolls* – in which you can roll up an unfinished jigsaw for another day

Cosmetics and skin-care products

- *Body Shop International plc* – vast range, as available in Body Shops locally
- *Allergy Shop* – send first-class stamp for details of skin-care and household range (includes odour-free disinfectant, vegetable-based furniture polish, etc) and useful booklets
- *Efamol Ltd* – skin-care products containing evening primrose oil
- *Cosmetics To Go* – catalogue's a highly entertaining read of an amazing variety of cosmetics and toiletries with weird and wonderful names, all non-animal tested
- *Yves Rocher* – plant-based beauty products
- *Woods of Windsor* – includes lavender, wild rose, lily of the valley, honeysuckle, wild orchid, forget-me-not perfume, soap, bath products, hand and body lotions, shampoos. Also special Woods of Windsor range for gentlemen plus pot-pourri and

home fragrances
- *Culpeper Ltd* – traditional skin-care and cosmetics range, also essential plant oils, herbal items, spices, pot-pourri, assorted gifts, etc
- *Avon* – armchair rather than mail order shopping. Products sold by local representatives visiting your home.

Fashion catalogues

These are small personal shopping, not huge agency-sized catalogues.
- *Zig Zag Designer Knitwear* – bright colourful original knitwear for all ages
- *Cotswold Woollens* – bright imaginative knitwear and leisurewear coordinates
- *Penny Plain* – beautiful but mostly pricey knitwear and coordinates, some jewellery
- *Rosalie Courage* – attractive picture woollens, shirts and skirts
- *Magic by Mail* – colourful easy-fitting casuals, some smart, all cheap, male too
- *Together (Rainbow Home Shopping)* – jeans and easy living, lively clothes and smart, all cheap
- *Hawkshead Countrywear* – stylish leisure- and outerwear (some men's), shirts, casuals, accessories. Cottons, canvas, leathers and woollens
- *Clothkits* – original and reasonably priced knitwear and clothing for all the family
- *Nightingales Ltd* – attractive, reasonably priced dresses, and separates, including several front-fastening designs, Victorian-type blouses and nightdresses
- *Sparklers* – quality shirts for women in pure fabrics (some ruffled necks)
- *Trading by Post (Edinburgh Woollen Mill Ltd)* – good quality, reasonably priced classic fashions, coordinates, and woollens, mainly women's, some men's
- *Robert Norfolk plc* – eye-catching coordinates and sweatshirts for all ages
- *Damart* – for women and men, wide range of underwear, especially warm thermals, more glamorous than they used to be. Also good selection of other clothes and outerwear (eg quilted jackets), shoes (some 'fur-lined' for winter), and gadgets
- *Selfridges* – quality fashions, pricey and glamorous
- *Laura Ashley* – clothes, separates, home furnishings and fabrics
- *Monsoon Mail Order* – glossy catalogue, ethnic clothes
- *Richer* – attractive clothes, underwear and shoes for women 5'2" and under
- *Woods of Morecambe* – packed into a tiny catalogue lots of underwear, nightwear, tights and stockings. Mainly for women, but some menswear. Traditional styles include pretty cotton, polycotton, and winceyette nighties, some front-opening bras
- *Mail to Male Ltd* – underwear, socks, pyjamas, etc
- *Bymail* – young fashion, male and female
- *Next Directory* – fashion and accessories for men, women, and children, plus home furnishings
- *Marshall Ward* – fashion and all manner of household and leisure items for all ages, male and female
- *Laurence Corner* – government surplus clothing and equipment
- *Carita House* – designer leisurewear, tracksuits, leg warmers, colourful tights
- *J D Williams: The Special Collection* – fashion, shoes, underwear for men and women, all ages, specially selected for ease of dressing and wearing
- *Jake Mail Order* – small, exclusive, quality clothes at reasonable prices in natural/almost natural fibres
- *Clifford James* – lots of men and women's reasonably priced leather, suede manmade and canvas footwear, some thermal lined, some with velcro® fastenings
- Three no-agency catalogues from Freemans: *Complete Essentials* – fashion; *Images* – elegant fashion; *Editions* – young fashion

Chapter twenty-four

OUT AND ABOUT

Though we YPAs have our fair share of mobility difficulties, and from time to time do let wheels 'take the strain', most of us aren't full-time wheelchair-users. I've written this chapter with that in mind, so if you are, on the contrary, wheelchair-dependent, please bear in mind you'll need more detailed, specialist information and advice. Your healthcare team will help you. So too will many of the other information sources I mention.

One book, *free* to disabled people, and well worth getting however mild or severe your mobility difficulties is *Door to Door* (A guide to transport for people with disabilities), available by post (no stamp needed) from the Department of Transport. It's packed with information – gadgets and benefits, walking and wheelchairs, cars, travel by taxi, bus, train, underground, air, sea, coach, and holiday travel, plus Dial-a-Rides and similar schemes – it could well start you solving problems you thought were insoluble.

The other key book is *Motoring and Mobility for Disabled People* by Ann Darnborough and Derek Kinrade, published by RADAR. It's weighty, but economically priced and jampacked with information on every aspect of getting from A to B.

Out and about on your own two feet

Let's look at the simplest things first, to help those of you who *can* get out and about on your own feet, after a fashion, anyway! However young and deceptively sprightly you look, you probably still welcome ways of cutting down on pain, fatigue, stiffness, plus the frustrations that go with them – call it all 'aggro' for short. Here are just a few ideas for cutting down on the aggro:

- Cut down ruthlessly on inessential activity but *do* do your prescribed exercises. – Strong muscles take the strain off delicate joints
- Don't leave things till the last moment. – Plan ahead so you don't have to rush to meet a deadline or have to make two journeys where one would do. Plan ahead too to avoid peak hours on crowded public transport.
- Accept any help available, whether it's people help or transport help. Remember that other people won't be able to guess how best to help you – you'll probably need to explain, difficult though that can sometimes be.
- The thought of falling can be alarming, especially if you look healthy but (a) can't get up by yourself and (b) already hurt so much anyway. Choose shoes without slippery soles, preferably ridged soles in winter. If you can't avoid leather soles, roughen them with a cheese grater before use. A stick or other walking support can help stop you falling, and also warns other people that maybe you *can't* get up by yourself. If you do fall, an ex-parachutist advised me that if you train yourself automatically to relax rather than tense up, you're less likely to hurt. Worth trying. (Drunks rarely damage themselves, because the drink relaxes them so much.)
- Lessen the misery of waiting in freezing bus shelters by wrapping up well and even using heated gloves or carrying a mini hand-warmer (eg from fishing tackle and sports shops or by post from the Raynaud's Association – see page 155 on keeping warm).
- If you regularly use pavement kerbs that aren't ramped, write to the local authority asking if they could ramp them. A polite letter really can sometimes bring results. – I speak from experience. Likewise, write letters to hard-to-access buildings suggesting

hand-rails by steps, less steep steps, ramps, etc. Join your local Access Group if there is one. Find out from the Access Committee.

● Heavy doors are often a problem. You'll work out your own tricks. If no one's around to help, try either pushing the door with your arm/shoulder, simultaneously jamming your foot or stick in the gap to help prise it open, or push slowly backwards against a door with your behind, having *first* checked that no one's about to pull it open from the other side.

● Think about the advantages of using a stick, however embarrassed or self-conscious you might at first feel. Even if you don't need one for support, just 'wearing a stick' can reduce invisibility problems, alerting people to possible difficulties: the bus driver/ conductor perhaps, so the bus doesn't start hurtling on its way with you only half on; or at a zebra crossing, as a warning to the traffic that you're not able to rush across. Using a stick can also cut down on maddening misinterpretations when people see an apparently healthy young person fall or stumble ('must be drunk or on drugs').

● Using a stick can also help create a 'protection zone' around you, to stop (or attempt to stop) people walking into you with painful consequences for your joints. Plastic carrier bags also create protection zones. I keep meaning to produce cards to hand culprits saying something like 'Please use your eyes to avoid walking into people. You may not realise that what's a mere bump for you can leave a person with arthritis in pain for hours or days afterwards'. Oh yes, and some sticks have a useful knack of accidentally-on-purpose prodding people who thoughtlessly get in the way...

● I know stick-using has its disadvantages too, especially if you don't need one for support – there'll be some Clever Dick who knows better than you and declares 'You don't need a stick at your age, etc' but the benefits might outweigh your wrath at such dumb remarks! If you've been advised to use a stick, do try to get over any qualms. It *can* help avoid worsening physical problems. Using a stick's a small price to pay for making a bionic hip joint last longer, for instance, or for putting off an operation as long as possible. Apparently, by using a stick properly, the loading on a hip can be reduced by 75%. More about sticks in a moment.

● For safety wear reflective bands (from cycle shops) in the dark, and fix reflective strips to sticks and crutches (electric scooters/wheelchairs too, if you use them)

● Read chapter 23, on shopping, for lots more ideas (including letting fingers do the walking, solving loo problems, stopping to rest).

● Disability Information Trust's *Arthritis – An Equipment Guide* and DLF's leaflet on *Walking Aids* include sticks and seat sticks, frames and trolleys, and crutches.

Choosing the right stick

Your doctor, physio or OT can advise on the best stick for you personally. Only a limited range is available under the NHS, and you might prefer to pay out a few pounds to buy a different one. A commercial supplier's leaflet (see page 144), or DLF's list will show what's available, but you should still get professional advice on its suitability for you.

I was amazed at just how much easier the right-shaped handle made things for me. It's a sort of 'mirror shape' of my distorted hand, so every twist and turn fits comfortably and helps spread the load. Don't forget to listen to professional advice on *which* hand to use the stick in. I was horrified to hear a lady say 'no one told me I was using it in the wrong hand'. It should be held at the side *opposite* the weaker leg, and moved forward *with* the weaker leg, so the leg gets all the support it needs. Get professional advice too on correct stick length; it makes a great difference.

A stick should always have a rubber end (ferrule) on the bottom. Avoid smooth ferrules. Choose one with the biggest road-gripping surface that will fit the stick. Keep it clean, and change it for a new one as soon as it starts getting worn down. Larger chemists (eg Boots) and walking stick shops sell them. Commercial suppliers on page 144 sell them by mail order, or you can ask for them under the NHS.

Sticks have minds of their own and easily fall. Maddening if you can't bend to pick yours up. By chance, I'm sure, my stick's handle is shaped so I can lever it up using my foot! But preferring prevention to cure whenever possible, I also fix a loop of ribbon or cord around the stick and loop it over my hand. Hand can then be used if necessary, without the need to work out where to rest the stick (but beware of tripping up over a dangling stick). You can also get special holders to support a stick when fixed to a table.

Try a folding stick if you only want one 'just in case'. You can keep it folded away in a bag till needed. However, closing and opening it up may be difficult, so try out someone else's before you buy, if you can. Chester-Care sell folding sticks; so do Cooper Care and Comfort (folding 'cumfy crutches' and walking frames too). Stick umbrellas are also available, and even walking sticks with an inbuilt shrill alarm (eg from Raymer Ltd).

A stick seat takes the weight off your feet when a seat's not available, and is usually more stable than the familiar shooting stick. Stick seats come in various sizes and weights, and with different types of 'grip'. However many are heavy to carry, and don't usually give as effective support for walking as an ordinary stick. In the right situation though, they can be a boon. I keep one at work to take with me when I have to visit another office where the seats are too low. My boyfriend carries one for me when we're out and about in seatless territories. Mine's made by Phillips of Axminster, with a canvas seat, and comes in four heights. (Also from suppliers on page 144.) G & C Products make lightweight 'Flipsticks', with a flick-down triangular seat you can perch on, and which pack into a neat carrying-pouch. You'd need to be sure you could balance comfortably and safely before you buy one.

Manual and electric wheelchairs

Most of us aren't full-time wheelchair users though might use one temporarily now and again. Sometimes it's the lesser of two evils – uncooperative legs either confine you to stay miserably at home alone, or you opt for the chair so you can face going out with the family around the zoo or to the seaside or whatever.

Self-propelled wheelchairs are difficult for people with weak hands and stiff shoulders, and satisfactory wheelchair pushers few and far between! Pushing's an underestimated skill. Educate your pusher by getting the booklet *How to Push a Wheelchair* by David Griffiths and David Wynne, from the Disabled Motorists' Club.

You might have other ideas. A powered chair or electric 'scooter' definitely makes you feel independent, and you don't need a driving licence! Scooters are attractive, and useful 'icebreakers'. Children love the jolly bright yellow scoota I use from time to time. You can even whiz round large exhibitions and superstores on them. Though some have special 'kerb-climbers', kerbs are usually impossible, so you need to be sure of ramped kerbs on your route, or have a strong muscle man to hand, as the scooter batteries make them extremely heavy to lift. Beware of losing your concentration: some can tip over if you don't watch where you're going. But advantages usually outweigh the disadvantages:

> *"For days out I have my 'Lark' scooter. My husband and I take it in turns to ride because I like to stretch my legs now and again. The scooter creates no end of interest when we are out and I've given several people a ride to try it out. On a good day I don't use it at all! I bought mine second-hand and find it very useful."* (Jacqueline S, who's had RA since her early 20s, now in her mid 50s.)

Jennifer Purple resigned herself to a very long wait when she heard how much she'd have to save to get a battery car, but a friend's mum got in on the act:

> *"Unknown to me she spoke to her daughter and about two weeks later they popped round. They suggested they raised the money towards my battery car and their aim was to raise £2000 in about 18 months. After letting people in the village know of their plans*

they started off with a garden party on a sunny day in May with lots of people there... At the end of the day over £300 was raised. This is how things went on, the villagers raised money with discos, jokes and sponsored events. After one year over one thousand pounds was raised.

"I had still been collecting Battery Car leaflets, etc. We asked for a demonstration, but unfortunately I found I could not manage the handlebars with the controls on. I was so disappointed, as I liked it so much. But all was not lost, the demonstrator suggested cutting off the handlebars and using a joystick control, something like a helicopter. So this was how it was produced, straight from the production line, brand new. One month later it was delivered...complete with joystick control and a seat belt." (*In Contact*)

Kay Jones bought her electric indoor/outdoor wheelchair with mobility allowance, after being a full-time wheelchair user for about four or five years:

"So has it been worthwhile you ask? Well it took a while to learn to drive, being very powerful, the battery capacity is that of a car, I kangarooed like a learner driver for the first few weeks! I was initially nervy at going out, crossing roads under my own responsibility being somewhat new and even now I don't like crossing major roads (we have quite a few death traps here!) if alone. Kerb climbing too requires nerves as although it is safe there is an art to it and you feel rather catapaulted until you get used to the effect. Also if you do not approach the kerb correctly, you won't get up it but it really only comes down to common sense.

"My first few trials I have been accompanied, as I've never been out alone. I thought I would be very panicky at the prospect of going out alone, but today, spring sun shining I ventured out alone and loved it! No doubt passers-by thought I'd escaped from the local asylum, as I kept trundling up and down, turning round, exploring unvisited roads, stopping to look at houses I'd previously been whistled past, but the feeling of being at your own command was wonderful! ...if you are faced with life in a wheelchair and a car is out of the question, as it was for me, think hard about buying an electric wheelchair, it's possibly the best thing I've ever done in my life and is certainly going to open up my life with the new freedoms I now have." (*In Contact*)

If you need a manual wheelchair, get expert advice from the doctor/OT/physio first. S/he can help you get a push-only or self-propelled manual one on temporary or permanent loan from the NHS Disablement Services Authority (DSA).

Powered wheelchairs are more difficult to get. – If you can't walk and can't propel a manual wheelchair, the DSA may supply a powered wheelchair, but only for indoor use. They'll only consider a powered chair for *outdoor use* if you can't propel a manual wheelchair yourself *and* if they agree (rarely) your attendant isn't able to push you instead. If, however, you need a manual or a powered wheelchair for work, then your jobcentre DRO can help.

The British Red Cross Society loans out manual wheelchairs for temporary use – useful if you're staying away from home on holiday, perhaps. *Motoring and Mobility* (see page 189) lists wheelchair hire firms.

Powered wheelchairs/scooters come in all shapes and sizes but are expensive (though VAT-free). DLF's *Wheelchairs* leaflet includes electrically operated wheelchairs and there's a useful guide *How to Choose a Pavement Vehicle*, available free from Banstead Mobility Centre. Chat to your OT/physio too. If you qualify for DLA mobility component, you can use it for buying a powered chair. Motability has negotiated special terms with some manufacturers. If money's no object all sorts of refinements are available, including a powered wheelchair with a seat you can raise to reach high shelves and lower as you wish!

You can see and try several types in one go at places like the Transport and Road Research Laboratory's Mobility Roadshow (see page 186), or at the NAIDEX shows (page 144) and some disabled living centres (see page 143).

Some are available second-hand. It's a good idea to seek advice on purchasing from the

British Association of Wheelchair Distributors. The DLF keeps lists, and Exchange and Mart magazine carries adverts. So does RADAR's monthly bulletin, and the magazines of the Disabled Drivers' Association and Disabled Motorists' Club. New and reconditioned ones are available from other places too, eg at the Keep-Able Centre (see *Motoring and Mobility*). Ask your DIAL what's available locally and try the *Yellow Pages*.

Pamela's solution − 'Get on your bike'!

Pamela Waterhouse developed RA in her early 30s, and was depressed and frustrated at not being able to get out of the house on her own. She couldn't drive. However...

"One day I was falling asleep watching 'Pebble Mill at One' when an item jerked me wide awake. They were demonstrating ordinary bicycles with battery run motors attached − a miracle designed for me, I thought. It took a long time to convince the family that it would be suitable but finally, in August, we travelled up to the factory in the Midlands for me to have a trial run. This proved to be quite an ordeal in front of the men of the factory and with the salesman running, puffing alongside me, especially as I hadn't ridden a bike for nearly twenty years! Eventually, they found a bike which could be adapted low enough for my short little legs and we travelled home with my newly acquired miracle folded up in the back of the car.

"The feeling of independence which the bike has given me is unbelievable. Of course, things haven't been all plain sailing. Like the time I had a puncture up a mountain and had to waylay a friendly farmer. And like the time the wind blew my hat off and a bus ran over it! ... But the pleasures far outweigh the tribulations. To be able to pop down to my mother's for coffee, to go to choir practice, fostering meetings all on my own with the wind blowing in my hair is a real joy. " (In Contact)

She couldn't at first use the bike on her 'worst' days because it had to be pedalled a few yards before the motor could be turned on. But:

"the firm which produce this miracle have been most helpful. They've adapted the motor now so that it can be used straight away without my having to pedal. This makes it even more useful because I can now restart on the steepest of hills... "

Electric tricycles are available for people who can't manage bikes. Neatwork is one company that specialises in adapted bikes and tricycles for disabled people and their families (even tandem trikes!). Or look in the *Yellow Pages* or *Thomson Directory*. The firm Pamela used no longer does bikes.

Public and community transport

Some areas, eg Edinburgh and London, operate special schemes so you can use ordinary taxis at special rates. Ask your local DIAL, CAB, or social services what's available locally, eg 'Dial-a-Ride', cars driven by volunteers (eg WRVS), wheelchair accessible buses. In London I use the Taxicard scheme for black cabs (for London residents only, details from LRT Taxicard Section). Black cabs aren't easy to get in. − My method is to back on to the tip-up seat, easing my legs round and into the cab, which avoids strain on the hip and knee joints. I stay on the tip-up seat (a little precariously!) for the whole journey. Recent cab models have tip-up seats that swivel out making the process easier.

The DRO/Employment Service will subsidise taxi fares to work if you're severely disabled, on the Disabled Persons' Employment Register, and having to pay extra travel costs because you can't use public transport.

Remember, do *plan ahead*. Find out all you can about your journey beforehand and work out how you'll cope. Tripscope (see page 277) could help − it's a telephone helpline (office hours), which can help you work out the best way to travel, taking into account your special needs. If you need help from anyone on your journey (eg BR) ask well in advance. Phone again shortly before you travel as a reminder.

For bus travel information, get the Bus and Coach Council's *Getting Around* (free). Ask too at the nearest coach station of the company or companies operating in your area, or at a local travel agent. For rail information look at *British Rail and Disabled Travellers* (from your local station) and *A Guide to British Rail for Disabled People* (RADAR), with details of access and facilities at over 400 stations.

For travel in London: contact London Regional Transport (LRT)'s special Unit for Disabled Passengers. Look at 'Visiting London' on page 276. In Newcastle-upon-Tyne, the Tyne and Wear Metro was designed to be fully accessible to all disabled people and has specially designed interchanges with parking for disabled people and access to bus stations. Manchester's new trams are also designed to be accessible.

For information on air travel: get the appropriate British Airports Authority (BAA) *Who looks after you at... Airport?* These outline facilities at Heathrow, Gatwick, Stansted, Glasgow, Edinburgh, Prestwick, Aberdeen. Contact other airports direct for information. Ask individual airlines about special arrangements too. Even if you can walk, but it's a real struggle, using a pre-booked wheelchair/electric buggy can make all the difference. Some airlines produce special information leaflets, eg British Airways, from BA Customer Services. Also useful: *Care in the Air – Advice for Handicapped Travellers* , free, from the Civil Aviation Authority (CAA).

Travel by sea: several ships now have lifts and toilets for disabled people, but find out for sure and make arrangements well in advance. Ask individual ports and ferry companies for information on access, eg assistance with parking your car near a lift. On some ships fare concessions are available for registered disabled people who are members of the Disabled Drivers' Association or Disabled Drivers' Motor Club.

Other useful travel information appears in chapter 34 on 'holidays', and in the publications mentioned on page 189. RADAR has a range of access guides available by post.

Using a car

Whether you're a passenger, a driver, or a would-be driver, the two publications mentioned at the start of this chapter, *Door to Door* and *Motoring and Mobility* will tell you far more than I ever could about subjects like choosing a car (new or secondhand), car finance, makers' discounts, DLA mobility component, Motability hiring and HP schemes, adaptations and accessories, assessment centres, learning to drive, taking your car on holiday, breakdown and recovery services, etc. ARC's *Driving and Your Arthritis* is worth getting too (free, but send SAE). Here are a few titbits to be going on with.

The Orange Badge scheme
Get a leaflet and application form from your social services department. With an Orange Badge you can, whether driver or passenger, park free and without limit at on-street parking meters and in time-limited waiting areas. You can also park for a limited period on yellow lines in England and Wales, and without time limit in Scotland, except in bus lanes or where loading and unloading is prohibited. You must park safely and cause no obstruction.

You qualify for a Badge if you get DLA mobility component, or if you have a 'permanent and substantial disability which causes inability to walk or very considerable difficulty in walking'. You don't have to be registered disabled. Your doctor may be asked to confirm the disability, and you may be asked to go for a medical examination. Some local authorities may make a small charge. (OB rules are under review as I write.)

Seat belts
There are gadgets to help with reaching a stowed seat belt. Birch Products' Pulla belt is a

removable, adjustable plastic clip which grips the seat belt, to form an extension handle. Beacon Associates' Clever Clip has a locking device which grips an inertia (self-adjusting) seat belt to stop it fully recoiling, thus leaving a longer end to catch hold of.

Specialised advice on car purchase and adaptations

If you're already a licensed driver who develops a disability lasting more than three months, you're required by law to inform the Driver and Vehicle Licensing Agency (DVLA). Don't despair if the arthritis starts making driving more difficult. Problems can often be overcome. Finding out about just two or three adaptations (eg hand-brake assistance, mirrors/lenses to overcome stiff neck problems reversing) could well be all it takes for you to continue happily driving your usual car. A disabled driver may qualify for exemption from road tax: check with DVLA.

If you're starting from scratch, you have to report any illness when you apply for a provisional licence. You'll be asked to fill in an extra form. Get *What You Need to Know About Driver Licensing* free from DVLA. Disabled people taking the driving test are allocated extra time to allow for explanation of adaptations and for getting in and out of the car.

Useful information and assessments are available in several places. MAVIS is the Department of Transport's Mobility Advice and Vehicle Information Service, and has a variety of adapted cars you can try out on a private driving circuit. Contact MAVIS or the Disability Unit of the Department of Transport for details of your nearest assessment centre. Banstead Mobility Centre runs a mobile assessment service which travels throughout Britain. Assessments can be made too by MIS, the Mobility Information service, a voluntary organisation (see page 187).

Getting a report from an assessment centre like Banstead on your ability to drive might give you useful additional evidence to submit to DVLA, and would give you ideas on suitable car and adaptations. However, some centres (eg MAVIS) say you need a provisional licence *before* they'll assess you!

Every two years, the Transport and Road Research Laboratory (TRRL) at Crowthorne holds a Mobility Roadshow, covering all aspects of mobility, including electric wheelchairs/scooters, various mobility aids and accessories, and a vast array of cars which you can try out on the test track there if you have a provisional licence. It's an ideal place for looking, trying out, and collecting oodles of useful leaflets.

Don't be shy of visiting local showrooms and, for a start, just trying cars for comfort, ease of access, and driving controls. Some manufacturers make a special point of catering for drivers with disabilities, but in the end it's only you who can really decide what's best. Keep a note of what you like and dislike about each car and take your time deciding. Janet Flower tried car after car after car. Eventually she found one so perfect she didn't have to pay extra for any adaptations, even though it was more expensive than she'd bargained for:

"My problem is not having much bend in my knees, making it difficult to get the seat in the right position, without being too far away from the steering wheel so my arms can't reach it... When I tried the Swift, I was amazed! It has an adjustable steering wheel as standard, *so having got the seat right, with my feet using the brake/accelerator comfortably and safely, I was then able to lower the steering wheel, and found I could hold and control that comfortably and safely too. It was unbelievable, having almost resigned myself to the process of having adaptations carried out...*

"All the features are easy to operate – the wing mirrors electrically adjust, the bonnet and tailgate lock and unlock from inside the car, it even has air conditioning as standard. It doesn't have power steering but is incredibly light to handle, and has power assisted brakes. I've had to have a strap attached to the tailgate, as being short I wouldn't be able to close it otherwise, but that's all that has been needed." (In Contact)

Second-hand cars should only be bought with the greatest of care. It's sensible to pay for an independent assessment by the AA or RAC. *Exchange and Mart* magazine has a section on 'Adapted Cars', but bear in mind that someone else's adaptations may not suit you.

Other useful organisations
The Mobility Information Service (MIS) is a voluntary organisation, which can organise assessments, and publishes leaflets on all aspects of choosing, buying and converting a car (and electric wheelchairs and 'scooters'). *Wheels Under You* is cheap, comprehensive, and specially for young or newly-disabled people. The *Mobility Information Pack* includes road tests on suitable cars.

Disabled Drivers' Association (DDA) produces an informative quarterly magazine and advises on all mobility matters such as vehicles, conversions, ferry concessions, insurance, legal requirements, etc. Has local groups nationwide, and a holiday hotel (see page 275).

Disabled Drivers' Motor Club Ltd has a similar service to DDA, and has lists of disabled drivers around the country willing to demonstrate their cars.

Finance
If you're awarded the DLA mobility component, Motability (see page 189) can help finance a new or used car. Alternatively, you don't have to have the mobility component to apply under the AVS Finance scheme (details below), or you might prefer the wider choice and flexibility a bank loan gives you, but check and compare interest rates.

Aid Vehicle Supplies (AVS)
Commercial company with large range of car types for hire-purchase (some on a no-deposit basis) and used car purchase. The scheme includes extras (eg life assurance cover) and claims to be more flexible than Motability. Finance is provided by the Greyhound Equipment Finance Ltd (a British subsidiary of the famous American bus company).

Motor insurance
See chapter 19.

The Disability Living Allowance (DLA) mobility component

The DLA mobility component, which replaces the old Mobility Allowance from April 1992, is paid at two rates, the higher to people who can't walk or are 'virtually unable to walk'; the lower to people whose disability means they can get about out of doors only if they're under the guidance or supervision of another person. You have to be likely to remain that way for at least six months.

Mobility component isn't means-tested or taxable, and you don't have to own a car or even be able to drive to qualify. You can spend it any way you want – on an electric scooter, on taxis, on a car, etc. It's awarded for a period of between one year (the minimum), and life. It might be awarded for, say, two or three years initially, and reassessed again later.

As I write, the details of how DLA operates are still being finalised. Read the section on DLA on page 130, but bear in mind that some of what I'm writing may have changed by the time you read it, so get up-to-date information from the sources on page 127, eg BEL, CAB, your self-help group (eg Young Arthritis Care, NASS) or the Disability Rights Handbook.

To apply for the old Mobility Allowance, you had to have a medical examination, but most initial claims for DLA components will, instead, be decided on a detailed self-assessment form completed by you. You can get free telephone advice from the DSS on completing the form (phone the BEL helpline, page 127), or get advice from your local CAB. See too my notes on pages 128 and 137 on completing forms.

Some applicants will still be required to have an assessment by a doctor, and you could still ask to have one if you feel it would help support your application. If so, the following notes may help you prepare for it, though they're based on the old MA medical examination, and there may be changes.

You'll be asked to go to a surgery near you. You can claim travelling expenses including taxi fares if you can't use public transport because of your disability. If you can't get to a surgery, a home visit may be possible.

The examining doctor will have to complete a form. It may request a statement from you, the claimant, on your disability and how it affects your walking, so go with prepared notes, based on the information here on how your eligibility is likely to be assessed. Read your notes beforehand as if you were the DSS assessor, who will know nothing about you except what is on your claim form. Ask yourself, does 'the claimant' have a good case?

The doctor will ask questions, and give you a physical examination. S/he may also ask you to go for a walk either in the surgery or in the street, to assess how far you can walk. Unless you obviously can't walk at all, what the doctor and the DSS will be looking for is evidence that you are 'virtually unable to walk' or 'the exertion required to walk would, in itself, constitute a danger to your life, or would be likely to lead to a serious deterioration in your health', or that you can't walk outdoors without supervision or guidance. Your physical condition is what counts, not how it is affected by external circumstances, so for instance where you live (eg far from the nearest bus stop) isn't taken into account. Nor is the type of work you do, nor your ability or inability to use public transport.

When assessing whether you're 'virtually unable to walk', the doctor and DSS check whether your 'ability to walk out of doors is so limited, as regards

–   the distance over which
–   or the speed at which
–   or the length of time for which
–   or the manner in which

(you) can make progress on foot *without severe discomfort*, that (you are) virtually unable to walk.'

Most of us spend our lives putting a brave face on things, grimacing inwardly while lying to the world that the pain's not too bad. You need to do the opposite when being assessed. Tell the truth and stress how much it hurts and how much you *can't* do (though don't overdo it). If the pain starts the moment you stand up, say so. An optimist describes a glass as being 'half full'; a pessimist describes it as 'half empty' – both statements are true, but you're assessed on the evidence produced by the pessimist, not the optimist.

'Severe discomfort' isn't the same as 'excruciating agony'. When walking with the doctor, don't be distracted into chatting, but concentrate on when you first feel severe discomfort, stop, and say so. Any extra distance after that is ignored. Your assessor is *not* assessing how stiff your upper lip is! Instead of arranging your assessment appointment for when you're at your best, make a point of going when you know you'll be at your worst, so the doctor sees just how bad you really are. If you happen to be having a 'good' day, explain what you're like on 'bad' days. You might want to take a friend or relative along for moral support, but if so make sure they're briefed, for once, *not* to say how wonderful you are at coping!

The DSS will also be looking for evidence that you're likely to remain 'virtually unable to walk' for at least six months. With something like RA, where walking ability varies from day to day, you may have difficulty qualifying on this count. You could try keeping an accurate diary to send with your claim form. Even though you might be able to walk on some days, that might not disqualify you, provided the DSS consider that, looking at your physical condition as a whole, it would be true to say that you're normally virtually unable to walk and likely to remain like that for at least six months.

Is there any other evidence that might help your case? If so include it either in a separate note with the self-assessment form, or, if you have an examination, in your statement at the doctor's. For instance, have you had hip or knee joint replacements which have since loosened, and walking loosens them further, causing 'severe discomfort'? How do steps and stairs affect you?

The decision will be posted to you, but don't panic if you're refused. You can appeal. For help with an appeal you'll need advice from experienced people, so contact your local DIAL or CAB and self-help group. If you don't appeal, or your appeal is turned down, you can still try claiming again at a later date if your condition worsens and you think you might then qualify. The new Disability Appeal Tribunal (DAT) will be made up of one legally qualified chairperson, one medically qualified member and one non-medical member who as far as is praticable should have professional or voluntary experience in the needs of disabled people or has a disability.

Motability

Voluntary organisation, set up on government initiative, and financed by the major banks, aims to help people with disabilities to use their DLA mobility component to buy or lease a new car, or to get an electric wheelchair or good used car on hire purchase. See their leaflets *Motability Car Hiring and Hire Purchase Schemes* and *Used Car Hire Purchase Schemes*.

You can use the scheme even if you're not able to drive the car yourself, but are nonetheless buying it for your benefit. This may however confuse the car salesman and/or the car insurance company! You and they will need to distinguish between the registered 'owner' of the car (you, the non-driver) and the 'keeper' of the car, the actual driver (who must be insured). DVLA Swansea will confirm the regulations if necessary (tel: 0792 782341 or 42091 or 72134).

Further Reading

- *Door to Door*, free from the Department of Transport
- *Motoring and Mobility for Disabled People*, by Ann Darnborough and Derek Kinrade (RADAR)
- In the Disability Information Trust's Equipment for Disabled People series *Arthritis – An Equipment Guide* has a well-illustrated chapter on various aspects of mobility, and other relevant titles in the series go into more detail: *Outdoor Transport, Walking Aids, Wheelchairs*.
- One or more of RADAR's Mobility Fact Sheets (small cost), and/or DLF low-cost Information leaflets, cover all aspects of getting out and about.
- The Department of Transport's *Ins and Outs of Car Choice* – simple practical advice on what to look for in choosing a car, includes sections on getting in and out. (From the DoT Disability Unit).
- In Michael Leitch's *Living with Arthritis* (Lennard/Collins) there's a chapter on 'Out and about', where five people with arthritis talk about their experience of travelling by train, in a wheelchair, by car, and getting a car adapted.
- Information from the organisations on page 187, eg MIS's *Mobility Information Pack*.
- Leaflets from the Office of Fair Trading eg *Credit Wise* and *Used cars*.

Chapter twenty-five

OTHER PEOPLE

"My favourite people are those who...
- *respect and love me as I am, just as I am, and not as they wish I were.*
- *boost my confidence and self-esteem with praise and encouragement, and who do not criticise or blame me for failures for which the arthritis is responsible, not I.*
- *never bid me to 'hurry up' and take my tasks from me, for often I need time rather than help.*
- *don't fuss, but are ready and willing to help, quietly, when I ask.*
- *ask for my help, for my greatest need is to feel needed.*
- *do me the courtesy of asking me what I need or want, rather than assume they know what's best.*
- *don't let me down when they agree to do something, however trivial or unimportant it may seem to them.*
- *make me smile and laugh and inspire my interest in the world outside myself, and whose presence reminds me that life is well worth living.*
- *let me know I need never feel lonely, yet understand my need at times to be alone.*
- *forgive me for not always remembering that other people have problems too.*
- *if I am snappy and miserable, unloving and feel unlovable, nevertheless give me a kiss and cuddle and say they love me.*
- *aren't embarrassed if there are tears, but are sympathetic and supportive, even joining in, if they want.*
- *don't say 'you'll just have to learn to live with it', but instead 'I'm here to give you help and support as you soldier on, and here to listen to your problems even if I can't always help solve them.'*
- *remember the arthritis is only a part of me, and who take an interest in the rest of me!"* (adapted and expanded from *DIALOGUE*, spring 1987)

As if pain and stiffness and an uncooperative body weren't enough, arthritis can sometimes be a dab hand at complicating relationships with other people, be they at home, at work, at college, in the street, in shops, on holiday, even, sometimes, healthcare and disability experts. If only they'd learn to understand the arthritis, and treat us as people, not oddities, life would be so much easier, and at no cost to anyone, even the NHS.

Surprisingly, most books written for people with arthritis by medical experts scarcely touch on its impact on relationships, and few non-YPAs understand the possible problems. One 12 year old girl, who launched a campaign for ARC to make people aware of children with arthritis described one problem:

"One thing that hurts is when people look at me as though I am different, as though I'm odd, and treat me like that as well, when I'm not different. It's hard to explain to people what I've got wrong with me. When I say arthritis they think that I am joking – they think it's an old people's disease."

An older YPA, who works in a bank, wrote a very perceptive article in *In Contact*:

"It's not easy, sometimes, because I have good and bad days. I feel the pressure to be like other people – to run up a flight of stairs to get something, to reach something down from a shelf, to use a typewriter keyboard. So many little jobs, that others take for granted, and don't seem to realise I can't do. How much of this pressure is deliberate I

don't really know. Some days I can see that people don't know how to react, what to say, how to help. Other days I get so fed up with explaining that I can't do something and fending off the (in my view at least) idiotic comments like 'Surely you can cope with this, manage to do that, reach the other', that I feel like screaming 'It's can't not won't, you stupid fool' (or stronger words to that effect). Then I'd like to burst into tears and run out of the branch, so that I'd never have to face these people again, who seem to flaunt their abilities in my face and make fun of me for doing things which I would love to do. Worst of all, are the 'helpful ones', who make comments like 'You can't blame us for your problems, don't take them out on us', when all the time I'm trying to cope as well as I can, and it's their actions which make it impossible for me to do so."

The experts on 'arthritis and other people' are YPAs themselves. There *are* ways of changing things for the better, though it may mean a tiresome process of trial and error for all concerned. Talking to other YPAs or reading what they've have written of their experiences can help. Look at some of the books in chapter 29, and at *Young Arthritis News*.

We can each do something towards putting things right, towards educating people, hard though it seems that *we*, not they, should have to be the ones to take the initiative, and hard, too, if we ourselves don't understand the arthritis or know what's in store for us next. The alternative is just to say 'Damn you', and turn away, in anger, bitterness, or silent misery. We each have our days when we do or certainly feel like doing so, but that doesn't solve anything in the long run. Instead, reacting differently might help all of us. Each of us is really an ambassador for all YPAs. It's not easy, but when we can, let's try to be positive instead of negative, and educate our fellow beings. Let's work to replace their disbelief or pity or fear with awareness and understanding.

"If people don't know WHY you can't do something, explain to them, as simply as is necessary. You aren't silly for not being able to do it, they are for not seeing why for themselves. If you don't explain, you aren't just penalising yourself (bad enough), you are also making life harder for every arthritic with whom that person comes in contact. That person will assume that because YOU haven't had any problems with the action, no other people with arthritis will have problems either. So explain, communicate, remove the folklore about arthritis (eg only old people get arthritis) – not just for yourself but for all of us..." (The same YPA again, who works in a bank.)

We first need to come to terms with ourselves, to boost our bruised self-esteem and self-confidence. If that's difficult, I hope chapter 13 will help you get started. A teacher who developed RA when he was 15, Roger Glanville, wrote:

"It is obviously a tremendous task to come to terms with oneself, particularly if the disability occurs after a normal life has been established. When at last one feels able to cope with a newly restricted pattern, resentment against the injustice, the 'big chip' has to be dealt with. One has to try to find one's real character, to deal with other people in a reasonable way, to react normally to all situations, to harbour no bitterness, to be ordinary and normal. On those days when coping is impossible, the barriers go up again; but when one finally succeeds in living with oneself, these barriers collapse completely because they are no longer needed to protect one from everyday high-speed life.

"During the period of adjustment one needs more than anything to feel that there is some meaning in life. Relationships with other people play an important part in finding this meaning, but in order to achieve mutual understanding, communication without tension is desirable. Yet, at the same time one's disability makes one feel not quite right, a little ill at ease, and therefore tense: so the primary task is to combat the tension and spread a little relaxation around. Fit people (the ones with duodenal ulcers, varicose veins, or blood pressure but no outward manifestations of abnormality) find it difficult to be normal with the disabled. They are tense before they start. The first thing they want to know is, 'What's wrong?' And then, 'How long? never! I thought...! My aunt...! Have you tried...? mud, codeine, turkish baths, vegetarianism, bee stings,

cortisone, corks in the bed, real leather shoes, ACTH, REST, EXERCISE, PRAYER?'
When these questions have been answered, they relax and sometimes turn out to be
quite nice people; just thought they were helping. " (In Paul Hunt's *Stigma*)

How does the arthritis create misunderstandings between us and other people?

1 The invisibility problem

One of the oddities of something like RA and its cousins is that it can be invisible, even
when it's at its most unbearable internally. Someone with early RA has no obvious joint
deformity, and unless you use a stick or wheelchair other people may not realise you have
problems. Worse still, they may even disbelieve you and think you're 'putting it on'.

Invisibility's a mixed blessing. It's lovely to blend in, to 'look normal', but sooner or
later something gives the game away. Like the times you get up in the pub after a mild
shandy or two, and wobble drunkenly (so it seems) all over the place! Like the time you
try to get on a bus and find you can't, and the conductor rings the bell and sends it lurching
off too soon. Difficult for someone with a visible disability to appreciate, but 'appearing
normal' can build up all sorts of tensions and frustrations:

"I often feel I'm in 'No-man's land' – not incapacitated sufficiently to receive any help
(physical or financial) and yet disabled enough for it to literally change my whole life.
To be honest, I found it easier to cope when I was at my very worst 2½ years ago. Every
one was so helpful and sympathetic and the constant pain was so all-consuming that
even ordinary tasks became sources of pride in their accomplishing. Now that the pain
is in the background and my joints only take it in turns to play up I try to live as normal
a life as possible. This is far more difficult, especially when people (including family)
start to treat you as a 'normal' person once more...When I'm busy bustling about moving
chairs in one of the many meetings I go to, for example, I often feel like shouting out
'Yes, I'm here. Yes, I may be working just as hard as you are. But can't you see I'm in
PAIN.' I never do shout it out of course. And one soon learns to hide the pain but I still
can't get over the unfairness of it all... "(Pamela Waterhouse)

To add insult to injury, someone with a bandaged finger may get more sympathy and
understanding than you, with your stiff, pain-wracked body. Hardly surprising if all sorts
of emotions build up inside, at the frustration of it all, but the invisibility problem means
other people are taken by surprise when our anger and exhaustion and pain erupt against
them, or turn us in on ourselves in misery. Leading, alas, to yet more misunderstandings.

2 The visibility problem

Arthritis becomes visible with joint or limb deformity, or clumsy body movement, or when
you use a stick or crutches or a wheelchair. You may then come up against *Does he take*
sugar? attitudes, when people may treat you as a 'non-person' and ask your companion
rather than you whether you take sugar, feel cold, or whatever. Some may recoil in
embarrassment or fear or ignorance, some may even think you're mentally deficient. They
can be patronising and condescending and insulting, even if they don't mean to be.

Arthritis distorts 'body language'. – The way we sit or move conveys false messages.
Inner pain can make me look forbidding or fierce, or might stop me walking over to
someone to comfort them physically, or bending down to join in friendly play with a child.
It's not that I don't care, just that my body's giving false messages. More misunderstandings to be overcome.

Skin problems in lupus or psoriatic arthritis can provoke absurd reactions, even though
neither's infectious or contagious. In Michael Leitch's *Living with Arthritis*, Cheryl
Marcus talks about her early days with lupus, before effective treatment started:

"To look at I was quite a sight. I was covered in a rash. I lost my hair completely...A lot

*of people were scared to come near me, and my son was not allowed to visit me because
we were worried about the effect it might have on him..."*

Fortunately, with treatment, things improved, though Cheryl now experiences misunderstandings because

*"I now look extremely healthy. A lot of lupus people do. We have nice round faces, some
rounder than others – an effect of the steroids we take. I have pink rosy cheeks. This is
because I have a rash, which I cover up with powder. I look suntanned. This is because I
take an anti-malarial drug which tends to make the skin look yellow. Looks are truly
deceptive. I know a lot of lupus people get very frustrated when people tell them how
plump and well they look, when all the time they know it is because they are on extra
steroids and in fact are feeling grotty."*

Both the Psoriasis Society and the Lupus UK Group can give lots of tips and support.
R H Phillips PhD's *Coping with Lupus*, (Avery Publishing), available through Lupus UK)
includes tips on coping with emotions, and 'other people'.

3 The youth problem

The oh-so-tedious disbelief that the younger ones amongst us could *possibly* have arthritis.
Even those who do believe us may find it hard to understand how devastating it can
sometimes be, physically and psychologically. Like one unhelpful doctor who chided me
"Stop worrying and go out and have a good time." Maybe he meant well, but the message
that came across was one of total misunderstanding, and only added to my misery.

Some people are blinded by preconceptions based on the older-type arthritis, OA, in
the over 60s age group, or the mild twinges type of 'rheumatism'. Even one arthritis group
organiser bluntly told a young friend not to bother going along to a local meeting unless she
was prepared to help out physically as all the members were 'elderly and arthritic'. In fact,
in terms of number of joints and extent of joint damage, and its impact on her life, she was
a good deal worse off than many of the elderly members.

Inside us youthful spirits and desires tussle with uncooperative, very elderly-feeling
bodies, and it's hard for contemporaries to understand that the carefree spontaneity they
take for granted is now often an unattainable luxury for us. It's hurtful to feel different and
unable to keep up with friends.

Usually, when you're young, bodies can be left to look after themselves, leaving plenty
of time and energy free for other concerns. But with arthritis, our bodies are 'too much
with us', reminding us constantly of their painful, uncooperative existence. Usually, too,
youth goes hand in hand with boundless energy. 1,001 things can be packed into a fragment
of time, and time's an unimportant dimension. Suddenly, though, with RA and its cousins,
time looms large, and the smallest tasks can take forever to accomplish. How many other
under 60s take at least an hour to get dressed, and have to spend most of that time
consciously thinking about the process? Yet another area where youthfulness makes having
arthritis *more* difficult, more liable to misunderstandings. Arthritis really is an appalling
waste of time!

4 The problem of how to explain its oddities

Samuel Johnson said, 'Those who do not feel pain, seldom think it is felt'. It's difficult
enough to explain where it hurts, how it hurts, and in what ways it restricts you. Even more
difficult for other people to understand something that's so variable and unpredictable:

*"what I can do today, I may not be able to do tomorrow (although I may be able to do it
again the day after)."* (A YPA, writing in *In Contact*)

If instead you'd lost a leg or an arm, say, after a while you'd learn the limitations and you'd
be able to explain your 'static disability' fairly easily. A once and for all process. But with
RA you could be in agony at 6 am, barely able to move, yet get to the office at 9.30 and
appear to move reasonably easily. One day you might feel lively enough to have a mad fling

at a disco, and yet next week be barely able to move across the room. A strange switchback existence, 'up and down like a perishing yo-yo'. Not surprising other people are baffled by this 'intermittent disability', but oh how cruel any disbelief can seem.

How can we explain another characteristic that causes many misunderstandings? Sometimes we're accused of 'not trying', of being unnecessarily clumsy. People don't understand it's something we can do little or nothing about.

We would if we could. One YPA described it as feeling as if you have to struggle through thick mud to do anything. Grace Stuart (*Private World of Pain*, Allen & Unwin, 1953) described:

"That strange powerlessness – so typical of the arthritic joint, so well known to the arthritic and so little known to anyone else...Beyond a certain point in this disease there is no question of endurance. You may endure all the pain you can or will, but if your wrist, lifting the teapot, gives way, you spill the tea or drop the pot. There is no argument! Only acquiescence! Useless to lift teapots!..."

"There has been no time when, if I could at all do something, at whatever cost, I did not do it. [Nonetheless, she had] *the bitter experience of not being believed – and the bitterer experience of not being able to explain...Often in those days I wanted to cry out 'I am doing more than my best. Please say that you believe me!' "*

Something else non-arthritics find hard to understand is what has been called 'the interaction of different disabilities'. Maybe you *can* do something, like dressing, or making a cup of tea, but at considerable cost in time, frustration, and pain:

"If one sets out to assess the functional ability of a person with severe arthritis in, for example, the kitchen, one is likely to find that many individual activities are within the sufferer's capacity. However, effective preparation of a meal calls for integration of these activities, particularly by ease of movement between one part of the kitchen and another, and it is especially at this level that the arthritic experiences serious difficulty. Similarly, affected individuals are usually capable of dressing themselves but the fact that the process may take well over an hour cannot help but distort organization of the day's schedule." (In the World Health Organization's *International Classification of Impairments, Disabilities, and Handicaps, a manual of classification relating to the consequences of disease,* Geneva, WHO, 1980)

These characteristics of 'intermittent disability' and 'interaction of different disabilities' can cause special difficulties if you're being assessed for a benefit: 'Can you dress yourself?' 'Yes, but...' How often does the assessor listen to your 'but'? *Make* them listen! Why not show them the quotation, above, and this:

"Insensitivity to these dimensions leads to arbitrary administrative distinctions; that arthritics are not totally lacking in the ability to move often renders them ineligible for benefits such as a mobility allowance, and yet in terms of effective mobility to allow integration in society they are as much in need of this type of help as many others. This failure arises from failure to distinguish between disability assessments, which focus on individual activities, and the overall handicap or disadvantage that may result from the interaction of different disabilities." (ibid)

Look back at page 89, at the way Carolyn Wiener described the 'uncertainty' of RA. Her description may also be worth showing to other people and officials who can't understand the quirks of chronic inflammatory arthritis.

Two poems, which appeared in *In Contact*, express in just a few words what it can feel like to be a younger person with arthritis:

Arthritis is no friend of mine, Arthritis is a pain.
He's never invited, but always delighted, to make me cry again.

You wake up each morn stiff as a board, and say to yourself 'O Lord, O Lord,
Why curse me with this dreadful disease, when all I want is peace and ease?'.

The weather gets worse, and so do you, and you wish the sun would come shining
through
To ease your pain and make you smile again.

Can't climb the stairs. Crippled in chairs. It really is a shame.
Arthritis is no friend of mine, Arthritis is a pain.

and the second poem:

Arthritis really is a bind; when I walk my joints all grind.
Sometimes I have to walk with sticks, it makes me feel I'm ninety six.

I rub in creams and take my pills, but these produce some other other ills.
Yes, arthritis really is a bind: osteo, or the other kind.

People wonder 'what has she got?' To tell the truth, not a lot:
Just worn-out bones that creak and groan, and oh the pain, it makes me moan.

Yes, arthritis really is a bind, but I thank God that I'm the kind
That sometimes sees the funny side, of this disease I can't abide.

5 The folklore problem

Folklore confuses inflammatory arthritis with those relatively trivial aches and pains, loosely called 'rheumatism' or 'arthritis'. People don't realise that there are over 200 types of rheumatic disorder, ranging from the trivial to the very serious, sometimes even fatal. Not only joints but almost any part of the body can be affected. Then they wonder why you're so put out when they compare your RA/AS/whatever with their elderly aunt's 'twinges in her shoulder' or their own occasionally 'rheumaticky finger'!

An even worse folklore is the belief, even among YPAs, that little or nothing can be done about rheumatic disorders, and the belief, too, that 'arthritis is just a part of growing old'. Such fallacies are very damaging, for much can and more could be done if these disorders were taken more seriously, and if far more resources were devoted to them:

> *"In one study it was found that 42% of arthritic sufferers could have benefited from specialist help that had not been made available to them. These deficiencies reflect low levels of demand by the public and insufficient appreciation of the problems by policy makers (or politicians), but they have been compounded by professional ignorance in some localities and this leads to perpetuation of neglect."* (*If You've Got Arthritis, Expert Advice is Badly Needed*, ARC, 1983)

6 The fatigue problem

The struggle to cope, and to 'keep going', can lead to tremendous physical and emotional fatigue, again difficult for other people to understand. All they may see is someone who spends a lot of time withdrawing from social relationships and activities, wanting time to be alone, seemingly anti-social. A YPA who works may give up other forms of social contact, merely to keep enough energy in hand to be able to cope with work. Or a YPA may have to give up work just to find enough energy to keep a marriage going.

Fatigue can make us lose patience, and get angry at innocent remarks. 'Can't you manage to pick it up yourself?' someone asks, in all innocence, only to be snapped at when in my exhaustion I interpret it as an unfeeling snide comment.

The struggle merely to get out of bed and face the day may so exhaust a husband with inflammatory arthritis that he does little for the rest of the day, only to be snapped at by an unthinking wife who sees only all the odd jobs around the house that need doing and an apparently lazy husband ignoring them. More misunderstandings to sort out...

7 Other people's handicaps

Many people genuinely would like to be helpful or react 'in the right way' if only they knew how. Others think they know how but end up being just the opposite! As Corbet Woodall wrote *"Handicap is experienced by non-disabled people when faced with a person who needs special consideration.."* Once understood, this is one handicap we can do a lot about.

Some people act oddly towards us, when they see something's 'not quite right'. A few are just plain bloody-minded, but more usually they're just afraid or embarrassed, or ignorant. *"They may be afraid you're going to fall in a fit or be eccentric in some way"* (Corbet Woodall again). Or they sense you need help but don't know what help to offer. If you feel upset at someone's odd behaviour, tell yourself that on the whole people are kind or understanding at least once they know you have a problem and are told how they can help, or something of the whys and wherefores. As for those who can't be taught, pity them and give them up as a bad job. They aren't worth wasting your precious energy on.

Our nearest and dearest, and our friends, may feel especially helpless when they see the person they love struggling and in pain. They can feel 'handicapped': something it's easy to forget. It's sometimes harder to be an outsider looking on, wondering helplessly what to do, than it is to be the actual 'sufferer'. We can take the initiative in showing them what to do, in making them feel needed and useful and encouraging their understanding of what's going on.

Sometimes the problem's just the opposite − other people thinking *they* know what's best for you. In the early days or bad times some of this mollycoddling may be welcome, but in the long run you'll need gently to educate them into accepting that *you* can take charge of your life and aren't just a helpless victim. *You* are the expert, but (important) they can still play a welcome part in making life easier for you.

8 The problem of needing help − sometimes, but only sometimes

A thorny area. You may need (or want) a lot of help one day, and very little the next. No wonder other people get confused! One moment their help's fiercely rebuffed, the next they're accused of being heartlessly unhelpful!

As you become more skilled at dealing with the arthritis, you'll learn in which areas you do regularly need help. In other areas your needs may be unpredictable. Try to come to a clear agreement. Explain the predictable areas and how help can best be given. Agree that, otherwise, no help should be given, *unless* you ask. Promise that you *will* ask for help when you need it. Do what you can yourself, even if slower and clumsier.

Explain that one of the best forms of help is not to '*hinder*': not to create *extra* work and difficulties, eg by leaving things lying around that get in your way, or have to be cleared up (see page 160). And implore them not to move anything of yours without first asking permission. We all know how maddening it can be to spend hours getting something into a manageable position only to find it's moved away again the moment we turn our backs...

Work out how to use other people's desire to help constructively, so they really *do* help and so you really *are* grateful. Direct proceedings tactfully so you don't end up worse than you started! Work out, too, how to curb any *over*-helpfulness! Ironically, though they don't realise it, people who are overhelpful can make you feel *more* disabled:

"Two races of men! Those who make disability more disabling and those in whose presence one may even, mercifully, forget." (Grace Stuart, in *Private World of Pain*)

We don't want to put people off offering help − I feel we need to encourage them to make the offer, but then wait, and *listen* to our response: if help is wanted then it needs to be provided as requested, no more, no less, and without fuss. That's definitely the best sort of help! We in turn need to avoid gruffly rebuffing the offer – another time that help may be desperately needed. We can say something like 'thank you for offering, but I'm fine at the moment', or 'thank you for offering; perhaps I can explain how best you can help me'.

Look back at 'Balance the giving and the taking' (page 100), for more thoughts on 'help', and at page 216 for thoughts on asking for and giving help within a relationship.

9 Minding about 'what other people think'
Have faith in yourself, and the courage to be different, if necessary. Don't let 'what other people think' influence you. More often than not, they're thinking only about themselves, anyway! It's not easy to be self-confident when you're laid low emotionally and physically, and long to be inconspicuously 'normal', but it'll come, in time. Remind yourself that *you* are the only person who can decide what's right for you. Don't let 'what other people think' dictate how *you* organise *your* very different, unique, life.

Minding about 'what other people think' may be one reason you won't use a walking stick, or gadgets that would make life easier. Why let 'other people' dictate that your life should be more difficult than it need be? Are you telling them how they should lead *their* lives? For tips on coping with minding about the arthritis, and minding about other people's reactions, look back at page 103, 'Learning to live with the minding'.

Some thoughts on dealing with these Joe Public v Arthur Itis difficulties

If you're naturally extrovert, you're lucky, you're already well on the way to overcoming problems, but many of us are shy and retiring, too 'bruised' emotionally to want to come out of our shells. I believe we need to try, though. Margaret Mayson developed RA in her 20s. In Paul Hunt's *Stigma* she wrote:

"In time one learns a technique in handling the well-meant but tactless remark, but I was surprised to find how long I remained sensitive to comment on my crutches. A typical instance occurred at a social function when an acquaintance, completely uninhibited herself, called out, 'Whatever is the matter with you?'. My immediate and ignoble impulse was to make a facetious reply, 'Oh, I enjoy walking like this.' But I muttered, 'It's just the arthritis', feeling thoroughly ashamed. I would have felt quite happy to be able to say I'd broken a leg skiing or riding, because a healthy body, temporarily maimed, is very different from a body affected by a progressively crippling disease."

Chapter 13 will help. Remind yourself to keep things in perspective. *Most* especially, keep alive your sense of humour. Remember too:
–   Other people are well-meaning but ignorant; they need educating!
–   It's other people who are handicapped, not you.
–   Other people can't mind-read.
–   You're not on your own in the Joe Public v Arthur Itis match, though it sometimes feels that way.
–   Overcoming 'other people problems' will help not just you, but all YPAs.
–   The person you're talking to may be disabled too one day. What you say or do now could be important to him/her in the future.
–   More flies are caught with honey than with vinegar.
Try, too, putting yourself in other people's shoes to understand their reactions, and how best to tackle any difficulty.

To explain or not to explain?
Have a few facts and figures, even a funny story or two, ready for the times you do choose to explain. Where possible, I try to explain, briefly. A taxi-driver looks puzzled as I contort

my way into his cab and says 'what have you been up to then?'. [Not again, I sigh, inwardly, and take a deep breath.] 'Oh, it's rheumatoid arthritis'. [I know what's coming next] '*Never*, not at your age!' 'Well, it's amazing how many younger people *do* get it, sadly. Even small children'. [Then, if he's looking interested, and hasn't already started to tell me about *his* twinges, I add a few impressive facts and figures] 'Hmmm, yes, there are actually about 200 types of rheumatic disorder. Amazingly...etc'

Long explanations aren't always appropriate, for instance with children. They're naturally curious and want to know what's 'wrong'. A friendly, unembarrassed response is important. Upon your reply will depend future public attitudes. 'I've got a bad leg' might do, or, if the child's older, you could add 'It's something called rheumatoid arthritis'. If the child's interested in your stick or helping hand or wheelchair, use that interest constructively, and show them how it works. The worst thing is a child who's hustled away and told off by an embarrassed parent...

Coping with questions/remarks (sometimes very silly ones)
–   'But you're so young.'
–   'But you look so healthy.'
–   'Drunk again, dearie?'
–   'What on earth do you find to do with yourself all day?' (As a senior nurse pityingly said to a very talented RA friend in full-time employment...)
–   People think because your legs don't work properly your brain's packed up as well. What idiots. Stun them with a long account of all your talents, and continue with impressive examples of what other YPAs get up to.
–   'You're *wonderful*. How *do* you cope. *I* couldn't'. Maybe you demur with a blush, say 'oh no, I'm not wonderful' or suchlike, but do also give yourself a quiet pat on the back. Writing this book has really brought home to me the incredible courage and achievements of YPAs who've worked out ways of 'living with' arthritis. Don't squirm!
–   'There's plenty worse off than you.' Well – yes and no. I loathe comparisons of disability. Just because someone's in a wheelchair doesn't mean they're 'worse off' than a non-wheelchair-bound YPA with active RA/AS/lupus/whatever; the former may be a pain-free strong-armed London Marathon winner, the latter possibly unable to get across the room to make a cup of tea, let alone raise it to her lips, even in a wheelchair... Besides, thinking of 'others worse off than me' doesn't make me feel better: at really bad times, I feel if what I'm going through is *this* bad, what must it be like for them? I end up feeling thoroughly depressed!
–   'Count your blessings' – Yes I do, over and over again.
–   'Isn't your husband/wife/mother/father *wonderful* ...' 'For putting up with you' is left more or less unsaid. Well, yes, they certainly *are* wonderful – but I do resent the implication that I don't contribute anything, or have anything to put up with (!) in return. The 'disabled' partner may even be the *stronger* half in many ways, in emotional strength, good sense, household management, etc.

However... On the whole I'd rather people asked questions, even silly ones! At least then misunderstandings can be got into the open and cleared up. Some people would like to ask, but hesitate to do so. We YPAs can each develop our own style of making such people feel 'comfortable' about asking. A useful spin-off if you're fund-raising is that it gives you the opportunity to answer questions about why you're doing it.

Getting over some invisibility difficulties
You look young and healthy but feel b- awful, and simply can't bend this or that way to do whatever has to be done. Nothing for it, alas, but to make the invisible visible, or audible.

You drop something standing in the bus queue, but can't bend down to pick it up. No need to go into details, but ask someone briefly to help; something like 'I've got a bad leg and can't reach to pick that up; please could you help?' I was temporarily flummoxed when a doddery old lady dropped her bag and doddery young me was the only one to notice. Luckily I had a voice I could use to ask an unobservant someone else to help.

Another time, voice and eyes again proved their superiority. Sitting in Outpatients, I suddenly noticed an old man silently keel over and sink to the floor. Of the 30 or so people nearer than me, not one noticed or moved. Doddery me had to raise the alert.

If you're getting a lift in a car or taxi, mention that you'll be a bit slow getting in. It'll stop them rushing off too quickly. If your hand won't turn or bend to take change in a shop, try holding your purse out firmly and ask the assistant to count it in. Watch carefully to see it's correct. I used to be too proud to do this, and got sworn at by an assistant when all the coins she'd 'put in my hand' fell straight out into every nook and cranny. Hurtful at the time, but she wasn't to blame. How could she know?

Maybe you can dance, after a fashion, but think you'll look a bit odd to the handsome stranger you've just accompanied on to the dance floor. No time (or need) for a detailed medical history – something like 'I'm just a bit tired' or 'I'm not the world's best dancer' will do for the time being. Or indicate a poorly shoulder or bad neck. Remind yourself of the most important thing – s/he likes you enough to want to dance with you!

Getting over some visibility difficulties.

Maybe your illness is all too visible. People stare. Rude, and maddening. But the stares aren't necessarily *meant* to be hostile. Most people stare at something; if it weren't you it would be something or someone else. Don't you ever find yourself staring or looking twice at something unexpected?

Glare in return if you must! But if you're able to give them the benefit of the doubt, try a smile instead. Show you're really quite a civilised human being! Be a good advert for the rest of us YPAs. You might even get a smile and a friendly chat in return. A stare treated the right way can banish prejudice and even lead to friendships which would never have started if something hadn't attracted the other person's attention. Even in unfriendly London I made friends like this along the way to work.

Smile and the world smiles with you

Someone said 'Rheumatics are always smiling'. I dislike generalisations, but if that's true at all, it's certainly not that we're always happy...I suspect it's sometimes a cunning device to get the world on our side. (No, I don't like being described as something akin to pneumatics, like the Michelin man...)

A sense of humour certainly helps tremendously. Marie Joseph has a lovely one, and her autobiography is well worth reading. She's even able to chuckle at the maddening unpredictability of RA:

> "It does...ensure that you never become a bore. If asked how you are, and you are foolish enough to answer truthfully, there is always a different part to complain about."

White lies are useful too, as she says:

> "I learnt quite early to answer 'fine', every time my health was enquired about, and I'm sure that was the way I kept my friends, and ensured the sanity of my family. 'How d'you do?' is one of the most hypocritical phrases in the English language. No one really wants to know how you do, however much they may love you; they have their own lives to be getting on with..." (One Step at a Time, Arrow Books)

Close relationships – family and partners

The best medicine is the love and support of a person or people close to you. For many of us, this is what keeps us going. But the closest relationships can also be the ones most strained by arthritis. Things that cause problems in relationships outside the home cause misunderstandings inside too, indeed can sometimes seem even worse because home's the one place you feel you should be understood without endless explanations.

YPA Janet Flower put into words some thoughts that may sound familiar. In an article that could have been called 'Should they nag me, leave me, or help me?', she wrote:

"Do you ever think that people, even those closest to you, just don't understand..? Have YOU ever stopped to consider what living with an arthritic is like?

"Just because our nearest and dearest live with us doesn't mean they'll automatically become experts on arthritics and their needs/behaviour. Knowing more than the average person about its nature and treatment is not necessarily any help when it comes to day-to-day normal life. No doctor could hand out a guide to parents/partners. WE all have varying arthritis and varying needs of sympathy/ nagging; THEY all have different levels of patience, encouragement, sympathy, optimism, etc. Yet most of us expect our family to be understanding at all times but do we really stop to explain our difficulties or consider theirs?

"For instance, I used to struggle at home to manage something and if no-one noticed I'd think 'typical – no-one bothers to help'. Then when one of the family came over to assist, what was my reaction? Grateful thanks? No. A terse 'I CAN DO IT!'. So, no wonder they never knew whether to help or not. Yet I wouldn't expect strangers to realise I was in difficulty, or if they offered persistent unrequired help, I'd politely decline or accept without any sign of irritation.

"Finally, I realised how unfair I was being to my family. That they weren't always aware of my problems unless I told them and that it was just as difficult for them as anyone else to know whether to nag me, leave me or help me.

"Now I try to anticipate and communicate as much as possible to everyone and not expect the family to be experts or psychic. Another revelation was the 'guilt factor'. Realising that my Mum, especially, at times blamed herself for my illness. This was why she tried to protect me from things (not as I'd thought, to stop me enjoying myself). And why, at other times, she pushed and nagged at me for my own sake, (not as I'd thought, because I was an irritating burden).

"So many other families who seem uninterested, or too harsh, or too over-protective...are acting in the way they think best, rightly or wrongly. What is not perhaps realised by the arthritic is the awful pressure of guilt, responsibility and uncertainty their families come under. Doctors can't always tell whether a family is being too harsh/soft, etc. The family probably doesn't realise – and the arthritic may not either. It does therefore rest with us to guide and help, not just the public at large, but our own families, to know best how to help us.

"Often I've come across fellow arthritics who are scared to attempt any independence, who get no encouragement from their family. Others are fiercely independent but left with bitterness at the harshness of their family's attitude. The great majority, of course, find a happy medium but even so, a great deal of us could really benefit from looking more deeply into the matter, and realising that caring for an arthritic can be just as draining emotionally and physically as it is for the actual sufferer." (In Contact)

In Michael Leitch's *Living with Arthritis* (Lennard/Collins) Phil echoes the worrying thoughts of many married people with RA:

"I was very concerned about my husband, and I think what I felt must be a fear with many women who have arthritis. He has always been very supportive, and I have been lucky in that respect; but in the early days I remember thinking, 'What am I going to do if he leaves me?' I didn't want him to go – of course I didn't – but if he had decided to leave us, I would have understood.

"The husband of someone with arthritis has a lot of pressure on him. He comes in the

door after a long day at work and he does not know what he is going to find. It may be all right: she may have felt OK and been able to manage. But supposing she had had a bad day, which had been a real struggle to get through – what then? I can imagine husbands standing outside the door and thinking, What's going to face me tonight?"

Arthritis brings changes that the whole family has to adjust to, not just the YPA alone. This topic really needs a book to itself... More in later chapters about special relationships. For a male point of view, read Corbet Woodall's *A Disjointed Life* (Heinemann 1980).

Existing friendships and the arthritis

PB: *"I'd no idea, until it got really bad, that I had so many friends, good friends, true friends, kind people who will put themselves out time and time again to help. I think I appreciate people much more now and understand them better – understand their pain, their sufferings, be they physical or emotional. Arthritis has forced me to feel more, see further, understand more fully than ever before."*

A recently separated YPA:

"Then one weekend all my (our) friends came over; everyone! – it was an exhausting few days and it wasn't until they'd all gone home again that I realised how lucky I was. I probably won't see any of them for two or three months at a time, which seems endless, but the value of their love and friendship brought me back and now I want to fight."

Real friends are worth their weight in gold, the ones who stick with you. A special friend can help offload some of the misery which you can't offload on your nearest and dearest and give you support and breathing-space to weather the storms:

"I was short and bad-tempered with the kids and hardly spoke to poor old F. Finally I became so screwed up that it was obvious even to me that something had to be done. Reluctantly (I hate having to ask for help) I forced myself to pick up the phone and dial the number of a very understanding friend. She helped me over the bad bit until things settled down again both physically and mentally.." (Mary*)

In the early days, friends probably react as they would with any other short-term illness. They'll treat you in a special way, and will quite accept if you can't do something. In time, when the short-term illness ends the 'special treatment' comes to a natural end too.

Arthritis, of course, just has to be different, and some friendships may suffer, even end, in puzzling and hurtful ways. As time goes on, some friends may tire of waiting for things to get back to normal. Others will try harder, but even so may find it difficult, and puzzling. They can't see the pain, can't understand why one moment you leap down the stairs, yet another time take an eternity, struggling down on your backside. So remember to explain things to them. To avoid monotony, vary the reasons why you can't do things, and don't over-do the explaining! Corbet Woodall wrote:

"I've talked to one or two close friends... and they have said that the worst part for them was their inability to help and thus their frustration. The fact that they were constant and loyal enough to want to help was more than enough, because it took away much of the sheer loneliness which a long-term disease involves." (In *A Disjointed Life*)

In time you and your real friends will adjust. Talking to other YPAs will give you no end of tips; other parts of this chapter will help too. Just a few ideas here to be going on with:

- Put yourself in their place from time to time and take a look at 'You' from the outside. Remember they may see a crotchety 'outside' you, they can't see what's going on inside, the pain and frustrations, etc, so explain, in moderation. Show them an ARC booklet too, maybe, to help them understand.
- Take the initiative in working out solutions to problems. Maybe someone suggests a walk on a bright sunny day, and you know your body won't cooperate. Could the walk be done with a slight change in plan? Suggest a flat rather than a hilly area, perhaps, or choose a spot where they can walk while you sit in the car and enjoy the view. Or – let

them go off and do what they want to do. You can still take an interest. They'll enjoy telling you all about it later. Put the time they're away to good use (eg read an interesting book, listen to a radio play, learn a funny poem, etc; all things you can chat about later). You'll all end up having had a stimulating afternoon.

- Find new areas of common interest. Counteract awful feelings of 'being left out', eg if friends and family seem constantly to be doing things you can't do, suggest things you *can* all do – playing board or quiz games, going to the cinema, driving around a drive-in zoo, etc. If you used to enjoy sports, there are still some you might be able to share with friends, either actively, or by spectating, or by becoming, say, a tennis umpire or cricket scorer. See chapter 35 on 'Pastimes' for more ideas. Peter West took up sports commentating when AS stopped a more active sports career.
- Don't clutter relationships with too many can'ts. Emphasise the can dos.
- Helping yourself will help relationships with other people too. Eliminate practical problems as much as possible, eg by using gadgets and eliminate anything making life and you more 'unfriendly' than need be.
- Look outwards: take an interest in other people and their activities. The less time you have to worry about your illness the better and the more likely people are to find you interesting, and to want to seek your company.
- Don't be too demanding. Let them do their own thing without feeling guilty about you.
- Try not to shout at friends over-anxious to help! Sort out potentially thorny 'help' problems. (Look back at page 196.)
- Ration moans and groans! No need to pretend the arthritis doesn't exist, but keep it in perspective. Even if it seems to be dominating your life, it has limited interest for friends as a topic of conversation. Concentrate on areas where you *do* have something in common. (You'll still need escape valves for your moans and groans of course – see page 102.)

Meeting new people, and making friends

When you're going through a bad patch it's easy to blame everything on the arthritis, especially if you're feeling lonely and finding it hard to meet people and make friends, but plenty of people without arthritis experience shyness and loneliness too. Arthritis can, it's true, create physical barriers which make it hard to get out to meet people, but if these can be overcome, then many of the remaining problems, like shyness and lack of confidence aren't so different from other people's. So reading something like Dr Phyllis M Shaw's *Meeting People is Fun* (Sheldon), and other books on page 206 can be helpful, even though most of the books listed aren't specifically 'arthritic'. Best of all, have a chat with another YPA, or a sympathetic somebody else.

Overcoming physical barriers

For ways of tackling any physical problems of getting out to meet people look back at chapter 24, 'Out and about'.

Keep your horizons as wide as possible. Meet other people through work (paid or voluntary), through hobbies, through evening classes, Open University, residential study weekends, through local special interest organisations or a multi-activity social group like Nexus (see page 292), and through organisations like PHAB and Arthritis Care. If you're shy about going alone, why not phone the secretary first, to explain? Maybe one or two of the members could come along first to meet you at home. See chapter 35, 'Pastimes', and chapters 13 and 33 for more ideas.

Many of us, when unattached, hope that in meeting other people we'll meet 'someone special'. Wonderful when we do. Many of us *have* been lucky and met someone special, as you'll see from the 'Marriage' chapter, for instance. But don't, please, limit your horizons by becoming over-obsessed with that hope. Simply meeting other people and making friends is wonderful too, and it's easy to lose sight of how precious friendship can be, whether you live a solo life or in partnership.

Who knows, meeting that 'special person' may happen when you're least expecting it. S/he could be the sister or brother or son or daughter of anyone you meet anywhere! I met my special person through work – he was the friend of a colleague's boyfriend.

Some YPAs, now married, met through a Young Arthritis Care meeting or holiday. At least one YPA, Mandy King, boldly tried computer dating. It was a bit nerve-racking to start with. Her first date was with Simon:

"We arranged to meet at a pub in Essex approximately mid-way between London and Southend...at this point I began thinking 'Hell, what about old Arthur-ritis?' You see, on the computer form there was no section about physical disability... I hesitated to put anything about it in my letters, because quite frankly some people have odd ideas about arthritis and it's hardly an asset when meeting members of the opposite sex. 'I'm blond, slim, with blue eyes and a pair of ravishing arthritic kneecaps...' Hmmmm!

"When I arrived at the pub...my knees were like pillars of jelly! Luckily, Simon had positioned himself fairly near the door so I didn't have to wander around the pub feeling conspicuous. I needn't have worried – we soon began talking and the evening passed really quickly...we enjoyed each other's company. The dreaded arthritis only came up in conversation when I found I was unable to undo the cream container served with the coffee! Simon had noticed my 'funny' fingers earlier but being a polite gentleman he hadn't liked to ask me what was wrong! I explained briefly and was secretly pleased to discover that it didn't seem to make a lot of difference.

"I was most impressed with my first date and this encouraged me to go out with several other people afterwards...The odd disastrous evening would occur...but really I found these occasions to be surprisingly infrequent. Some months and several dates later I still thought about my original meeting with Simon and realised that I liked him quite a lot. One day, on impulse, I rang him and we decided to meet yet again...

"I know a lot of people are put off by the 'contrived' aspect of computer dating agencies, but basically, all they do is put you in touch with individuals whom you are most likely to get on with – after that of course it's up to you...Don't make the mistake of thinking that anyone who can't find a boyfriend/girlfriend in the normal way must be a bit odd; members can be people moving to a new area looking for friends, or separated people getting over relationships... All I can say to anyone thinking of doing likewise is go ahead...you've got nothing to lose!" (*In Contact*)

Not long ago, Mandy and Simon got married.

The computer dating agency called Dateline produces the glossy *Dateline magazine*, for anyone, not specifically for disabled people. It's available in shops, or on subscription.

Even if you can't get out much, there are ways you can communicate with other people from home, for instance by becoming a Citizen's Band follower, or playing chess or scrabble by correspondence, or, like Janet Mason, writing to penfriends, by cassette if that's easier:

"Up to now I have got five actual Pen-Pals (people who I write to regularly and have never met), three female and two male, and then I have four or five friends who I met either at school, college, or in hospital and live too far away to see who I keep in touch with regularly. Then...I have 'annual' friends as well, if you see what I mean so I am kept quite busy. [And] I often write to television stars, pop stars, etc, asking for their autographs. I love doing it.. Easier than talking on the phone I think, and cheaper!!..."

You could help run a DIAL information service, or invite people round to you, for musical or book-reading/discussion evenings, or card games, or organise a birthday card reminder service, or whatever...!

Overcoming emotional barriers

Arthritis can sometimes create emotional barriers when we meet other people, when, for instance, we feel self-conscious and ill-at-ease with our bodies, and out of touch with healthy contemporaries. Or when other people feel ill-at-ease with us. In *Meeting People is Fun*, Dr Shaw reminds us that other people experience similar feelings:

"Some people who have never regarded themselves as particularly shy discover at some stage following a crisis in their life that it is difficult to make relationships with other people or even to approach them. Sudden bereavement in early or middle life, the arrival of a congenitally handicapped child, redundancy and other events which change circumstances may bring on a form of shyness or social anxiety."

We can start to do something about this once we understand why it happens. Look back at the section on page 192 onwards on 'How does the arthritis create problems between us and other people?' Dr Shaw, again:

"You have to remind yourself time and time again that other people are well-meaning but ignorant. They do not know how to cope with your situation, they realise how grave it is and would like to help but are frightened all the time of interfering and putting a foot wrong. This is why bereaved, separated or divorced people sometimes complain of being shunned or avoided...

"Other situations include physical catastrophe from outside, such as assault, burglary or an accident, and although these might seem obvious cases where friends and neighbours could rally round, yet again we find the familiar problem that they are frightened of interfering and worry that they will say the wrong thing. Once again, the sufferer has to make the first move."

Encouraging other people to relate to us in a friendly and comfortable way comes, with time and practice. The old tricks really work, like taking a warm, friendly interest in the *other* person, asking them about themselves, and cultivating hobbies and interests which you can share, taking your mind and theirs off the arthritis. After all, arthritis *isn't* the most important thing about you, so keep it in its place!

Sometimes the way we react to the arthritis can indirectly put people off. Pride and a fierce desire to be independent may make us appear gruff or aloof. An over-obvious craving for reassurance can be off-putting too. Insecurity may make us mumble, creating other misunderstandings. Try to appear calm and quietly self-confident, even if that's not how you feel inside.

Please, for the sake of the rest of us, don't fall into the trap of becoming a 'professional arthritic' or 'professional moaner'! A mention now and again's OK, and we do want to educate people. It's a part of your life, yes, but only a part. Please avoid giving the rest of us a bad name!

For more tips look at the books mentioned at the end of this chapter, and look back too at chapter 13. You may sometimes wonder if it's worth making the effort at all, but that's normal:

"By and large, in our society where there are few rules and little is taught in the formal way, we have to learn by trial and error. This means it takes quite a lot of courage and it is not easy for any of us to learn social confidence easily. Knowing this will perhaps help you be more tolerant of your own shortcomings." (Dr Shaw again)

Feeling lonely

It's all too easy to feel like Anne Ryman, when she first had RA, in her teens/twenties:

"I felt a lot closer to my mother and grandmother's friends than those my own age. My contemporaries were all racing round going to all-night parties, and getting engaged in their droves, and I felt as if I was on another planet."

Yes, but try not to let loneliness get to you or make you bitter. Bitterness doesn't help with making friends. Work at feeling happy alone, hard though it may be at times. Loneliness and being alone are different. The latter can be enjoyable and does have its advantages. You can get up and go to bed when you like, watch what TV you like, and be as messy as you like. No one else's mess to put up with, and there's a *lot* to be said for being able to do things at *your* pace, knowing that you'll find things exactly where you left them! Paradoxically, the happier we are at being alone, with ourselves, the happier we're likely to be in relating to other people.

If loneliness is getting you down really badly, don't forget the Samaritans (known worldwide as Befrienders International) who are *always* only a phone call away. Give them a ring. Look back at chapter 13 on working towards a positive philosophy, and at chapter 14, the section on 'talking therapy'. Look too at all the ideas in chapter 35 for developing interests which you'll be able to share with other people. Look back at page 117 for the benefits other people found from joining a self-help group: join Arthritis Care/Young Arthritis Care, NASS or another self-help group, and try Nexus and/or other clubs mentioned on page 292 and elsewhere.

The non-profitmaking Portia Trust was set up about 20 years ago to help people in trouble or distress. They produce a monthly magazine, called *Future Friends*, 'with one thing linking all its readers: genuine loneliness. We refuse salacious or suggestive advertisements... some readers are searching for companionship, some want pen-friends, some seek marriage, and so far as we can ensure it, all are genuine.'

Boyfriends/girlfriends

The worries of being lonely may idiotically be replaced by other worries the moment a boyfriend/girlfriend comes on the scene. Some, it's true, may be put off by the arthritis – but those are the ones not worth bothering with anyway. If it wasn't the arthritis, there'd be some other paltry excuse. Take heart from a 25 year old girl with RA:

"I would like to tell young girls who have arthritis not to give up and not to think boys don't want them. I was engaged to a boy for three years who knew from the beginning about my complaint. Just one day he broke it off because I had arthritis. I was heart-broken, but some months later I met Steve, my husband. I have been in hospital many times, but he has always stood by me. I think I am very lucky." (*Under 35s News* no. 10)

And another writer, in *In Contact*:

"...what is awkward, in my experience, is when you get the feeling the person wants to ask you about it, but doesn't like to ask. Or when they do ask it is a question of telling them enough without going into your whole medical history. I have had people ask me out merely because they 'felt sorry for me' and on the other hand not asking me out because yes, they were 'put off' by the arthritis. On the whole though most blokes do simply accept the arthritis, and naturally this is better for both parties and means 'problems' can be dealt with at the time, together, and without embarrassment or feeling you've got to keep up an image..."

Those of us who developed arthritis very early on may find we missed out on what Peter Nightingale, in Michael Leitch's *Living with Arthritis* calls 'the social growing-up bit',

"Everything takes longer if you have arthritis, which is why at the age of 32 I am still living at home with my mum and dad. This is not unusual among the people with arthritis that I know, but it is unusual among the population as a whole...I never used to mix with anyone after school. I went to a single-sex school, I was picked up in the afternoon and taken home, and that was it...The result is that you need more time to grow up and mature..."

So finding someone special might take an extra long time. I didn't find him until I was 32. Other people I know have suddenly discovered him/her in their late 20s, or 30s. At least by then you've learnt better how to deal with the arthritis and its wily ways.

A word of warning on the boy/girlfriend scene. Some of us have been in the situation where we're so desperate for a boy/girlfriend we've allowed ourselves to fall for someone we wouldn't normally have looked at twice, and regretted it. It's a difficult situation to extract yourself from. Be choosy, arthritis or no arthritis. Watch your motives as well as theirs! Reginald Ford warns about another stumbling block for some young men:

> *"Many women, especially those of a certain age and experience (or lack of it), think they are perfectly safe in mothering or sistering anyone suffering from apparently incapacitating disablement. They are genuinely embarrassed and shocked when they find that the protégé has normal masculine feelings – perhaps even stronger because of enforced suppression. They feel he has let them down if he reacts in a normal way, and many a beautiful friendship has ended in protestations of injured innocence and misunderstandings on one side, and on the other deeper bitterness and disillusionment. Pity is no basis for any but the most temporary or superficial relationship."* (Writing in Paul Hunt's *Stigma*, Geoffrey Chapman, 1966)

Happy relationships with other people

I seem, alas, to have talked an awful lot about problems with other people in this chapter. Sorry! That's *not* the whole picture. But I do believe that it helps to understand the problems, before then pushing them away where they belong, into a corner.

Let me reassure you there's plenty of joy and love and happiness and fun out here in our relationships with other people, be they family, lovers, friends, or neighbours, work colleagues, acquaintances, or whatever. For me certainly the most important thing in coping with the arthritis has been the support of a loving, imaginative, and understanding family and some wonderful friends. We've had our problems, but many can be overcome. So get what problems you can out of the way, then relax, have fun, and make the most of the brighter side of life.

'Laugh and the world laughs with you; weep and you weep alone.' Maybe sometimes you *will* weep, but remember you *don't* weep alone, because we other YPAs also know what the problems are. Remember there'll be good times too, when you *will* be able to laugh. Laugh and we and the world will happily laugh with you.

Further Reading/Contacts

The books here barely, if at all, mention chronic illness or arthritis, but they're nonetheless worth looking at. Look too at the books in chapter 29, 'Personal accounts of arthritis'.

- Dr R H Phillips' *Coping with Rheumatoid Arthritis* and *Coping with Lupus* (Avery Publishing, Garden City Park, New York, USA), latter available through Lupus UK.
- *How to start a Conversation and Make Friends*, by Don Gabor (Sheldon Press)
- *The Relate Guide to Better Relationships* by Sarah Litvinoff (Ebury Press). Helpful even if you're not in a relationship, eg sections on dealing with anger, overcoming communication difficulties.
- *Human Relationships*, by Steve Duck (Sage publications)
- *A Woman in Your Own Right*, by Anne Dickson (Quartet) and *Assert Yourself* by Gael Lindenfield (Thorsons) deal with assertiveness. Learning to be assertive can help you cope with expressing difficult feelings, eg anger, anxiety, in a positive way, building up self-confidence and self-esteem. The Young Arthritis Care Personal Development Courses include help in developing these skills.

You'll find other helpful books (all available by post) on the booklists from Relate, Healthwise, the British Holistic Medical Association, the Sheldon Press and Thorsons Publishing. Some publications concentrate specifically on a solo life, eg:

- *Living Alone: A Woman's Guide*, by Liz McNeill Taylor (Sheldon). The writer's a freelance journalist, widowed in her 40s, with four children. Assumes you're fit, so some of it's irrelevant, but has useful ideas, nonetheless, for women and men too.

Chapter twenty-six

MARRIAGE AND PARTNERSHIPS

"Being an arthritic...is not romantic...*What man is there, who would want to plight his troth to a woman who sits with her feet in a bowl of Epsom-salted water four times a day? Or to one who can't get her right arm high enough to wind it lovingly around his neck?..."* (Marie Joseph, in *One Step at a Time*, Arrow Books)

Plenty of men, fortunately, do plight their troth. Including, despite the Epsom salts and RA, 'Mr Marie Joseph'. Most of us know what Marie means, though. Married or unmarried, we worry about the effects arthritis might have on a partner.

Any setbacks due to the arthritis will test the strengths and weaknesses in a partnership. Male or female, if the arthritis has laid you low, your spirits may be low, and your love life/marriage/partnership all too easily laid low too. You may worry about becoming a burden, about your body's ability to make love, worry your partner may walk out, etc. Added to which, alas, it is often our nearest and dearest who take the brunt of frustration and anger due, not to them, but to the arthritis. More setbacks...

It's true that any problems will test the love and strength of a relationship, but, as the experts on relationships, Relate Counsellors, point out:

"Meeting problems together and in the right way deepens love, and couples who learn to tackle differences positively can survive even serious crises." (*The Relate Guide to Better Relationships* by Sarah Litvinoff, Ebury Press, 1991, a really excellent book.)

How do partnerships that already exist cope, survive, even flourish when arthritis appears on the scene? And if the arthritis arrives beforehand, how does a successful partnership ever start?

When arthritis is on the scene before a partnership starts

The good news is that many of us who are unattached (except unwillingly to the arthritis) *do* find someone special to share our lives with. I was flabbergasted when my Special Person turned up, in my early 30s, and flabbergasted too that he actually had the patience to put up with the arthritis quirks which had long ago exhausted *my* patience. Even more amazed that he actually fancied me and my far from perfect body. Oh yes, and that I fancied *him*!

I know plenty of other YPAs too who've forged great relationships. How reassuring it would have been for spotty and doddery adolescent me to know all this *was* possible. Maybe you *will* meet that Special Person, and form a married or unmarried partnership. Maybe it'll take longer than you imagined. Or maybe you won't. Maybe, instead, you'll live a solo life, which need be no less happy and satisfying.

The important thing, whatever happens, is to value yourself and to keep the arthritis in its place, as only one of the very many things that make up the unique and special 'you'. When you feel comfortable with yourself, other people will feel comfortable with you, and you'll be well-prepared either for a successful relationship with that Special Person when s/he comes along, or for a successful solo life if Fate, or you, choose otherwise.

To get hitched − or not?

What happens when you do meet that Special Person, and a long-term partnership is in the air? You may have some misgivings:

"My deep love for Evan heightened my depression, for I felt I could be of no possible use to him in the future and I ought therefore to end our engagement. However, despite the many traumas, Evan stood by me as a tower of strength and I came out of hospital some 13 months after admission...Within four months of leaving hospital I was married and I must be the only person who has gone on honeymoon with a large bag of extra arms and legs [ie splints] *for luggage..."* (Carol J, with RA)

"When I was 26 I was going to get engaged but felt through my condition it was not fair to burden myself on a girl several years younger, because if I was ever to become really ill, by the time I was 30 she would still be a young woman and I don't think it would be fair on her." (YPA, with RA)

Doubts and worries like these are understandable. But it's appalling that other people should sometimes add yet more. When I was in hospital I was horrified to meet a girl who told me her fiancé's parents had stopped him marrying her when she'd developed RA. How dare they? (On second thoughts, maybe it was for the best: if he couldn't sort out his parent-problem what hopes were there for other black spots, inevitable in any marriage?).

Don't, for goodness sake, be put off by people like his parents. We've just the same right to love and be loved as anyone else. Even the right to be emotionally hurt at times, too. Plenty of people come to mind, physically fit, but totally disabled in their emotional relationship with each other. That's one way in which we *don't* have to be disabled!

True, other people, especially parents, may worry. That's understandable. Encourage them to air their worries, and to help you think through any problems and work out solutions together, rather than to create more by any antagonism. Don't though be dictated to about what you should or shouldn't do. You and your Special Person need to work out what's uniquely right for you two. Would living together be better than marrying, or vice versa, for instance? Here are some thoughts to mull over, when the two of you are thinking about a married or unmarried long-term relationship:

- Marriage is a mighty big step, arthritis or no arthritis. Just as you need to sort out your thoughts and expectations on money, for instance, or on children, so too sort out your thoughts on the arthritis. Make sure you both understand what you can about your type of arthritis, and that you both express and discuss any doubts and fears. Read, for instance, any relevant ARC booklets, and talk to your rheumatologist.

- Accept and admit to each other that there may be problems to be overcome. Try jotting down separately what worries you, then talk them through. By bringing fears into the open they can be dealt with and kept in perspective. Find out where you could get help if necessary.

- Though some worries are understandable, try not to be too negative. To my mind, some YPAs actually make the same mistake as many ignorant Jill and Joe Publics. They see themselves only as 'disabled', as 'burdens', as arthritis and nothing else, forgetting all the 'disabilities' and quirks, odd ways and habits, so-called *non*-disabled people bring to relationships, and forgetting completely their 1,001 other qualities and abilities. Write at least some of *these* down, to remind yourself and your partner!

- Coping with other people's misgivings. You could ignore them; or remind them that 'the able-bodied of today may be the disabled of tomorrow', which could include them, one day. Perhaps the best option is first to give them examples of successful 'arthritic partnerships'. Get them to express any worries; but make sure they know the *true* facts about your type of arthritis. They may think *everyone* with RA/its cousins will end up wheelchair-bound – *very* far from the truth. Or they may be unaware of all the help available to overcome problems. Don't be modest about your talents and abilities – make sure they hear *all* about those, too, *not* just about the arthritis. Remember that in the end what really matters is what you and your Special Person think and feel.

- Don't be so obsessed by the arthritis that you forget everything else! Look at some of the books and leaflets written for *anyone* contemplating marriage (eg on page 217, especially the Relate book). Think about what they say. Agony Aunt advice on 'giving and taking', on the importance of 'communicating' with each other, even tips on how to put up with his smelly socks/her chatting all through his favourite TV programme will all help to keep your partnership on a happy, even keel.

- Your sex life. Read chapter 27. Sex-plus-arthritis can go well or badly, just as it can for anyone. When it goes well it can be wonderful, and go a long way to making up for arthritis-induced difficulties in other areas of your life.
- Pregnancy and children. Get facts straight. Read chapter 28. Work out your thoughts on the subject together. For me, before I'd commit myself to a long-term relationship, it was essential my partner knew I'd decided long ago not to have children, and essential to hear his thoughts on the subject, and to be sure they were genuine.
- Might advice or counselling from a 'third party' help you both? For instance, a rheumatologist, an enlightened OT, a nurse specialising in rheumatology, or a Relate (relationships) counsellor? Or a Young Arthritis Care Contact? Besides giving you practical tips, it's sometimes easier to bounce ideas and worries off a third person than face-to-face in a twosome.
- Don't be so obsessed by any problems *you* might be bringing to the relationship that you forget to think about whether your partner might have any that need thinking about!

Some inspiring thoughts from Dr Wendy Greengross:

"No one is perfect, and the happiest marriages are between people who realise this, recognise each other's limitations and can express and accept their mutual feelings of inadequacy and their particular needs and anxieties. Communication is the key word in any discussion on relationships, sex and marriage; because the ability to put those very personal feelings into words and deeds not only helps a couple to understand and appreciate each other, but also helps them *to grow as individuals, and the marriage to develop into something worthwhile and lasting.*

"Where many marriages go wrong – particularly among the young – is in ignoring the fact that communication is not only communicating one's strong points. It is showing that there are weaknesses and vulnerable spots too. For the disabled contemplating marriage, the fear of being unlovable is reinforced by the fear that if they reveal their weaknesses they seem even less attractive. If they go into marriage concealing their real emotional needs and bottling up frustrations and depressions and putting a brave face on it, they will be heading for trouble. It is knowing that you will be loved warts and all that makes marriage a rewarding experience. No marriage can survive on false pretences..." (In *Entitled to Love*, J M Dent)

What about when arthritis invades existing partnerships?

Yes, partnerships *do* weather the storms, and they *do* thrive. Take, for example, a lovely lady I met in hospital. She's in her 50s now. She'd led a full and active life, working hard as a hospital sister, and enjoyed lots of sports too. RA struck in her early 20s, when she'd been married just a few months. The doctor told her she'd be in a wheelchair in no time and shouldn't even think about becoming pregnant. Soon afterwards she *was*. She produced two lovely daughters, now grown up, and, some 30 years and several operations later, she is still gallantly weathering ups and downs in the same happy marriage.

A good partnership has to be worked at, and will always have its ups and downs, but the ups are wonderful, and better than any medicine. Sadly, for some of us, there's the other side of the story too. The walkouts, even divorces, when the going gets too tough for some partners:

"My husband could not deal with the problems of my disability at the end of the day and so opted out. That I could have understood to a certain extent if he hadn't chosen to

opt out with my best friend. It must be difficult being on the other side of the coin, coming home from work..and to more problems and sometimes despair. I'm sure he felt unable to help any more; for that I don't blame him...The person who has helped the most is my mother-in-law. She should be nominated as a saint! Her support and my father-in-law's have been wonderful."

Maybe, alas, a break-up would have happened anyway. All sorts of things conspire to cause difficulties in any marriage, not just the villainous Arthur Itis. Hardly surprising if his uninvited appearance is more than some relationships can take. *Some.* By no means all. It's crucial to remember there's lots that can be done along the way to weather any storms, to avoid break-up, and to encourage calmer, happier days to appear.

Some outsiders find it surprising that so many marriages *do* survive and flourish, but they do:

"I must give credit to my husband who has shown infinite patience with me during the trying times. Now of course we can laugh at a lot of problems but it hasn't always been like that." (Jacqueline S, now in her mid 50s, developed RA in her early 20s)

"My husband really is so helpful now. At the beginning I don't think he understood how bad I was. Since then he has been attending the hospital with me and seems to be a lot more understanding. We both get on really well, and somehow we both have to work just that little bit harder at our home, children, marriage, etc. Maybe that is what keeps the marriage sparkling!" (Bernadette Sparks, 28, with RA, married nine years, two children)

In this chapter I'm looking particularly at the emotional strains on a relationship, but interwoven with those there may be others, too: social and financial strains, for instance, and sex. Sex I'll deal with later, in chapter 27, for:

"sex is only part of the marriage relationship, and... if a couple are not satisfying each other's emotional needs then a wild sex life is not going to make up for it." (Dr Wendy Greengross, *Entitled to Love*, J M Dent)

Although the partner with arthritis is the one suffering the pain and stiffness and exhaustion firsthand, others in the family may suffer and need to readjust their lives too. Like us they have to learn to understand what's happening and to work through their feelings. Think of your own reactions to the arthritis. Fear, anxiety, depression, frustration, anger, guilt? Your partner may have similar feelings, and worry about you and the illness and the future, wondering what to do for the best, how to help you, and so on. Other family members, too, in varying degrees. Or they may feel totally unable to handle the situation, and shut themselves off from you.

In the early days, when there's so little to see, they may even disbelieve that there's anything wrong with you. Who's to say you're not just being lazy or making it all up, being wilfully slow and clumsy or just bloodyminded, apparently deciding you can do the ironing and cooking one day and next to nothing the next? The pain and stiffness of something like RA may be bad enough, but its invisibility, variability, and unpredictability are particularly nasty extras, seemingly almost guaranteed to produce misunderstandings and communication problems in the best of marriages. It may seem to threaten everything those idyllic Mills and Boon or TV soap opera marriages would have you believe are essential (they aren't, of course) – an attractive body, expressive 'body language', spontaneity, energy, self-confidence, and the wonderful, wonderful glow of health.

OK, yes, alas, there may be problems, especially in the early days. But do, please, hang on in there, both of you. Be patient. Remember what Jacqueline and Bernadette said above? They did have ups and downs, but things got better. Take heart from knowing that others have been through it before. It'll get easier to handle, and any struggle will be worth it in the long run. A happy relationship that you work at together will help put all other problems in perspective.

To understand something of the mixed feelings of you both, read again Sandy

Burnfield's comparison of the onset of chronic illness with a bereavement, on page 90. Read too, both of you, the rest of this chapter, and chapters 25 and 27. As Sandy Burnfield explained, both partners (and other family members) need to 'mourn their loss', and adjust to changes in their relationship. Sandy's own illness is multiple sclerosis (MS), medically totally different from rheumatic disorders, but emotional reactions can be similar.

Both partners in the relationship need support, though may find it difficult to give it to each other, as Sandy (in *Multiple Sclerosis*, Souvenir Press Ltd) explains:

"...if they become depressed at the same time, it will not be easy for them to help each other. Instead they may feel unsupported and resentful towards one another. Wives and husbands may feel uncertain about how far to push the partner who has the MS, and may not be able to distinguish between difficult behaviour which is really due to the MS, and behaviour which is due to normal selfishness or bloody mindedness!"

"...A caring partner may feel overwhelmed and exhausted by the constant demands made on her...and may feel trapped in the relationship. She may find it impossible to cope with her partner's depression, irritability and self-pity and may desperately need someone to care for her, too, sometimes, and to understand her needs."

What can you do about any relationship problems?

What really does make a happy marriage? How much of it really does depend on glowing physical good health? All marriages are different, but most people would probably agree that the recipe for a perfect marriage should include give-and-take, tolerance, good humour and a sense of humour, the ability to communicate with each other, the ability to accept differences and clear up misunderstandings, the willingness to share feelings about the ups *and* the downs, and shared friendship, too, over and above the original 'zing' of love and attraction. You don't have to be physically fit to have *any* of these qualities!

True, having arthritis in the list of ingredients can mess up the recipe. But cooks can learn skills to avert disasters, or lessen them, at least. There are skills you can use together to handle problems, and others you can work on individually. First, some you can look at together.

Essential skills for both of you

● *Learn about the arthritis, together*   Tackle the medical problems first and you're well on the way to sorting out emotional difficulties. With the help of your doctor, try to understand what the arthritis is doing to you physically, and how best to deal with the symptoms. Encourage your partner to join in the finding out process. Remind yourselves that various treatments *are* available to help keep the symptoms manageable, though it may take a while to work out what best suits your particular body.

● *Sort out practical problems, even the tiniest*   Molehills can so easily grow into mountains. Depending on the severity of the lurgy, you may need to deal with bigger changes to your lifestyle. Tackle changes, together. You would, wouldn't you, if you were moving house, changing jobs, or planning a family? A chronic illness in a partnership needs to be dealt with the same way. You *both* need to take stock and work out where changes are needed; rethink your use of time, money, physical strength, energy, social life, hobbies, etc. Look back at chapter 22 for starters. Put your heads together and work out how you can each/all best contribute to running the home. Think separately about it beforehand, before pooling your different ideas. Make sure everyone has their fair share of suggesting *and* being listened to!

You, the YPA, can still be an important part of the family by taking charge of the non-physical side of household management, eg planning meals and the shopping list. Some physical tasks may still be possible, like preparing the meal, with careful forward planning, or if others put everything ready in the right place first.

● *Understand the peculiarities of chronic arthritis, together* Try looking back at chapter 25. Discuss it together, and discuss what bits do or don't apply in your partnership. Tackle misunderstandings before they get out of hand. Get outside help, if necessary, eg from your doctor, OT and social worker, supportive family and friends, and from other people who've been through similar experiences, especially old-hander YPAs. Don't hesitate to try Relate (the former National Marriage Guidance Council), perhaps, CARE, or the Catholic Marriage Advisory Council, even the Samaritans, or any counsellor or support service your doctor can recommend. Look back at page 110, 'talking therapy'. An outsider can often help defuse an otherwise explosive situation. Take heart from knowing that others have been through it before, and there *is* light at the end of the tunnel.

● *Communication – keyword to success* It means each of you saying what you think, at an appropriate time, and each of you in turn listening, really listening, to what's said, not mind-reading it, and acknowledging and respecting the other's opinions and feelings even if they're different from your own. Listening means allowing the other person to say what s/he really wants to say, without feeling under attack. *The Relate Guide to Better Relationships* is the best written source I've come across of practical, really excellent advice on understanding and dealing with communication difficulties.

Many arguments start because one partner misunderstands what the other says and takes offence, unreasonably. Think before you speak. Misunderstandings can happen all too easily between two people tired of coping with a chronic illness.

Be wary of misreading 'hidden messages'. For instance, the fit partner may misinterpret an angry or critical comment by the YPA to mean 'I'm not a bit grateful for what you do' or 'I hate you', when it really means 'Can't you see how miserable I am? – I desperately need your help and support' or 'I'm really afraid of losing you, so I'll make sure I *don't* like you then I won't miss you when you've gone'.

You'll both need to handle misunderstandings with all the skills of a diplomat, and like a diplomat you may need at times to negotiate through a third party. *Do*, as I said before, make use of outsiders like doctor/counsellor/Relate/Samaritans/priest/special friends, etc, to defuse potentially explosive situations.

● *Anger in the partnership* Again, the *Relate Guide to Better Relationships* has lots of really helpful practical tips. Look too at page 86. Psychiatrist Sandy Burnfield also has helpful thoughts on handling what can be a very destructive emotion in a relationship under stress from chronic illness. His own illness is multiple sclerosis (MS), medically totally different from rheumatic disorders, but emotional reactions can be similar:

"Sometimes it is difficult for the caring relative to be angry with a partner who has multiple sclerosis. This can be because she feels guilty, and because she does not want to hurt someone who is already vulnerable and dependent, through no fault of his own. On the other hand, the person who has MS may also feel angry, he may have lost his role as 'the bread winner' in a family and may resent being dependent and having to rely on his partner. He, too, may feel unable to express his anger, in case he is rejected by the person who has control over him. This anger can gradually build up until it either explodes or turns into severe depression....

"The very thing that people hope to avoid – violence – can become more likely to happen when they are unable or unwilling to admit their angry feelings towards one another. The opposite is also true. Once we can openly say to someone, 'I am angry with you', this can lead to deeper honesty and love in a relationship. But saying that we are angry is not the same as saying 'You make me angry', or 'It is your fault that I am angry'. These responses are destructive and are made by a person who is not taking responsibility for himself. He is trying to force another person to feel responsible or guilty for his own feelings.

"We all need to realise that anger is not necessarily bad or destructive. It is a

natural reaction to frustration or misunderstanding, and admitting this to ourselves is often the best way of putting things right. By doing this we can help other people to take responsibility for their feelings and behaviour, and some sort of adult solution will be found to the problems. Usually there are misunderstandings and mistakes on both sides, and each person needs to give as well as take in a relationship.

"By treating anger in this way we are behaving as adults. I am not suggesting that we go to extremes and shout and scream as soon as we feel under strain! This would be a childish response; we have to be mature enough to choose the right time and the right way to express our anger, not any old place at any time. Self-control is just as important as freedom of expression, and they must go together if we are to get the balance right. Perhaps I can compare it to fire. Fire and anger are similar; they are not in themselves good or bad, it all depends on what we do with them."

- *Blame Arthur Itis, the intruder, not each other*   Giving the arthritis a name and personality can be helpful. It means you can blame 'him', the real villain, and not each other. You can talk about him angrily, or with a touch of humour. Unite against him as your common enemy. Agree to support each other against him/it, not to blame each other for problems that *he* causes.

- *Turn towards each other, not away*   When we're unhappy we may turn inwards, in a way that may put other people off trying to get close physically and emotionally. Both of you need to understand this and make a conscious effort to turn towards each other rather than away.

  Work out how and when to give and take help, when to give each other space and freedom, and when to give each other extra love and attention. Give each other encouragement too, and respect and courtesy. Avoid taking each other for granted. Above all keep alive your sense of humour!

  Talk together; laugh together. Just take things day by day, step by step, tackling problems as they arise. Talk about them. Better still, laugh about them, together and with other people: it all helps reduce the tension and keep things in perspective. Remind yourselves of what you've got, don't get over-obsessed with the losses. Remember you're not 'just an arthritic', not just an illness; there's so much more to you than that.

- *Make time for fun and enjoyment, together*   Shared laughter, especially, is so important. Arthritis doesn't mean life stops still. Though you may have to change what you do and share together, make sure you substitute other activities, which you can share and enjoy and laugh about together. Otherwise it's all too easy to fall into the trap of sharing only arthritis-related activities, such as helping the YPA to wash and dress or make a meal. Even if it's only setting aside an evening a week to eat a take-away together, while you watch an eagerly anticipated TV programme or video, do it, share it, enjoy it, together!

- Try Ogden Nash's advice!
  "To keep your marriage brimming
  With love in the loving cup,
  Whenever you're wrong, admit it.
  Whenever you're right, shut up."

(From 'A Word to Husbands', in *I Wouldn't Have Missed It*, André Deutsch)

More ideas for you, the partner with arthritis

- *Think 'self-help' as much as possible*   Avoid leaning on your partner for everything, emotionally as well as physically. That happens in the most able-bodied of partnerships, with sometimes dire consequences. Don't expect your partner to solve all your problems for you; solve as many as possible yourself. OK, you won't always be able to handle the changes on your own, but keep working on your self-help programme. Doing almost anything is better than nothing.

- *Keep your independence of mind and interests*   Help your partner do the same. Give your partner 'space' and freedom to keep up interests and recharge inner batteries. For instance if s/he enjoys a regular night out playing darts, or squash, encourage him/her to continue, without feeling guilty at leaving you.

  Try not to waste the time your partner's out feeling sorry for yourself on your own. Make the most of it, if only just to rest and to recharge *your* inner batteries, or maybe to read a new book, or to listen to a funny radio programme. Share the jokes later with your partner, and take an interest in their outing too. If the arthritis is giving you a really bad time you might find it helpful sometimes just to be by yourself for a while. Encourage your partner to understand your need, without worrying about it, or resenting it.

- *How's the voice?*   It's going to have to work harder in asking for help, in getting things done for you. But it's so horribly easy to sound like a nagger! Work on the voice, so it's softer, so it doesn't whine or nag.

  Cut down on requests for help, by (1) doing more of what you can do, even with difficulty, (2) by writing some, at least, down on paper; then discard or postpone the non-essentials, (3) by producing checklists for your partner for things which crop up regularly so s/he has doesn't have to listen to you repeating the same old things! (eg do a 'How to make the tea list', 'Having a bath list').

  For irregular requests, for instance shopping, or essential cleaning, why not use 'stick-up' notices. That way you can write them when convenient to you, and he'll read and do them when convenient to him. Timing's important! Amazing how long it took me to realise if I waited till the TV adverts were on I'd get a much less grumpy response than when I interrupted his TV viewing (not so easy if it's BBC).

- *Too self-critical?*   Throw out self-doubts. Not easy, but worth trying. Do you worry about what you can't do, about what your partner's having to do instead, worry about becoming a burden on the relationship? Are you perhaps losing your self-confidence? Well, be reassured there *is* still a lot you can do, once you start using the various sanity-saving gadgets and tricks available, and brain-power rather than body-power wherever possible. (See chapters 20 and 25 for tips).

- *Or not self-critical enough?*   The arthritis can, alas, sometimes make us seem very unwelcoming. Be wary! Keep your partnership a welcoming one, to which your partner looks forward to returning when away. Think back to what attracted you to each other in the first place. Are there things you've now let slide, like laughing together, taking a real interest in each other? Re-awaken them!

  Step outside yourself from time to time and ask yourself if you'd be happy to live with You? Do you moan? Do you always seem miserable? Have you let yourself go? Given up making an effort? Would you want to come home after a hard day at the office to You? Do you say please, and thank you? Or do you take your partner too much for granted? Are you taking life too seriously? How fit is your sense of humour? Or, on the other hand, are you too self-critical? Sorry if I seem to be going on. It's probably all totally unjustified. Stick pins into a wax model of me instead if you want!

  If you do seem to moan too much, to your partner, try to find an 'escape valve' for at least some of the moans (see page 102).

- *Too critical of your partner?*   Minimise the criticism, maximise the encouragement and praise. Use the carrot not the stick approach. Not always easy, but always worth trying. Stop being a perfectionist and believing the only way to do something is your way. – Live dangerously and see what other ways your partner can come up with!

  If you feel you do need to criticise, choose the right time and way. Try not to moan about the mess in the kitchen, when he's just spent hours concocting a shepherd's pie for you. Never bring problems up the moment s/he gets home from work. Plenty of time later, after a relaxing interval and on a full stomach. Make a habit of saying only *nice* things when s/he steps in through the door. Above all, remember to give your partner your *good* side as well as your bad. Don't save it for outsiders only!

- *Is s/he the one who's a real old misery?* When your partner's irritable and grumpy, and you're feeling low and full of self-doubt, it's easy to assume you and the arthritis are the cause. Remind yourself there are 1,001 *other* possible causes. Maybe s/he's just tired? Maybe there are problems at work, or some bureaucratic idiocy in a bill just received, maybe s/he's hungry or has a painful corn? You aren't the only one with invisible problems! Be ready with a shoulder to lean on, when necessary.

- *Remind yourself of all the non-physical ingredients of a successful relationship* Look back at those I listed on page 211. You can still give plenty, as well as taking. However bad the arthritis, you can still give love and care and time and support to your partner.

- *'Thinking of opposites'* is an exercise I sometimes find helpful in dealing with difficulties, especially in relationships. For instance:
  - Do you always seem to be on the receiving end, and hate it? Think, instead, about what you can give. However bad you feel you can still give warmth, moral support, understanding, inner strength, and share smiles as well as tears.
  - Think 'independent' instead of 'dependent'. For instance if you're going through a bad patch and need masses of help and attention, bully your partner now and again into taking a break and going out for a change of scene.
  - If the 'can't dos' are obsessing you, force yourself to spend at least half an hour, regularly, thinking *only* of 'can dos'.
  - Mad at what you can't achieve physically? Think of your mental skills and voice, eyes, etc. Can they achieve what you want instead?
  - Maybe you're used to solving emotional crises physically? For instance by stamping your foot and rushing upstairs to get it out of your system? Practice non-physical alternatives (eg look at chapter 14).

More ideas for you, the partner without arthritis

- *Find out what you can about Arthur Itis's wily ways* Then you're halfway towards stopping him/it upsetting your relationship. Your first difficulty might well be believing there really is anything wrong with your partner, when s/he's fit as a fiddle one minute, and miserably stiff as a board the next. That's Arthur for you – invisible and unpredictable, and *not* easy to understand, almost guaranteeing to create misunderstandings. Find out too about things like joint care and rest and exercise and energy conservation. Don't, please, make the mistake of thinking your partner's simply being lazy, or 'giving in', when resting. Dealing with the arthritis means so much more than just 'taking the tablets'. Why not try going along with your partner to the doctor's sometime? You'll both benefit if you look on the arthritis as something you deal with together.

- *Be patient* It'll take both of you time and effort to work out how best to cope, but agree to tackle any difficulties together, united against a common enemy. Some or most of the jigsaw pieces in your life may have to come apart and be put together again in a different way. You need to give each other unselfish love and support and patience while you sort things out together.

- *How do you feel?* Do you wonder how to cope? Does your partner grumpily rebuff you one moment and accuse you of being unfeeling or helpful the next? Do you try to ignore what's happening, hoping any problems will just go away? Do you want to shout angrily at your partner one moment and feel guilty the next? Do you feel sorry for yourself? Ignored or overburdened? Do you fear the future?

   All perfectly understandable feelings. Try explaining some of them to your partner; s/he can't mind-read and may not realise *you* have problems that need to be worked through too. Avoid implying that your partner's to blame; say 'I feel...' not 'You make me feel...' Remember the cause of your problems isn't your partner; it's an enemy intruder some people call Arthur Itis. Talk too to other people who will understand and may also be able to suggest sources of practical help, eg doctor, Samaritans, Young Arthritis Care members/and their partners.

● *How best can you help your partner?*   Just 'being there', just constantly reminding him/her of your love and loyalty and support is the best possible thing you can do. Someone with arthritis may instinctively turn inwards and through sheer misery or self-doubt appear outwardly unwelcoming and unloving. Arthritis can make us feel unlovely and horribly unlovable inside. Please don't be put off, but reassure us of your love, in words and in touching. A loving smile or touch or gentle hug is wonderful medicine. If you're worried about causing pain, why not explain 'I'd like to give you a cuddle, but don't want to hurt you' and see what happens?

Please, too, help bolster our self-confidence and self-esteem, so easily bruised by the arthritis. If we can no longer do everything we used to, please value what we can do. Encourage us not to feel useless. See pages 190 and 196 for some more guidelines.

In practical terms, how can you best help? Some partners may do too much, and end up making the YPA much more of a helpless invalid than necessary. It can be hard watching someone you love struggle to do something rather than doing it for them. Others may take the opposite, 'snap out of it approach' – unkindly or unthinkingly offering little or no help to someone whose body simply won't *allow* him/her to snap out of it.

There's really no easy answer – you'll both need to keep readjusting to fit in with the arthritis ups and downs. In general, when it's not at its worst, I do believe it's best for the YPA to try to do as much as possible for him/herself, while making use of every sanity-saving gadget or trick your combined efforts can unearth. But you must gently *encourage* your partner, not bully! And accept that with some things and at some times your help most definitely will be needed. Agree between you that when help is really needed the YPA will ask for it and the help will be there. Corbet Woodall described his wife Ingrid's attitude to him and his RA as

"*hard to put into words but, roughly interpreted, meant that she was saying to me: 'Sink, and you'll sink alone; try to help yourself and I'll be the first to back you'. This, with amazing consistency, she has done.*" (In *A Disjointed Life*, Heinemann)

Please don't be reluctant to seek outside help. If, for instance, your partner needs lots of help with washing and dressing, why not see if any help's available through your doctor/OT/social worker, or through organisations like the Crossroads Care Attendant Scheme? Outside help can ease practical *and* emotional burdens on both of you.

Remember too, you can give *so* much help simply by *not hindering*, by *not creating* more work or more obstacles. Do for instance always clear up after yourself! And don't move things without checking first that you're not thus complicating life for your YPA. Make a point, now and again, of simply saying, 'is there anything you'd like me to do?'

● *Don't let the arthritis dominate your lives completely*   *Do* make sure you share plenty of other things besides, including laughter and love, and shared interests and activities. Make sure too you allow each other 'space', space for being alone and recharging your batteries and keeping up with individual interests and relaxations.

Marie Joseph told a psychiatrist what had helped most in her fight against RA was her husband – he'd actually helped

"*by* not *helping me...He has never allowed me to feel that I am anything but a normal woman. He knows that if he stretches out a hand to help me, I am more than likely to knock it away. He boosts my morale by telling me I look good when I am tired and he praises me when I complete a task that other normal women would take for granted...He doesn't rush forward to help me out of chairs, because he knows I would hate it. And he swears that my hands aren't noticeable, so that just occasionally, if someone does mention them, and wonder aloud how I cope, I get a shock because quite honestly I never think about their shape.*" (In *One Step at a Time*, Arrow Books)

Further reading and helpful organisations

Look back at the list on page 206. Send for booklists from Relate (ask for their *Marriage and Relationships* booklist), Healthwise, and the British Holistic Medical Association. Though few if any of the books listed talk specifically about arthritis or chronic illness you'll often find helpful tips on coping with general stresses in relationships, in, for instance:

–   *The Relate Guide to Better Relationships*, by Sarah Litvinoff (Ebury Press, 1991), subtitled 'Practical ways to make your love last from the experts in marriage guidance'. Barely mentions chronic illness, but is really excellent, sensitive yet realistic, and full of tips to help you understand and tackle emotional and relation-ship problems, whatever their cause, and whether you're in a married or an un-married relationship. Particularly good on dealing with anger, and communication difficulties. Many tips may be helpful even if you're not in a relationship.
–   Dr Paul Hauck's *How to Love and Be Loved* (Sheldon Press)
–   Dr Tony Gough's *Couples Arguing* (DLT)
–   Laurie Graham's *A Marriage Survival Guide* (Chatto and Windus) is amusing but thought-provoking too
–   The British Medical Association's low-cost booklet *Marriage – Making or Breaking?* by J Dominian (from BMA House)

Reading books by other people with arthritis or other chronic illness may help (see chapter 29). And I've mentioned before psychiatrist Sandy Burnfield's book *Multiple Sclerosis, A Personal Exploration* (Souvenir Press): he includes the impact on his marriage of his own chronic illness, MS, very different from chronic arthritis in its *physical* effects, of course.

–   Dr Wendy Greengross's *Entitled to Love* (J M Dent) deals with the sexual and emotional needs of handicapped people.

Several books focus on 'the carer', the 'non-disabled' partner in a relationship. You might find helpful ideas in something like *Taking a Break* – a guide for people caring at home (details from Taking a Break), or *Keeping Fit While Caring* which includes information on moving and bathing someone with disabilities, basic muscle exercises for the carer, etc by Christine Darby, (published by the Family Welfare Association). There's also a self-help group, the National Association of Carers.

Organisations

Relate (formerly the National Marriage Guidance Council)   Whether you're married or unmarried, counsellors can help you work through relationship difficulties. Some have made a special study of physical disability and relationships. Don't delay contacting them, as there may be a waiting list for an appointment. Look too at Sarah Litvinoff's Relate book mentioned above. In Hilary Edwards' *Psychological Problems. Who Can Help?* (Methuen and British Psychological Society), a Relate counsellor explains:

"Our service is free. Clients are asked to make a voluntary contribution, but there is no obligation to do so. About half our clients refer themselves directly, and half are recommended to come by a professional worker or by the Citizen's Advice Bureau. We have a waiting list for counselling, but we do see people for an early first appointment within a week of them contacting us. This is to get an idea of the problem, to give an idea of what counselling involves, and to make sure we are the right service for them. We meet clients in our offices, or in their local health centre, surgery or CAB. If the person

is severely disabled we may see them at home..."
There are some special religious counselling groups, too, for instance the Christian Action Research and Education (CARE Trust), the Catholic Marriage Advisory Council (CMAC) and the Jewish Marriage Council.

The Institute of Family Therapy offers counselling to couples and family groups (no referral necessary). Fees are based on what the client can afford.

The Advice Unit at *MIND* can put you in touch with projects, groups or organisations offering psychotherapy, counselling, or self-help groups in your area who might be helpful. See too 'Talking therapy' on page 110.

Gemma is a national organisation of lesbians of all ages, with/without disabilities.

If the worst comes to the worst...
I hope it doesn't. But if it does...Some organisations who can help:

Relate and the other organisations mentioned above. Also *Citizens' Advice Bureau* (see page 118), for advice on financial and legal aspects, legal aid information, etc.

Solicitors Family Law Association provides a list of solicitors who take a conciliatory rather than confrontational view of divorce. *National Family Conciliation Council* too can help when a couple (married or unmarried, separated or divorced − or plan to be) disagree over important issues, especially those concerning their children. Trained counsellors help both partners work together, cooperatively rather than competitively, to sort out an agreement for themselves, the future, and the children, rather than just communicating through a solicitor. They have a helpful publications list, some available by post, some to help parents, some for children.

Organisations offering advice and support to single parents include *Gingerbread* (over 300 groups nationwide) and the *National Council for One Parent Families* and *Scottish Council for Single Parents*. *Families Need Fathers* advises on access and custodial matters for both parents. See also page 236.

Get Relate's booklist on *Divorce and Remarriage*, which lists several books available by post, including some of these:
−   *On your Own*, by Jean Shapiro (Pandora Press). How to deal with living on your own again. (Available from Relate)
−   *Going it Alone* by Anne McNicholas and *A Woman's Place* by Sue Witherspoon. (By post from SHAC, the London Housing Aid Centre)
−   *Divorce: Legal Procedures and Financial Facts*, Consumers Association, (Hodder and Stoughton, available from Relate)
−   *How to Split Up − And Survive Financially*, by Tony Hetherington (Unwin)
There are some books written specially to help children of divorcing parents, many available from Relate, and tThe National Family Conciliation Council has a list. Examples:
−   *How It Feels When Parents Divorce* by Jill Krementz (Gollancz), for over tens.
−   *Mike's Lonely Summer* by Carolyn Nystrom (Lion), for five to ten year olds.
−   *When Parents Split Up* by Ann Mitchell (Chambers), for teenagers
−   *Voices in the Dark* by Gillian McCreadie and Alan Horrox (Unwin), for seven year olds to teens.
−   The Children's Society publishes helpful, very cheap leaflets *Divorce and Your Children* and *Divorce and You* (written for children and young people).

Chapter twenty-seven

SEX AND ARTHRITIS

Write to ARC for the booklet *Arthritis: Sexual Aspects and Parenthood* (enclose SAE). It's worth reading, even though it deals with pregnancy *before* looking at contraception! I'll tell you about other relevant publications later.

So many books, especially those 'for disabled people' launch straight into the doom and gloom of problem sex. So let's start, instead, with the *joys* of sex. By 'sex' I mean 'making love', high quality sex, where the coupling of the genitals is only a part (not necessarily always an essential part) of a whole mass of psychological, emotional and sensual interactions between two lovers.

OK, so arthritis may mean you need to rethink and reorganise your sex life, just like other aspects of your life. Pain and stiffness and fatigue may sometimes cause difficulties, especially in a flare-up, so too may your psychological reactions to the arthritis, but if you *can* get your sex life right, even just occasionally, what a tonic. Marvellous medicine:

"It is not only the physical pleasure of orgasm that's so important. Equally valuable is the pleasure that comes from giving pleasure, the psychic boost of being acknowledged as a lover and experiencing the satisfied response of a loved partner. This is a real basis of femininity and masculinity...Sex is not just a physical act, it is a means of telling your partner your feelings, your love, and your joys; of sharing a deep unconscious pool of real individuality. " (Dr Wendy Greengross in *Entitled to Love*, J M Dent)

Even if you have to cut down on the quantity, there could well be an improvement in its quality! As psychiatrist Sandy Burnfield says, in the book about his own chronic illness:

"Sexual experimentation can lead to new ways of giving one another pleasure and there is some evidence that people who are disabled often enjoy a sex life with their partners that is more variable and imaginative than that of many able-bodied people. Those who are disabled may have to make adjustments and to experiment!" (In *Multiple Sclerosis: A Personal Exploration*, Souvenir Press. Multiple sclerosis is medically *very* different from RA and its cousins, but there can be similarities in impact on lifestyle.)

Incredible though it may seem to the ablebods of this world, the very fact that certain problems need to be overcome may well lead you and your partner to discover more about yourselves and about lovemaking than you did before. Normally, it's easy to lose sight of all the things *other* than basic sexual mechanics which go towards making a warm, caring and satisfying relationship.

Reading what some 'sex therapists' write makes me wonder how they'd cope if their sex lives were suddenly complicated by chronic arthritis. Having trained themselves to be aroused only by the most exotic methods, can they ever really know the intensity of arousal that can come from the simplest of things – the sensuality of the hair on a man's chest, the sensitivity of an ear lobe, the softness of a woman's skin? If pain and fatigue ruled out full intercourse for them, could they fully appreciate how much pleasure two people could still bring to each other?

Being fit and healthy doesn't guarantee a wonderful love life. Look at all the well-publicised messes some 'healthy' people make of their love lives. Outwardly healthy people may well be emotionally disabled inside. Vice versa, too: outwardly disabled people may be wonderfully healthy inside... In both cases, the disabilities, inner or outer, can be dealt with. Maybe not always completely eliminated, but certainly understood, and reduced to realistic proportions.

What sort of problems might arthritis cause?

Yes, there may be problems, made worse if you find them difficult to talk about and share. In a perceptive chapter called 'The Image of Rheumatic Disease', in *Altered Body Image – The Nurse's Role*, edited by Mave Salter (John Wiley and Sons, 1980), Rheumatology Nurse Practitioner Jan Maycock reminded her colleagues that sexual drive can be reduced by chronic pain, feelings of lethargy, changes in self-esteem and body image, and, some-times, depression; some medicaments used in treatment may also reduce sexual drive. She pointed out that although a patient with a rheumatic disorder may be worried about sexual adjustment, it's something that's not often discussed openly by health professionals.

Please don't be depressed by this. It's just to show you that you're not alone if you *are* having difficulties. Problems *can* be overcome, not least through simply letting any worries come to the surface. With time and patience, understanding and adjustment, and outside help if necessary, the joy and tonic of sex *can* replace sex-and-arthritis worries.

As you'll know from other parts of this book, there are few instant solutions, so do be patient. The early days, when it's all a new and unwelcome experience, may be the worst, for you and your partner. Be caring and comforting to each other. Keep touching and being affectionate even if anything more energetic seems, for the time being, out of the question.

In *Towards Intimacy* (Eurospan Group, 1978) a woman with RA says:

"We don't do much 'hard-core sex', but find our greatest fulfilment in slow, deep touching and holding. We can't seem to get enough cuddling. It's different I guess... cause we can't do much moving, but that doesn't seem to detract from our pleasure."

Take heart from the assurances of old-handers, that you *can* put the jigsaw pieces together again, maybe not in the same pattern as before, but in a good pattern even so.

Seeking outside help

Thoughts follow on self-help, but do seek outside help, if necessary, however difficult taking the first step might be. Many problems can be solved quite simply by talking them over with an unbiased and independent 'third party'. The underlying causes of some problems may well be the same as those which cause problems for *anyone*, arthritis or no arthritis, due perhaps to a lack of communication and unsatisfactory relationship with one's partner, or sexual inexperience or inhibitions, or maybe a poor self-image and poor self-esteem.

You could seek help (counselling) either alone, or together, from your doctor, from a Relate counsellor, from a family planning organisation, or from SPOD, which is specially for people with a disability: SPOD's full name is the 'Association to Aid the Sexual and Personal Relationships of People with a Disability'), and there's a phone helpline (see page 225). Some GPs are specially trained to help people with sexual problems, or may refer you to an NHS sex therapy clinic or some other counsellor. Look back at page 110, the section on 'talking therapy'. Some OTs and rheumatology nurses may also be able to help. There are books and leaflets you can read, too. Details on page 225.

Some self-help ideas

1 Dealing with emotional and psychological problems

- *Good communication between you is important*   Look back at chapter 26. Feelings of anger and misunderstandings can easily develop in a couple who have to cope with chronic arthritis. Unless these are dealt with, their sex life may suffer:

   "Psychological and emotional responses are an integral part of lovemaking. They awaken desire and influence performance, and it is these that need to be looked at if a couple are experiencing sex problems. Impotence and frigidity are nearly always caused by unacknowledged emotions. Jealousy, resentment, anger, insecurity and

feelings of inferiority, both conscious and unconscious, can prevent and block the communication that should take place during intercourse.. " (Dr Wendy Greengross, *Entitled to Love*, J M Dent)

Talk together about your feelings, listen to each other, and show that you care about the other's feelings. Avoid blame and criticism. Substitute praise, cooperation and understanding. Work on the other ideas in chapter 26. The Relate book, too (page 217), gives lots of really helpful practical advice. If you can't overcome communication blocks through self-help, seek outside help.

A common worry, of both partners, may be of causing hurt. The fit partner may avoid touching or caressing for fear of hurting the other, and pain and stiffness may make it difficult for the YPA to be loving in turn. The YPA needs to be able to say 'come over here and give me a cuddle', or 'I like you touching me this way' (rather than another). The partner shouldn't hold back from finding out what gives pleasure rather than pain.

- *Sexual inexperience or inhibitions* may inhibit the flexible, openminded approach you'll need for working through any problems. Upbringing or religion may give some people rigid ideas of what is or isn't appropriate or pleasurable, and some may think sex is indecent or shameful or something to be ignored. Such ideas will, alas, only add to any problems caused by the arthritis. Think and learn about sex afresh.

Ideas can also be too rigid in the opposite direction! If you consider yourself *very* sexy and expect great athletic performances and great orgasms every time, it'll be difficult to come to terms with any failures or problems.

Both sorts of people need to open their minds and bodies to things like non-coital pleasuring in all its many forms, to the pleasures of mutual or solo masturbation and stimulation, and to the pleasures of 'simple' bodily senses and feelings, as well as to alternative positions for full sexual intercourse. So widen your ideas and information on sex! The idea *isn't* to make you miserable about all the antics you can't accomplish, but instead to loosen any inhibitions, any preconceptions about what is and isn't possible and pleasurable, and to contribute to your fantasies!

Read, for instance, books like *The New Joy of Sex, Men and Sex*, and others mentioned in this chapter (by post from Healthwise/FPA is a nicely unembarrassing way to get them). The books don't concentrate exclusively on weird and wonderful Kama Sutra positions, but do emphasise emotional and psychological aspects, as well as sensuality generally, for instance erogenous zones and the pleasures of touching and using other senses. Books like these may be reassuring too in showing you that much of what you feel applies equally to people without arthritis.

- *Poor self-image and poor self-esteem* Sadly, an arthriticky body can undermine self-confidence and make you feel less of a man or less of a woman. Non-disabled people may experience similar feelings if they feel let down by their body, by breast or penis size, for instance.

With arthritis, washing, making-up, doing your hair, dressing attractively, may become difficult or just too much bother, and if you feel like a doddery and ancient so-and-so inside anyway, it's hard to believe anyone might find you attractive or lovable. Similarly, a man who equates masculinity with a strong, active, virile body may wonder how his weakened body could ever be attractive to a lover. How the arthritis affects other areas of your life can undermine your self-image too, for instance if as a man your career or role as breadwinner is threatened, or if as a woman at home your homemaking and childcare roles suffer.

Feeling unlovable may even lead to the partner with arthritis consciously or unconsciously *making* him or herself unlovable or unapproachable, and rebuffing approaches by the other partner. Sadly, if the latter doesn't understand, s/he in turn may draw back and become aloof, leading to a 'vicious circle' of misunderstanding and apartness, at the very time when you both could gain so much comfort from each other.

Instead, with patience and understanding, the fit partner could do much to boost self-confidence and self-esteem, to show the partner with arthritis that s/he really is loved 'warts and all'. In *Towards Intimacy*, someone with RA explains her feelings:

> *"My knees are the ugliest part of me cause the arthritis has really deformed them − I want my partner to acknowledge them in a tender, loving way, rather than to avoid them."* (Eurospan Group)

The book doesn't say if her partner knew what she wanted. Quite possibly he might have been too embarrassed or worried about hurting her, or simply at a loss to know what to do...Or he might not even have noticed her knees! But if she could get the message across, he would at once know how to respond, and how to give her pleasure. Her knees would become a positive asset to their love-making.

However difficult the arthritis makes it, try to take a pride in being 'nice to know' and avoid neglecting your personal care and appearance. Looking good, and feeling good, are an important part of a good self-image and sex life.

If you're a man with arthritis, with doubts about your attractiveness to women, read something like Bernard Zilbergeld's *Men and Sex* (Souvenir Press Ltd), especially the chapter 'Some Things You Should Know About Women'. Non-disabled women talk about what they want in men − none excluded by arthritis:

> *"We want men, not supermen; lovers, not beasts; and intelligent, warm companions, not Hollywood handsomes stroking their egos at our expense.*
>
> *"I like a man who feels free to be vulnerable, to give up his masculine stereotype, who can be gentle and sensitive and passive, as well as aggressive. A man who allows me to do the same. A man who can relinquish control of the lovemaking and allow it to be a shared experience. A man who can tolerate imperfections in himself, his penis, and me... A man who appreciates and enjoys women's bodies − even the not-so-perfect ones.*
>
> *"Actually, the things I respond to most in men are qualities which are traditionally considered feminine: tenderness, gentleness, caring, touching, and sensitivity to emotions."*

2 Overcoming physical problems caused by arthritis

- *Plan your daily activities* to avoid becoming too tired and try to keep some energy in reserve for your love life. Don't despair if that's not an everyday possibility. Now and again will do just as well so long as you don't overlook it completely as a part of your life to be planned for. Try if possible to time love-making for the part of the day when you and your body feel at their best.
- *Exercises − don't neglect them* Keep muscles in trim with a sensible exercise programme recommended by your physio. If possible, ease stiffness and tension before making love, perhaps by having a bath or shower. Luxuriate in some exotic fragrance. Hot or cold packs may help ease painful joints and muscles, too.
- *Medication* Try to time your love-making for when your painkillers are at their most effective. Some medication (eg for insomnia or depression) may dampen your libido (sexual urge) and interfere with ejaculation, cause impotence, or lack of sexual satisfaction. Check with your doctor, pharmacist, or SPOD if necessary.
- Make sure your bedroom's *a comfortable temperature* Make sure the bed's firm and comfortable too. Don't get rid of the double bed:

> *"It is because physical closeness and the caring touch can bring so much comfort and reassurance to a marriage that it is most important to sleep in a double bed. I am against single beds for almost any married couple, because I believe that the psychological as well as physical gulf between two singles is so great that it can eventually result in a couple drifting apart themselves. Even for the able-bodied who sleep separately, getting out of one bed and into another, especially in winter in a*

cold bedroom, takes such an effort of willpower that many people think twice before bothering. And that is how the physical expression of love can begin to disappear completely. How much more likely that the disabled will abandon the initiative, if the effort to move from one side of the room to the other is hazardous and even painful. If you are already in bed together, even if sexual intercourse is rare, you are still close and can communicate feelings of love and tenderness just by touching an arm or stroking a limb. It keeps a couple in touch with each other. And touching with no clothes on, even without sexual intercourse can be extremely comforting and pleasurable. Sex can disappear only too easily out of the life of a married couple if they turn their backs on each other too often.

"If a disabled partner finds there are times when he or she suffers particularly from pain or discomfort, and is likely to disturb the other by a restless night, then obviously a move to a single bed is sensible. In that event it might be advisable to have two singles that zip together, or a double with a spare single somewhere else." (Dr Wendy Greengross, in *Entitled to Love*, J M Dent)

- **Take the initiative** It may seem paradoxical to ablebods, but often it's the *disabled* partner who needs to take the initiative. The fit partner can't tell how you feel inside and may be too worried about hurting you to touch you. So you need to help your partner verbally or physically to know what's pleasurable for you, and when, and what's best avoided. When things *are* going well, do let your partner know how good it feels. S/he will be only too pleased to be giving you pleasure in place of the miseries of arthritis, which s/he *can't* do anything about.

- **Don't ever criticise** Either of you. If you want change, suggest it at the right time in the right way. Instead of saying you don't like something, emphasise how much you like something else, or guide your partner to something preferable.

Don't mope about what you *can't* do together. No one *has* to copy the Kama Sutra in every detail! Enjoy what you *can* do. And remember love-making isn't only about taking pleasure, it's also about giving pleasure. If you, the partner with arthritis, are in too much discomfort to want full intercourse, maybe you can sometimes still muster enough energy to bring your partner to a climax? You can both get a lot of pleasure, even orgasm, from giving each other pleasure without full intercourse.

- **Why not try spending more time on 'emotional foreplay' if physical foreplay is difficult?** For instance by reading erotic or romantic books that turn you on and get the juices flowing. Read them separately, or aloud, together. Psychologist and author of a sex therapy manual, Dr Patricia Gillan, talked in a *Times* article by Liz Gill (10.9.1987) about erotica for women. She explained she didn't mean hard-core porn that women find offensive, but artistic and tasteful erotica to increase the sexual imagination. Her list would include paintings, films like *Belle de Jour* and *Emmanuelle*, books like *My Secret Garden*, and some music, particularly reggae and Indian ragas.

Try too books like *Delta of Venus* or *Little Birds*, erotica by Anais Nin (Star books, W H Allen), or love poems, for instance in *The Penguin Book of Love Poetry* edited by Jon Stallworthy, eg John Donne's *To His Mistress on Going to Bed*. Maybe you prefer raunchy Jackie Collins, Jilly Cooper or Judith Krantz novels, or Mills and Boon type books? Many books are in paperback, and available by post, eg from J Barnicoat (page 115) or Healthwise (page 114).

- **Try different positions** to get over physical problems, for instance stiff hips. Penetration doesn't have to be from the front, but can be from the rear, or side; and partners can experiment with standing, kneeling, sitting or lying across each other to find the best solutions. ARC's *Arthritis: Sexual Aspects and Parenthood* gives some examples for a man with arthritis:

"The man lies on his back while the woman sits or lies on top of him, either facing him or with her back to him. This could make a positive difference if the man cannot

move without pain, or finds it difficult to support his weight on his arms, shoulders or knees.

"There are also a whole series of positions involving the husband sitting on a chair or on the edge of a bed while his wife gently lowers herself on to him. Alternatively, there is the position called 'spoons' where the woman lies on her side and the man lies behind her.

"There are now many respectable books available which explore this area more fully — many with photographs or drawings that greatly help the explanation."

For a woman, support under the legs with one or more firm cushions or pillows may help. Or penetration from the rear, with the woman lying on her front, may overcome some hip difficulties. After a hip operation you should wait several weeks before trying intercourse; check with your surgeon how long. Once you start again you might still for a while want to avoid having weight placed on the new hip: Professor Hardinge suggests a position which could also be tried for a non-operated stiff hip:

"the female lies on her back and her partner lies alongside on the opposite side to the operated leg. The operated leg is moved out to the side and the non-operated leg is lifted upwards so that the partner, lying on his side can make a satisfactory entry. If for reasons of bodily dimensions, entry cannot be made from this position, it would be wise to wait a few weeks until the female can tolerate bearing her partner's weight on top of her." (In *Hip Replacement: The Facts*, Oxford University Press)

SPOD produces various leaflets that may help you work out other positions, eg *Useful Diagrams for Positions for Sex for either Men or Women Suffering from Arthritis*.

Contraception

You can get (by post) leaflets and books explaining different methods from the Family Planning Association (FPA), for instance the BMA's *Contraception: Choice not Chance* by Dr Barbara Law, John Guillebaud's excellent *The Pill* (Oxford University Press), and Robert Snowden's *IUD: The Woman's Guide*. SPOD have an advisory leaflet on contraception for people with disabilities, and a phone counsellor (see page 225). The FPA also have a phone counsellor; a family planning nurse and information who can talk you through your options. One of the College of Health's phone tapes (page 119) is on contraception.

You could go to your doctor for contraceptive advice, or you might prefer a family planning clinic. For the address of the nearest look under 'Family Planning' in the phone book. The FPA can supply some contraceptives by post, eg condoms, diaphragms and spermicides for people who find frequent visits to a clinic for supplies difficult. Details from Family Planning Sales Limited.

Some methods, eg the cap, may be difficult if your hands are bad; don't be shy about saying so. If you choose 'the Pill' make sure your GP and any other doctor who treats you knows you're on it. Interaction with other drugs will need to be thought about, eg some antibiotics, barbiturates and anti-convulsant drugs may reduce its effectiveness. You should be aware too that its effectiveness may be reduced if you have a 'stomach' upset, eg vomiting or diarrhoea. And if you're due to have surgery you'll probably have to stop the pill beforehand; ask your surgeon's advice. For contraception in lupus patients the oestrogen-containing pill isn't recommended, as it may cause greater disease activity.

Masturbation

Masturbation's the stimulation of the sex organs to produce pleasure, even orgasm, by means other than sexual intercourse. It can be enjoyed by anyone, whether in a relationship or not. If arthritis causes problems with masturbating, perhaps because of uncooperative hands, you might wonder about using sex aids, eg vibrators and electric masturbators. SPOD comments helpfully:

"Using sex aids is an idea that some people find hard to accept, but they can provide a lot of pleasure; part of the problem with aids is the lurid nature of most brochures. Work is in progress on producing a more sober version, of aids suitable for those with physical handicaps: SPOD will be able to advise on its availability."
One of the College of Health's phone tapes (page 119) is on masturbation.

Helpful organisations and publications

Relate   See page 217, and send an SAE for their *Sex and Sexual Problems* list of books available by post.

SPOD   SPOD's full name is the 'Association to Aid the Sexual and Personal Relationships of People with a Disability'. It's a charity, founded in 1972 by a group of professional carers. It provides an information service on sexual aspects of disability, and an advice and counselling service for disabled people in sexual difficulty. Write, with SAE, for SPOD's publications list. A telephone counselling line for people with sexual or relationship problems is open on Monday and Wednesday mornings, and Tuesday and Thursday afternoons (071 607 8851, ask for the counsellor).

Family Planning Association   For general information on relationships, sexuality, birth-control, etc, send an SAE asking for their Healthwise mail order catalogue.

Brook Advisory Centres   Brook Centres offer free birth control advice and supplies to young people, and also help with emotional and sexual problems. Centres open on weekdays, and some open in the evenings and on Saturdays too.

Other publications:
- ARC's *Arthritis: Sexual Aspects and Parenthood*. Free, for an SAE.
- Young Arthritis Care have produced a booklet on sex and sexuality
- Ann Darnbrough and Derek Kinrade's *The Sex Directory* (Woodhead-Faulkner, 1988) includes sex and disability. Expensive – try your library.
- *Towards Intimacy. Family Planning and Sexuality Concerns of Physically Disabled Women*, by the Task Force on Concerns of Physically Disabled Women (Eurospan Group/Human Sciences Press)

There are masses of other 'non-disabled' sex books on the Relate and FPA/Healthwise booklists, which can be bought by post from them, including these:
- Sarah Litvinoff's excellent *The Relate Guide to Better Relationships* (Ebury Press) (details on page 217) includes sex.
- Dr David Delvin's *How to Improve Your Sex Life*
- Derek Llewellyn-Jones' excellent *Everywoman*, a Gynaecological Guide for Life, and *Everyman*
- The BMA's low-cost booklet *Knowing About Sex*, by Eric Trimmer, answers lots of embarrassing questions that people are often loath to ask or answer about sex. It doesn't deal specifically with 'disabled' or 'arthritis' aspects of sex.

Chapter twenty-eight

HAVING CHILDREN

"Having arthritis in its acute form, and with two small children to look after...is a bit like trying to climb Mount Everest in winkle-pickers. There are some days when you don't get very far."

So says novelist Marie Joseph! She produced one infant before developing RA, and one after. Both are now grown-up, and to judge from her entertaining autobiography, *One Step at a Time* (Arrow Books, now out of print, sadly), both flourished despite any mountaineering problems. On the plus side, they probably learnt a lot of valuable lessons about life along the way, and brought Marie and her husband a lot of joy. For many parents with arthritis children are a real incentive to keep going.

Those of us with arthritis but without children face a choice that may be difficult, and raises lots of questions. Is arthritis hereditary? How would pregnancy affect my arthritis and vice versa? How could I give birth with hip, knee, etc, problems? With stiff, aching joints and enough difficulties already looking after myself how could I cope with a helpless, wriggly baby, an energetic mischievous toddler, and the countless physical and emotional demands of a schoolchild and temperamental adolescent? What about my partner, too?

Deciding whether or not to have a child

Anyone, with or without arthritis, considering whether or not to have children needs to make that decision carefully, taking into account not only the feelings and circumstances of both partners, but also those of the prospective newcomer to the world. Every newcomer needs and deserves love and security and commitment by its parents for 24 hours a day for year after year. Sadly, too many children are born without careful prior consideration, or for questionable reasons: to patch up a rocky relationship; 'because everyone else has them' and would-be grandparents apply pressure; because they're cute and every other magazine and TV picture shows wonderful mother-and-baby pictures where nothing ever goes wrong; because you want someone to love you and make you feel needed; because you want to be 'normal'. Or it just simply 'happens'. The consequences of such questionable reasons for having children are, alas, only too visible around us.

There's usually no reason why the arthritis itself should stop you producing a child, but you need to think things through extra carefully first. Even if you're fit, child-rearing is a tough and exhausting job physically and emotionally and you'll need to base your decision realistically on your own particular circumstances and abilities. If you decide to go ahead, then it's crucial that you don't just 'let it happen': forward-planning, for instance stopping or altering drugs (even before conception), and making practical arrangements, is essential.

For some of us, as for people without arthritis, the decision may be to remain child-free. That was my decision. Arthritis wasn't the only reason by any means, though it was arthritis which made me think twice about it. I made the decision before I met my partner, so had to make sure any conflicts in our feelings were aired and resolved. For me, my abilities and skills most definitely lie in areas other than housework and childcare and I much prefer to concentrate on what I *can* do rather than having to struggle constantly with things I'm not good at. I'm fond of children, and enjoy other people's (in moderation!), but am glad that ours remain happily unborn, and happily unaware of what can be a depressing and cruel world.

Deciding to be child-free isn't *easy*, arthritis or no arthritis, but there *are* other ways of fulfilling maternal or paternal instincts, or finding a 'purpose in life'. People who don't have children, through choice or infertility, are sometimes thought freakish and given a rough time by others: I do think it would help if everyone were reminded of how much child-free people give to the world and its children without producing a child themselves. Several of the nicest people I know haven't had children. Instead they've been vivid examples to me of how full and unselfish a life you *can* have without children: so many others have benefited from their abundance of love.

BON (British Organisation of Non-Parents) is a support group of and for people who believe in 'responsible parenthood', and who believe that the choice to be child-free should be respected and unpressured. BON provides information and moral support on the choice of being child-free. Send an SAE for leaflets *You Do Have a Choice, Am I Parent Material?* and *No Regrets*.

For childless people (those who want them but are unable to have them) there's the National Association for the Childless.

How can you help yourselves reach a realistic decision?

● Jean Shapiro's *A Child: Your Choice* (Pandora), subtitled 'an honest, everyday guide to the pleasures and perils of motherhood', is written to help people who are undecided about having a baby, or those who've decided to go ahead but want to weigh up any problems. C Howland's *The First Time Parents' Survival Guide* (Thorsons, 1986) takes an entertaining look at the negative as well as positive aspects of having a child. Though neither book looks at 'disability' or 'arthritis', they could help you both weigh things up generally. BON's free (for SAE) leaflet *Am I Parent Material?* is a quiz to help people think about the choice.

● Discuss questions of arthritis and pregnancy and childrearing with your doctor and specialist. What effect would pregnancy have on your condition, and vice versa? And see page 228, 'Taking the arthritis into consideration'.

● Talk to other people who've had children or thought about having them: friends, relatives, and other people with your particular type of arthritis. Your Young Arthritis Care Contact may help put you in touch, and so too the National Childbirth Trust (NCT), who keep a register of disabled mothers willing to talk to others. Bear in mind that everyone's different, of course. And meet as many real babies and children as possible, too!

● Read everything you can get your hands on. Much the best book is:
  - *The Baby Challenge* by Mukti Jain Campion (Routledge, 1990), subtitled 'A handbook on pregnancy for women with a physical disability'. It's friendly, full of information, and includes a section on arthritis, with the experiences of three mothers with RA.

For plenty of practical information on equipment, etc, look at:
  - *Parents with Disabilities* (Disability Information Trust – see page 142). There's also a section in DIT's *Arthritis – An Equipment Guide.*
  - *The Emotions and Experiences of some Disabled Mothers* (National Childbirth Trust (NCT), 1985)
  - ARC's *Arthritis: Sexual Aspects and Parenthood*

Read too personal accounts such as Marie Joseph's autobiography; chapters in Michael Leitch's *Living with Arthritis* (Lennard/Collins); and the excellent chapter 'Coping with a Young Family: a Personal Experience' in Heather Unsworth's *Coping with Rheumatoid Arthritis* (Chambers, 1986). Other personal accounts appear later in this

chapter. Don't forget 'standard' baby books, too, like:
- *The Marks and Spencer Book of Babycare*
- *Good Housekeeping Baby Book*, by Margaret Carter (Ebury Press)
- Sheila Kitzinger's *Pregnancy and Childbirth* (Penguin)
- Dr Miriam Stoppard's *Pregnancy and Birth Book* (Dorling Kindersley)
- Angela Phillips' *Your Body, Your Baby, Your Life* (Kegan Paul)
- Andrew Stanway's *The Baby and Child Book* (Pan)
- Penelope Leach's *Baby and Child* (Penguin)
- G Chamberlain's *Pregnancy Questions Answered* (Churchill Livingstone)

- Talk to anyone who might get involved in giving you support if you have children – doctor, OT, social worker, and friends and relatives. Find out what practical and emotional support you could expect.
- Above all, discuss *everything* thoroughly with your partner. The final decision has to be a joint one, and a realistic one. What about the financial, practical, job, social aspects? Does your partnership offer the love and emotional security a child needs, not only when the going's good but when it's tough, too? Remember the tedious unpredictability of RA and its cousins. Is the partner without arthritis willing and able to take on extra childcare and household responsibility, especially during bad patches?

   How will you cope physically? How would you cope during pregnancy and after with tiredness, frustrations, and isolation? How would you cope with the demands of a new-born baby? The first few weeks are exhausting even for healthy mothers. Write down, step by step, everything you'd need to do, from feeding and changing the baby, washing, lifting him in and out of cot, pram, bath, etc, comforting him when he cries, etc. Any baby book will help you remember everything that needs to be considered! What help can you count on?

I don't want to seem *too* negative! Though some marriages may suffer under the strain of arthritis-plus-baby, other people *do* cope, and *do* believe the pros outweigh the cons. It's how you cope with the difficulties that really matters: forward planning's crucial, plus support from other people. If you can cope with problems in an atmosphere of courage and love, your child will learn valuable lessons. But it's only realistic to appreciate that it's not going to be easy. Children do bring joy and happiness, but are you prepared to take on the stresses and strains involved in return? Some of us say 'no', however great the rewards. There *are* other ways of getting and giving joy and happiness.

Counselling, from your doctor or a Relate or SPOD counsellor, might help you both discuss this complex decision rationally and realistically. Try to get a counsellor with up-to-date knowledge of your form of arthritis.

Taking the arthritis into consideration

Get ARC's *Arthritis: Sexual Aspects and Parenthood* (free, but send SAE) and remember, if you want to start trying for a baby do first, discuss your plan with your rheumatologist. Some drugs should be stopped even *before* a baby is conceived, and you'll need to think through between you any other implications. Make sure from then on that any other doctor who treats you knows about your plans too.

Is it hereditary?   Haemophilia is really the only type of arthritis which is clearly inherited. Gout tends to run in families. ARC's booklet says: *"There may be a small tendency for many other forms of arthritis to appear slightly more commonly in some families than others (for example, rheumatoid arthritis, ankylosing spondylitis, psoriatic arthritis). But the chances of an affected parent directly handing on the disease to his or her children is very small indeed."* Discuss worries with your rheumatologist. A list of genetic advisory clinics appears in RADAR's factsheet *Access to Paramedical Services*.

How might pregnancy affect your arthritis and vice versa?   Again, do discuss this with your rheumatologist. If you have RA conception may be delayed slightly. During pregnancy itself, many women find the RA magically improves. Symptoms may settle down or completely disappear. Unfortunately the RA may flare up again *after* the birth, as it did for Mary*:

> *"I had difficulty coping with him. Mum came along once a week to wash out anything that needed to be done by hand and to do all my ironing. When S was two months old we went to stay with Mum and Dad for two weeks and ended up staying for five or six. I simply couldn't cope. I couldn't pick him up; put him down, feed him solids, bath him or change him. It was like a nightmare and it just got worse instead of better. We went home eventually not because I was any better but because it was becoming obvious that the problem was not just temporary and we'd have to learn to live with it.*
>
> *"Mum came over two or three times a week. F went into work only when he was actually teaching. I struggled with pain, putting more effort into the simple act of changing the baby's nappy than most people would put into spring cleaning."*

(Mary's two sons are now grown up and flourishing.)

With AS your back may play up more during pregnancy. Remission is much less likely than it is with RA, but, again unlike RA, ARC says *"the arthritis is rarely aggravated after the baby has been born"*. NASS spring/summer 1990 newsletter had an article on pregnancy and AS.

In *Lupus, a Guide for Patients*, Dr Graham Hughes summarises what's known about pregnancy in women with lupus (SLE):

Facts	*Pregnancy is usually uncomplicated in lupus.*
	There is no increased risk of lupus flare in pregnancy.
	There is little risk of lupus in the infant.
Problems	*Higher risk of miscarriage.*
	Increased risk of lupus flares after *delivery.*

St Thomas' Hospital in London has a special Lupus in Pregnancy Clinic, and the specialists there recommend a visit *before* pregnancy is attempted. It's essential that treatment is individualised, as some mothers are more at risk of complications than others. The Clinic can give advice on which drugs it's safe to continue with during a lupus pregnancy – patients and non-specialist doctors are often surprised to learn how many are considered safe. Psychologist Robert H Phillips includes pregnancy in *Coping with Lupus* (Avery Publishing, 1984, available from Lupus UK).

Drugs and pregnancy   In February 1981 the Committee on Safety of Medicines concluded that 'it is impossible to prove beyond a shadow of a doubt that any drug is absolutely safe in pregnancy' and 'drugs should not be given during a pregnancy unless they are essential'. Consult your rheumatologist about your drugs *before* you become pregnant. Some drugs (eg gold or penicillamine) should be stopped even before conception. S/he may advise continuing others, for instance steroids for someone with lupus, but perhaps with altered dosage (see the note above about St Thomas' Hospital).

Consult your doctor too before buying any 'over the counter' drugs (including aspirin). *Don't* fall into the trap of thinking that herbal remedies are any safer (see page 75). Remember to cut out alcohol and smoking too. If you're thinking of breastfeeding, remember that drugs can pass through the milk to the baby, so you shouldn't breastfeed while taking a drug unless your doctor tells you it's safe to do so.

Men with arthritis: you too should check on your drugs with your doctor before trying for a baby! In *Living with Arthritis* (Lennard/Collins), Alan Rogers, who has AS, explains:

> *"I remembered someone saying that the drug I was taking could affect the male sperm and cause damaged babies. I checked this out with the manufacturers, asking them for any research papers they had. I got a whole load of literature from them addressed to*

'Dr Alan Rogers'! I read it and, sure enough, discovered that the drug can affect the sperm. I saw my doctor about it and switched to another drug. Later my wife gave birth to two boys and they are both fine."

X-rays   Avoid X-rays during the first three months of pregnancy. Make sure your rheumatologist knows if there's any possibility you might be pregnant, so X-rays aren't done. That's why radiographers usually ask when your last period was, as a check.

Giving birth   Discuss this with your doctor. S/he may recommend a Caesarian section for delivery, for instance if you have stiff hips or small pelvis. If you have AS it's important to get mobile again as quickly as possible after giving birth or a Caesarian section.

Emotional adjustments   Does your arthritis make you tired and irritable? Do mobility problems make you feel socially isolated? Be prepared, alas, for such difficulties to become worse after the birth of a baby and do what you can to anticipate them and work out ways of coping. Though Sarah Litvinoff's *The Relate Guide to Better Relationships* is a 'non-disabled' book, it looks helpfully at the possible emotional impact a first baby may have on a partnership.

Ante-natal classes   If mobility problems make it difficult for you to get to these, there's a cassette called *Happy Birth Day* which covers things they'd tell you at the classes, like relaxation, breathing, exercises (from Professional Educational Training Aids Ltd). Some NCT teachers can give home tuition.

Fostering and adoption

After RA struck, Pamela Waterhouse was miserable at no longer feeling *"a useful, capable adult"*, despite magnificently looking after her own family of two sons and a husband. Challenges enough for anyone! She persuaded them to agree to her taking on the extra challenge of being a foster mum. After six months' questioning by social workers and fostering officers she was finally accepted: *"Family and friends thought I was mad. And they were probably right!"*

She wrote a lively article about her experiences in *In Contact* spring 1987, and pretty challenging they were too. She had to cope with some very difficult children, as well as her family *and* the RA. It was *"rewarding"* but *"like hitting your head against a brick wall – it's so nice when you stop!..."* Well worth reading if the thought of fostering crosses your mind. Another funny and touching account ('non-arthritic') for anyone thinking of fostering is Beth Miller's *Room for One More* (John Murray and National Foster Care Association).

The British Agencies for Adoption and Fostering (BAAF) has a range of leaflets and booklets. Send an SAE for information. **Parent to Parent Information on Adoption Services (PPIAS)** is a self-help support and information service for people already adopting or thinking of adopting.

Parenthood: some personal experiences

Talk to someone in a similar situation. The NCT or your Young Arthritis Care Contact should be able to put you in touch with someone. Next best is reading the experiences and tips of other parents with arthritis. In *In Contact*, a few years ago, Tracey Boardman described how she coped with her daughter aged 9½ months. It was hard work, and her RA flared up after Carly was born, but she was lucky to have help and support from husband and relatives. Her OT, Emma, was marvellous, too:

"My RA affects all my joints, my hands being the weakest. I have four replacement

knuckles in my right hand, so lifting Carly conventionally was out of the question. To overcome this a sling was fastened using two terry towelling nappies for strength with webbing for handles. Carly would lie on the sling in her carrycot and when I needed to pick her up, I would slip the handles around my neck and lift. Simple and safe...

"Emma and the team designed a trolley to hold the carrycot at the right height to ease the strain on my back. The trolley had wheels, each with its own brake, which meant I didn't have to carry Carly around the house, I could wheel her there. I am in a bungalow which also helps. A similar trolley was fashioned for Carly's baby bath to the right height for the bed. I can sit and bath her and afterwards put her straight on to the bed. I feel safer like this as the time she is wet and in my arms is only a few seconds. It gives me plenty of elbow room and space for Carly to roll too. The height of the mattress in her big cot was raised, which again saved my back and was ideal for nappy changing. Some cots do have a two position fixing for the mattress when you buy them.

"Nappies – using nappy pins was out of the question. I cannot open or close them. So I hit upon the idea of using velcro on terry nappies instead. Emma arranged for one to be made. However, this proved impractical, it was too bulky, they had to be folded the same way each time, and with repeated washing the cotton bits would stick to the velcro rendering it useless. The answer then? Disposable nappies. Still not so simple, as we were carrying out all these experiments before Carly was born and at that time the tapes on these nappies were such that once stuck they stayed stuck. Quite a bit of force was needed to wrench the tape from the nappy as it pulled the plastic nappy outer with it. This is when my teeth came into use – the day I need dentures, I'm lost! – By biting the end of the tape with my teeth and pulling I manage to undo them. Thankfully shortly after Carly was born the manufacturers brought out 're-sealable' nappies. Now I can just pull the tape from its second cover quite easily...

"From the nappies to clothes. Buttons – yes, poppers no. How many button through babygros have you seen? My answer is velcro. Sewn over the poppers it means I have no problem. Carly has it on babygros, vestpant suits, dungarees and pyjamas.

"This brings me more or less up to date. Carly has a high chair which sits on a platform with wheels. The tray also has large handles so I can remove it easily. I can take the chair to Carly wherever she is and I don't have to lift her far. As I cannot get down to the floor either to put Carly down or lift her up, Carly has been restricted to her carrycot or our bed and has not learnt to crawl. So her latest acquisition, a raised playpen, with the base at hip-height is marvellous. One side opens like a gate to give me easy access. She has room to move around and play with her toys. There I know she is safe and I now use it to dress and change her in.

"All these aids are priceless to me. They mean I can keep my independence and look after Carly as I want, without having to rely on others to do everything for me. This doesn't mean I don't want or need others, because without their help and support, life would be very hard indeed. My husband in particular was irreplaceable those first few months, as Carly's night feed, colic and my flare-up all came together. My mother and mother-in-law were a great help too, dealing with housework and meals. These days things are easier and I do the work myself. I will admit though, I appreciate the rest once a week when mum comes over. Hard work – yes, but when I look at Carly I wonder what I did all day without her before."

Unlike Tracey, Phil's RA was diagnosed after the birth of her son. Four years later she had a daughter. In *In Contact* she gave some tips on coping:

"Really what you need to do is get a bit more organised than you would be normally – and if you are normally so organised that everything has to be done on a certain day at a certain time then you'll just have to learn to relax a bit. Your baby really won't notice if it's Wednesday and the windows haven't been cleaned, and no, your friends won't notice either...

"Take some rest breaks during the day to save you from getting overtired. One way is to take a nap at the same time your baby has a sleep, at least for one session. Don't try to get all your jobs done while the baby sleeps or you'll be shattered. You can do odd jobs while the baby is awake, it will help keep it amused to watch you. And I'm sure that your partner could be persuaded to give you a hand with some jobs in the evenings and at weekends. You don't have to do everything for this little mite of yours, just to prove to yourself and others that you can cope. The baby is your hubbie's too, and of course, you may have some doting grandparents or family, even friends nearby who would like to help − let them.

"When you have visitors (and you'll have loads in the early days) don't pass the baby over if it's feeding time, if you are not breast feeding. And don't rush round making tea, cakes or sandwiches because you feel they need to be entertained...Get your visitors to make the tea (it will make them feel useful).

"Nappies. These are a problem for most mums. If the hospital or your health visitor has suggested you change your baby before a feed, then think again. It really doesn't hurt them to keep their nappy on for another 20 minutes or so, and once you have started to feed, they'll forget any discomfort in the joy of getting some grub and a cuddle to boot. Anyway, most babies choose to wet or soil their nappy during a feed, so you'll have wasted your time and energy and you'll still have to put another one on...

"...Can't manage to bath your baby, don't worry. Most of them scream all the way through it, well at first anyway. Just make sure you give the baby a nice wash morning and night to keep them cool and comfortable and smelling fresh and clean. Save bath-days until there is someone to give you a hand and make it a family affair..."

What about when the child or children get to the mischievous, into-everything, stage?

"As soon as Christopher started to crawl, I knew there would be trouble...that stage was a nightmare; we both experienced a great deal of frustration. Getting down on the floor with him was agony for me, so I tried to adapt. I found myself telling him off more than I wanted to, but I had to rely on words to restrain him because I couldn't keep up with him physically. I could not chase after him and retrieve him from the fireplace, or the wires...or the Christmas tree..." (Phil, again, in Michael Leitch's *Living with Arthritis*)

In OT Heather Unsworth's *Coping with Rheumatoid Arthritis* (Chambers) there's an excellent chapter, 'Coping with a Young Family: a Personal Experience', written by a mum who developed RA when her youngest son was one year old. Here's how she lifted him:

"For a child that can stand I devised a method of lifting which puts the weight on to the forearm instead of on to the shoulders and hands. Stand behind the child and put your arm between his legs. Put your other arm around his waist and draw him back so he is sitting on your forearm. Draw him closer to your body as you lift so that your arms and body take the weight with the encircling arm just steadying him and stopping him from falling. After a while the child becomes used to this method and helps..."

Another challenge was how to harness the baby in his buggy :

"I used a Mothercare safety harness to which a rein could be attached and used it for the pushchair, highchair and for walking. However, these have to be attached to two small anchor points in the seat of the chair. They are awkward to get at and fitted with dog-lead clips which are too stiff for a rheumatoid patient to operate. We solved this problem by making a single purchase which gave me total freedom. Go to a shop selling climbing or sailing gear and buy some carabina clips in a fairly modest size. These are used for clipping ropes together. They remain firmly closed in use but are opened easily by simply pressing down lightly on one bar. These we attached to the dog-lead clips and they remain permanently in position on the harness, to be clipped to the anchor points on anything I need or simply to attach the walking reins."

Resting's crucial; but how to fit it in?

"It is really worth ignoring the chores and having a set time every day to put your feet

up. We made it a rule even when my little one grew past much sleep that he and I went to lie on our beds for half to one hour every day and I found this invaluable for recharging batteries before the school age ones arrived home. We did this immediately after lunch. Now there are no day-time rests, but I try to ensure we put our feet up on the sofa for a while after lunch and read a book together or watch children's lunchtime programmes. I certainly notice the days we don't."

If you have more than one child, you may find that one may help out with the other, and look on it as fun. A youngster may enjoy picking up the toys flung down by his baby sister from her pram or pushchair, or chasing off to retrieve a straying toddler. Some children enjoy repetitive but helpful jobs, too, like passing pegs to mum who is hanging out the clothes, or careering happily around pushing a shopping trolley. My nine year old godson thought one of the best things about his day trip to the zoo was being able to push me around in a wheelchair! But of course few children are angelic all the time. Mary* describes her youngster's antics on a bad day for her:

"S always seems to reserve his most throttling, boneshaking kisses and cuddles for days such as these. Then he insists on playing games which involve grabbing me round the knees in a fair attempt at a rugby tackle and swinging on me. The pain is bad enough, keeping my balance is practically impossible and the whole thing is aggravated by S's shrieks of delight at, what constitutes to him, a good game. I ought not to shout at him so much at times like these but it really does get me furious that he should find it so funny to inflict all this pain on me. Of course that's unfair because it's not that he finds funny. He isn't even aware that he's hurting. But the sight of him laughing is like a red rag to a bull. I'm sure it does him no great psychological harm anyway when I shout at him. He just shouts back. (Another good game)."

As children grow older you may miss being able to do some things:

"Your physical range of activities is limited, but your vocal chords remain intact. I discovered some time ago, when my footballing and cricketing talents were diminishing rapidly, that a good story laced with kisses and cuddles makes a very acceptable substitute." (PB)

How do you deal with a child's reactions to your arthritis? If they ask questions, children need honest, yet simple explanations, that don't make them feel worried, or ashamed about asking. They may worry that you might die, or might not be able to look after them any more. And they may need your guidance in dealing with curiosity and questions from other children. Margaret Mayson wrote:

"A child's remark, 'Why is that lady in a push-chair?' did not worry me, but my son at eight years of age was embarrassed. 'Silly nit', was his terse comment. I sought to mollify his feelings at being singled out as a child whose mother was 'different', and in doing so, became myself less sensitive to my disabilities. I found it a good plan to make fun of my 'wooden' legs and knobbly hands and to laugh at my struggles with girdles and tight fitting dresses – this in private of course; in public we behaved unostentatiously. One time, feeling very much aware of my limitations, I asked my son what he thought mothers were for. 'Oh, to make food and be there', was his reply. Truly masculine philosophy, but it helped me feel less useless. One of the doctors made a similar comment when I was lamenting my inability to dash about and how it affected my family. 'Well, there's one consolation, they know where you are and that's more than can be said of some mothers.'" (In Paul Hunt's *Stigma*, Geoffrey Chapman, 1966)

Older children might be interested to see Dr John Shenkman's *Living with Arthritis* (Franklin Watts, 1990), which explains rheumatic disorders in simple terms, with plenty of illustrations. Psychologist Robert H Phillips' *Coping with Lupus* (see page 27) includes comments for parents on dealing with reactions and worries of children and adolescents.

Helpful people and organisations

Discuss medical aspects with your rheumatologist. Plan with your OT how to overcome practical problems and minimise strains on your body and on your family.

Social services departments   Services available vary considerably, and may not be widely publicised, so keep ferreting about. One YPA was particularly lucky:

> *"I have a Family Aid who comes four times a week...she takes us to Playschool in the car and on Mondays we go to Toddlers with my two year old daughter. The Aid stays with me so she can run after R and generally help me should my hip decide to be more awkward. On E's playschool days we go shopping, and do any other jobs I can't do while I am by myself. The Family Aid can work flexible hours, such as hospital appointments, which never seem to be on time. She's a great friend to all the family..."*

Another mum going through a very bad patch paid out a fortune in taxi fares taking her son to and from school only to find later that her social services ran a service called Home Care which would provide different people to take and fetch him from school each day.

National Childbirth Trust (NCT)   is a charity offering support and advice for mothers, on topics such as breastfeeding, ante-natal classes, post-natal and mother and toddler groups. Write with SAE for their useful publications list, plus Maternity Sales catalogue (mail order of all sorts from nighties and nursing bras to gadgets to help with baby care).

NCT runs a national Parents with Disabilities information/contact register that can put a mum or mum-to-be in touch with another with the same disability for support and information. And there's a resource list for disabled parents covering pregnancy, birth and early parenthood. One young mother with RA explained how NCT helped her:

> *"I still find it difficult to cope with vast hordes and for this reason we did not persevere long with 'mums and toddlers' although certainly my son enjoyed the rough and tumble. Instead we joined the NCT which has branches in most areas and runs good supportive services, social events and regular coffee mornings. This introduced my son into groups of children which were not too overpowering in number for either of us."* (In Heather Unsworth's *Coping with Rheumatoid Arthritis*, Chambers, 1986)

Meet-a-Mum Association (MAMA)   Post-natal support groups for mothers, specially any feeling tired or isolated after the birth of a baby. There's a network of groups who can arrange for two or three mums to offer practical support to another in their area.

Play Groups   for three to five year olds. Contact the Pre-School Play Group Association for details of theirs. Others are run on a voluntary basis. Social services and health visitors have lists of registered child-minders and local mother and toddler groups.

Self-help support groups for parents under stress   OPUS (Organisations for Parents Under Stress) runs a confidential telephone helpline (Parentline) for parents, can offer a sympathetic ear and, if you want, put you in touch with local contacts and groups. Parents Anonymous is a support group run by parents for parents having problems with older children. Look in your phone book, or contact the London branch for more information.

Maternity Alliance   is a charity which helps pregnant women and parents of young babies with queries about benefits and practical support. Your local Citizen's Advice Bureau (see page 118) will be able to help with benefits queries too.

Home Start Consultancy is a home-visiting scheme run by parent volunteers offering support, friendship and practical help to families with pre-school children. Ask if there's a Home Start Scheme near you (there are over 130 schemes in the UK).

If you want to search further, Fiona Macdonald's *The Parents' Directory* (Bedford Square Press) lists around 800 voluntary organisations able to give help, advice and information to parents on a wide range of topics.

Publications

Don't forget to look at the pregnancy and baby books listed on pages 227-228. Some of the organisations listed above produce useful publications too. Beg, borrow, or buy these key books: they'll in turn lead you to other sources of information and help:

- *Arthritis – an Equipment Guide*, which includes a section on parents with arthritis, and *Parents with Disabilities* are both in the *Equipment for the Disabled* series, produced by the Disability Information Trust. Really excellent, and full of problem-solving products and tips. Your OT should have a copy if you don't want to buy your own.
- Mukti Jain Campion's *The Baby Challenge* (Routledge)
- ARC's *Arthritis: Sexual Aspects and Parenthood* (free, but send SAE)

Other books listed here don't deal specifically with arthritis/disability, but may be helpful. The *Healthwise* booklist has a section on pregnancy, birth and childcare. Many books listed in this chapter can be bought by post from Healthwise. Relate has booklists on 'fertility, pregnancy and birth, adoption' and 'children and teenagers'.

- Useful DSS booklets include: *Babies and Benefits* (FB8), *Bringing up Children* (FB27), *Child Benefit* (CH 1), *A Guide to Maternity Benefits* (N1 17A), *Employment Rights for the Expectant Mother* (PL 710), *One Parent Benefit* (CH 11), *Help with NHS Costs* (AB 11). From DSS offices, post offices, or by post from the DSS Leaflets Unit.
- Nancy Kohner's *The Parent Book* (National Extension College/BBC). Lots of help and information for coping with life and babies and small children and where to get more help and information, plus tips from parents based on their own experiences.
- Ivan Sokolov and Deborah Hutton's *The Parents' Book – Getting On Well With Our Children* (Thorsons) is a practical book on communicating with children of any age, from babies to adolescents. Helpful and reassuring, with plenty of experiences from other parents and practical exercises.
- Johanna Roeber's *Shared Parenthood: a Handbook for Fathers* (Century). Written by an NCT counsellor. Good idea if father's going to have more on his plate than usual, thanks to the arthritis.
- T Bradman's *The Essential Father* (Unwin) – also for men new to fatherhood
- The British Medical Association's low-cost *Fathers-to-be*, by Ruth Forbes (available by post from BMA Family Doctor Publications).
- *Supertot: a Parent's Guide to Toddlers* by Jean Marzollo (Unwin)
- *Pre-School Play* by Kenneth Jameson and Pat Kidd (Unwin)
- *Until They are Five* by Angela Phillips (Pandora)
- Libby Purves *How Not to be a Perfect Mother* (Fontana)
- Laurie Graham's *A Parent's Survival Guide* (Chatto & Windus), funny but informative guide to parenthood
- Vicki Lansky's *It Worked for Me*. Over 1000 tried and tested tips passed on by other parents (Exley)
- *It's More Than Sex! A Survival Guide to the Teenage Years*, by Suzie Hayman

(Wildwood House), and *Help! I've Got a Teenager!* by R T Bayard and J Bayard. Yes, cuddly babies grow into difficult teenagers.

Magazines: *Parents* and *Practical Parenting contain useful news and tips. The NCT publishes a quarterly newsletter, Newsletter for Parents with a Disability.*

Some publications to inspire you in planning non-physical activities with your children:
- Geraldine Taylor's *Be Your Child's Natural Teacher* (Penguin)
- *Learning Through Play* by Jean Marzollo and Janice Lloyd (Unwin)
- Piccolo's *Early Learn Together* colour books for the under fives, and, for four to 11 year olds, *Learn Together* and *Practise Together*
- The Home and Schools Council publish low-cost booklets for parents and teachers on various aspects of schooling. (Send SAE for publications list)
- Look at Ladybird's *Puddle Lane* reading series.
- *Bringing School Home* by R Mertens and J Vass (Headway, Hodder and Stoughton)

To keep you in touch with books being published for children:
- A magazine for teachers, but good for parents too is *Books for Keeps*, on subscription from Books for Keeps. (Send SAE for leaflet).
- John Rowe Townsend's *Written for Children* (Penguin)

See also the Book Clubs in the last section on this page.

Bringing up children on your own

Get information, support and advice from Gingerbread (see page 218) and the National Council for One Parent Families (NCOPF), whose publications (many free) include relationship breakdown, housing, benefits and legal rights, and *We Don't All Live with Mum and Dad* (£4 inc p&p, 1991), which lists over 100 publications aimed at children and adults in one-parent families. Another book (non-arthritic) that may be helpful
- *Bringing Up Your Children On Your Own*, Liz McNeill (Fontana)

Some shopping by post addresses

- Send for NCT's *Maternity Sales catalogue*, which I mentioned on page 234
- Mothercare do a mail-order catalogue, and both Boots and Mothercare have a free home delivery service for their own makes of nappy
- *The Bear Necessities Directory* by Bridget Spowart (Pandora) – mail-order products for the under-fives
- The two *Equipment for the Disabled* books mentioned on page 235 include lots of postal suppliers of useful equipment
- Red House produce *Baby Book News*, a book club for expectant first-time mothers with books on childbirth and babycare. Subscribers have to take four books a year. They run a similar Children's Book Club for children. You agree to take at least three books in your first year.
- Books for Children – book club of recommended selections in four age groups. You agree to purchase at least four selections in your first year.
- Back to School – mail-order uniforms, equipment, stationery, sportswear
- Pooh Corner Book Club: for all things 'Pooh'!

Three mail-order firms for wonderful toys, hobby materials, etc, for children of all ages:
- Early Learning
- ¡Tridias!
- Stockingfillas Ltd

For children's party goodies by post (besides the three firms above):
- *Parties by Post catalogue*, from Frog Frolics
- Red House do a catalogue too

Chapter twenty-nine

PERSONAL ACCOUNTS OF ARTHRITIS
AND FAMOUS PEOPLE WITH ARTHRITIS

.

Several people have written about their experiences of arthritis; all well worth reading, and items by YPAs appear regularly in *Young Arthritis News*. One particularly good book, *Living with Arthritis*, by Michael Leitch (Lennard/Collins, 1987), is a collection of accounts by 27 people with arthritis, talking about different day-to-day aspects. The foreword's by Terry Wogan, whose mother has RA. Here are some other books to get your teeth into. Some of the older ones are now out of print, but ask your library to get them for you through the inter-library loan system (see page 115). My own favourite comes first:

Marie Joseph's *One Step at a Time. Living with Arthritis* (© Arrow, originally published by Heinemann, 1976, though now alas out of print)   Read this even if you don't read any of the others! Shows you can keep your sanity and sense of humour even after thirty-plus years of living with RA. It's the wonderfully lighthearted autobiography of the famous novelist. She was just 24, with her husband back from the Air Force, and a young baby to care for, when she was told she had RA. Her tales of family, hospital stays and other people's reactions and all the ups and downs sound so familiar, yet are told with a highly entertaining sense of humour. When she was 40, Marie wrote and sold her first story, about a mother going into hospital and leaving her children behind, and she's since published masses of books, short stories and humorous articles.

Norman Cousins' *Anatomy of an Illness* (Bantam, 1987)   Fascinating. He knew that negative emotions could have a negative effect on body chemistry, and when he developed severe AS he wondered if the opposite might be true. Could positive emotions, like love, hope, faith, laughter, confidence and the will to live, produce beneficial effects? With his doctor's support, he tried 'laughter therapy' (see page 110), with excellent results. He became senior lecturer at the School of Medicine, University of California at Los Angeles, and consulting editor of *Man & Medicine*, published at the College of Physicians and Surgeons, Columbia University.

Roger Glanville's *When the Box Doesn't Fit* (one essay in a collection called *Stigma – the Experience of Disability*, edited by Paul Hunt, publisher Geoffrey Chapman, 1966)   Now out of print. Roger was born in 1935, and developed RA at the age of 15. He went to the local grammar school, then after a year in hospital, to Bristol University where he edited the students' newspaper and was Vice-President and Honorary Secretary of the Union. He became a teacher, and taught in Nigeria, before returning to Britain to teach Liberal Studies at Slough College, when he acquired a wife, two children and a mortgage.

Roger describes particularly well the psychological and practical aspects of RA. He talks too about maddening tussles with unreasonable insurance companies. Fortunately the medical examinations for jobs went much better: *"It is very encouraging to be given the benefit of the doubt when doubt exists"*; each doctor *"understood my physical difficulties and understood the need for me to be allowed to try to do my work."*

Also in *Stigma* are Judith Thunem's essay *The Invalid Mind*, and Margaret Mayson's inspiring *Mind Over Matter?* Judith was born in Norway in 1918 and developed RA when she was 17. Margaret became aware of her RA on her son's fifth birthday. Other essays in *Stigma* are by people with different disorders, eg polio, cerebral palsy.

Cordelia Jones' *The View from the Window* (André Deutsch, 1978)   Fiction. Irene is 18, has had RA for six years, and is now, in the late 1960s, in hospital for a long rest. She vividly describes her loneliness at being cut off from ordinary everyday life and how her RA creates misunderstandings with other people. Most of the other patients are over 60. She feels like the Lady of Shalott in Tennyson's poem, who is 'half sick of shadows' and sees the real world only reflected in a mirror. An unexpected outing brings a friendship which helps her analyse her attitudes towards other people and her RA.

It's a thoughtful and perceptive book, even though Cordelia Jones doesn't herself have RA. She herself was an artist, and learnt about RA while helping in the art room in a local hospital where she got to know one of the patients very well.

Pamela La Fane's *It's a Lovely Day, Outside* (Gollancz, 1981)   Moving and inspiring autobiography. Depressing too in its picture of the plight of a young chronically ill girl in the past. In 1939 when she was 11, Pamela was evacuated to Oxfordshire, where pains in her legs and wrists heralded the arrival of RA. It worsened until she could do nothing for herself. Horrifically, for some 30 years, she was institutionally confined and bed-ridden, all too often condemned to a régime where a clear locker top was thought more important than the books and writing materials she fought for to keep herself mentally active. Eventually she taught herself to type (tapping on the keys with a stick), enrolled in a correspondence course in journalism, and through articles and a TV programme made contacts whose help at long last enabled her to leave hospital and move to an adapted council flat. Her story's brought up-to-date in Michael Leitch's *Living with Arthritis*.

Cheryl Marcus's *Lupus in the Family*   Another of the accounts in Michael Leitch's book. Cheryl's the founder of the Lupus Group, now Lupus UK. She was 21, and newly married, when she was diagnosed as having lupus (SLE). This was before the better diagnosis and treatment available today and the physical and emotional impact on Cheryl was shattering. Fortunately her husband and parents were very supportive, and later she even went on to produce two sons.

Frances Parsons' *Pools of Fresh Water. A Story of Healing* (Triangle Books)   Frances developed RA in her 20s, and is a past winner of the Dista Award (for YPAs). The book's a moving account of her life from its early days through school and marriage to Stephen, a vicar. A story of sadness, happiness, trauma and triumph. Other YPAs will understand many of the feelings and experiences she describes, especially young mums with young children, like herself. She and her husband now exercise a healing ministry together.

Alice Pearl's *No Leg to Stand On* (out of print)   Alice lived with RA for over 40 years, since she was 18. Her sensitive autobiography describes how she married, had a daughter, became a lay preacher, British Red Cross Commandant, Transport Officer for the local branch of what's now called Arthritis Care, and later faced widowhood. She has an inspiringly positive philosophy of life, despite many setbacks. There's a contribution from her too in Michael Leitch's *Living with Arthritis*.

Grace Stuart's *Private World of Pain* (1953, George Allen & Unwin, now Unwin Hyman of HarperCollins Publishers Ltd)   Alas, long since out of print, but try to get hold of a copy. When Grace wrote the book, she'd lived with RA for 33 years, since the age of 19. I learned a tremendous amount from this thoughtful and sensitive lady, particularly about coping with the psychological ups and downs of RA.

Rosemary Sutcliff's *Blue Remembered Hills – A Recollection* (Oxford University Press, 1984) Autobiography of the well-known writer, who received first the OBE then in 1992 the CBE for services to children's literature. Many of her novels are set in Roman Britain and the Dark Ages (with at least two disabled heroes, in *Warrior Scarlet* and *The Witches' Brat* – a nice change!). She developed Still's disease when she was 2½, and describes how it affected her physically and emotionally as she grew up, her studies to become a painter, her writing, and the love affair which left a lasting impression. *Blue Remembered Hills* ends in her late 20s, but two items in Michael Leitch's *Living with Arthritis* tell us how she lives and writes now, in Sussex, using a fountain pen, as always, despite the arthritis.

Corbet Woodall's *A Disjointed Life* (Heinemann, 1980) Autobiography of the former TV newsreader and broadcaster, who developed RA at the age of 38, while on the honeymoon of his second marriage. Refreshing to read a *male* account of the physical and emotional impact of RA on life, marriage, and career. It's a very honest, often self-critical account of his struggle to adapt, and many people will identify with his experiences and reflections.

Some famous people with arthritis

Two famous writers, Rosemary Sutcliff and Marie Joseph, developed juvenile chronic arthritis when young. Dennis Potter, the controversial TV playwright (*Pennies from Heaven*, *The Singing Detective*, etc) has suffered from psoriatic arthropathy since he was 26 and newly married. His hands are badly crippled, but he still writes, rather than dictates, his work in printed letters. Labour MP Jo Richardson has had RA for nearly 30 years. She has described her experiences in Michael Leitch's *Living with Arthritis*.

On the sports field, AS put paid to a physically active career in rugby and cricket for Peter West, but he became a TV sports commentator instead. Former golf Ryder Cup player Michael King has AS, so too do the young actor Michael Mello, who appeared in TV's *The Bill*, and Lord David Ennals, energetic member of the House of Lords. 'Mac' McEvoy was 23 when he developed AS. He went on to become Air Chief Marshal Sir Theodore Newman McEvoy KCB CBE, a veteran fighter pilot. After his retirement from the RAF, aged 58, he became vice-president of the British Gliding Association.

In 1978, at the age of 30, cancer specialist and TV personality Dr Bob Buckman developed the rare auto-immune disorder dermatomyositis. He was seriously ill for two years, but then returned to work. Another rare rheumatic disorder, sarcoidosis, may have caused Beethoven's deafness, joint pains, and other health problems, according to consultant rheumatologist Dr Tom Palferman.

Did you know that Auguste Renoir, the famous French painter, whose pictures are so full of the joy of living, had RA? It developed after a bicycle accident, in his 50s. That was at the turn of the century, when little could be done, alas, to treat it, and he became crippled and eventually confined to a wheelchair. He resolutely carried on painting, producing such masterpieces as *Les Grandes Baigneuses*. His fingers curled inwards and he could no longer pick anything up, but family and friends would fasten the brush into his fingers for him. (Described in his son's biography *Renoir – My Father* by Jean Renoir, Collins, 1962). Three other famous artists also developed rheumatic disorders: Peter Paul Rubens and Raoul Dufy had RA, while Paul Klee suffered from scleroderma. An article in *The Lancet* in 1987 compared the pigments all four artists used with those used by their contemporaries, and found that the four with rheumatic disorders tended to use much bolder colours. Researchers concluded that the four were slowly poisoning themselves with poisons like mercury, lead and arsenic, contained in the pigments.

Many well-known people have had hip replacements – writer Leslie Thomas, journalist Marje Proops and actress Thora Hird. Actress Sheila Mercier, who plays Annie Sugden in *Emmerdale Farm*, has had two knee replacement operations.

Chapter thirty

STUDYING FOR PLEASURE
OR FOR A PURPOSE

By 'studying' I mean both academic *and* non-academic skills — anything that broadens the horizons. Anything that expands and emphasises abilities, not *dis*abilities. When the brawn's not what it used to be, let the brain take the strain.

Some of us have had our schooling interrupted by the arthritis, but determine to make up for it later. It's never too late. Others of us manage to notch up sufficient qualifications and schooling to go straight on to further studies of some sort — vocational training, or further and higher education at a college, polytechnic, or university.

Some of us develop arthritis later, and decide we need to retrain in order to continue working. Others of us, after bringing up a family and more or less stabilising the arthritis, decide it's time to get the grey matter fully operational again. Or maybe we just opt, for fun, to learn a new skill like family tree researching, singing, even lace-making (yes — despite weak fingers). Some good reasons for studying:

- to train for a job
- to learn new skills
- to gain qualifications
- to prove to a potential employer you've been making good use of your time when unemployed, stuck at home, in hospital, or wherever
- so you can help the children with their homework
- to meet people and make friends
- to boost your self-confidence
- to show yourself and other people there's something you *can* do, that you're a person with *abilities* despite any disability
- to give yourself a sense of purpose
- to overcome boredom
- to stop yourself having too much time to dwell on pains and problems, or get depressed
- as an alternative to a job — something to do at your own pace, in your own time
- to brush up your basic skills, so you can write letters, deal more confidently with officials, etc
- just for fun, mental stimulation — for the sheer pleasure of learning!

What you do depends on you. I can only give a few signposts here to all the opportunities around. Don't stick exclusively to advice and advisers for disabled people. They can certainly tell you about things like access to colleges, study aids, and financial assistance. But, well-meaning though they may be, some have limited ideas about 'what disabled people can do', and may have limited knowledge of the vast range of opportunities open to *anyone*, much of which might suit you, give or take a modification or two here and there.

They may know little or nothing about your type of arthritis, too, the difficulties it causes and how to overcome them. You might be discouraged from aiming high because they don't want you to be disappointed if you fail, or simply because in their limited experience disabled people have been able to achieve very little. Alarming, and not true.

It's even more important that we should have all the education and training we can get. I for one prefer to try something and fail, rather than not be allowed to try. You might need to explain that 'brains don't get arthritis'. Nor does it affect hearing, speaking or vision (except for a rare few people with certain types of arthritis, whose vision *is* affected, but even that need be no barrier to judge by the achievements of some YPAs).

Seek as much information as possible from non-disabled sources, including ideas in schemes for other people with special needs, eg for unemployed people, mature students, or women returning to education/work after child-rearing.

One specialist organisation you can rely on to help you aim as high and as wide as possible is 'Skill' (National Bureau for Students with Disabilities). Skill does sterling work helping people overcome disability barriers in further education — be they physical, information or attitudinal barriers:

"People with disabilities often have to deal with others who do not understand their needs, or may feel they know best what is right for the disabled person. It is often difficult to understand, let alone accept, that the person with a disability is usually the best judge of their own capabilities."

Skill offers information and advice to students and staff. However, their resources are limited, so do do your own detective work first, especially on non-disability related questions. Send an SAE for a list of Skill's various publications. Skill's 1986/87 report explains what they deal with:

- *"Requests for information on courses, physical access to colleges, specialist provision and support services. Very often students do not know where to go for careers guidance or how to obtain the information they need. We can usually refer them to specialist careers advisers, coordinators for disabled students in their local colleges, or other professionals in their home area. Sometimes we can help students directly or liaise with people in their region.*

- *"Financial assistance: Students with disabilities generally incur additional costs whilst at college. They may, for example, need to buy special equipment, pay for personal care help, readers or interpreters, have additional travel costs, and need to buy extra books. [They] do not usually know where to go for the extra money they need, while social security regulations and rules relating to benefits are complicated...*

- *"Many students with disabilities have followed unconventional education and career patterns. Rules and regulations are invariably framed with the non-disabled in mind, with the result that careful negotiation is often required before the needs of people with disabilities can be accommodated."*

Another helpful organisation is the Educational Guidance Service for Adults (EGSA). EGSA gives free and independent educational guidance on courses, admission requirements, and grants to anyone (not just disabled people), over 19 (not school-leavers), who's interested in returning to or continuing in education. EGSA has computer bases on all sorts of courses throughout the UK. Counsellors can help with questions such as which course to choose? Will it meet your needs? Will you be able to cope with it? Some enquirers may only need one-off information, but EGSA helps other enquirers too who need regular support and encouragement, eg people with learning or study difficulties, or people with particular personal or domestic problems.

Some ways of overcoming study problems caused by the arthritis

● *Reading and writing problems*   See the ideas on pages 148-149. Other ideas: use micro-cassette recorder for note-taking, get someone else to write for you while you dictate (an 'amanuensis'), use electronic typewriters, request extra time in exams. Modern technology (computers, word processors, modems, etc) can overcome many problems, be they in or outside the home. BT, for instance, has donated several workstations to the Open University for use by disabled students. Each workstation has a telephone with loudspeaker, a multi-number directory with memory dialling, a word processor, and links to Prestel and Telecom Gold so students can talk to tutors and other students.

- *Access* Many colleges are now willing to see how they can help (eg by providing ramps, allowing the use of side lifts, special enrolment and parking arrangements). Skill can advise and RADAR has a handbook *Access to University and Polytechnic Buildings for Disabled Students*.
- *Variability/unpredictability in your arthritis* One YPA got depressed at the physical difficulties of coping with her college course. She eventually told her tutor who arranged for her to do half the work at home, which improved things tremendously. For other solutions look at courses in 'modular form', flexible learning, open learning, residential study weekends/weeks. Studying based totally at home (distance education) is flourishing, enabling you to study at your own pace, as and when the arthritis lets you. Look at schemes aimed at women with small children – they too need flexibility.
- *Disrupted early education* You can study for basic qualifications at any age, even skills like reading, writing, arithmetic. You can sometimes go straight on to further education without basic qualifications, instead, perhaps, being assessed on an essay and/or an interview. Bridging courses may be run as a preliminary to, say, an OU degree, for people with insufficient qualifications.
- *Negative attitudes in other people/colleges* Defy them by showing what you *can* do, and what others *have* done. Enlist the help of Skill/a good social worker/your GP/consultant/the DGCIS and ADP (see pages 260 and 261).
- *Eye problems* Some rare types of arthritis may cause sight problems/blindness – consult the Royal National Institute for the Blind for advice.

You may need perseverance and determination to overcome any barriers, be they physical or other people's discouraging attitudes. But don't be discouraged – take heart from all those who've done it before.

YPA tales to spur you into action

JCA in early childhood meant long stays in hospital for one YPA, but he later went on to get six A grade and two B grade O level passes and five Highers (in Scotland), and then the Pitman's typing exam. Another, now in her early 30s, developed RA at the age of 16 but managed to pass O levels in hospital. Later, while she worked, she studied for an ONC in Business Studies at evening class, and qualified as an Associate of the Chartered Insurance Institute. A works accountant developed RA in her 30s, which meant rethinking things, and retraining to work from home, running an accountancy and book-keeping service. She needed a new computer: Arthritis Care helped with some of its cost. Another 30 year old, with arthritis since childhood, gained four O levels and the RSA typing exam. She worked for five years but was made redundant. Undeterred, she successfully studied for the RSA Private Secretary course.

Glyn Barney missed a lot of schooling when he developed RA at the age of 15, but went on to take a foundation course in art and photography, followed by a three year diploma course at West Surrey College of Art and Design. He now works as a freelance photographer. Ken Porter was part-time manager of a band when he developed RA in his early 20s. He studied for an accountancy qualification, mainly on his own, and is now a senior manager in a leading firm of auditors.

Carol Cambridge (with JCA) and I (also JCA) both managed to get Honours degrees in modern languages, Carol at Reading University, me at Kent University, and we both did the compulsory year in France. Carol's just added the Diploma of the Institute of Personnel Management to her qualifications. We managed at university with only minor concessions to the arthritis, eg I was allowed extra time to write my exams, and lived on campus the whole time. A very good time it was, too!

When Peter Nightingale (30s, RA and diabetes) was a manager with a local authority, his employer financed his part-time studies for the Diploma in Management Studies, at Ealing

College. One YPA in her 20s has had arthritis since she was two, and lost her sight (a rare few people do, sadly, with some types of RA). Nevertheless, she studied at college and got nine O levels and three A levels, followed by studies at Leeds University in data processing, with the help of a team of volunteers (Community Service Volunteers have a special scheme). Another, who went on to become a computer programmer with the RAF, graduated from Leeds with a 2:1 Honours degree. She too had earlier lost her sight.

Carol J started off on a Youth Training Scheme working for the Civil Service and was then made permanent. Martin Ellingford (with AS) studied A levels in his 20s and went on at 26 to obtain a social sciences degree at Hatfield Polytechnic. Open University students and graduates abound – Mandy King, Pamela Waterhouse, Jennifer Purple, Janice Simons, etc. More about the OU on page 247.

Another YPA developed severe AS at the age of 14. After nearly a year in hospital he had to attend a special school, where you couldn't do O levels. He left at 16, was advised to go to a 'disabled' college, but decided instead to go to the local Tec to study O and A levels. Then on to university, where he got a psychology degree...Alas he couldn't get a job. Demoralised, he decided he had to do something to keep his mind occupied, and ended up deciding to study law full-time! Yet more obstacles appeared. His mum described in *In Contact* what happened:

"He enlisted the help of the Disablement Officer, who thought he would be eligible for a special grant. To apply he first had to obtain a place at a college. He was already halfway through the first term at a London polytechnic when he learnt that he had been turned down for the grant. He appealed, to no avail. The only reason given was that he could not guarantee that he would have a job at the end of the training.

"By then I had seen for myself the enormous improvement in his morale, and there was no way I could bring myself to say 'we just can't afford for you to do this, you'll have to give it up'. We tightened our belts. Then we discovered a clause in the DHSS rules which said that unemployed disabled people are exempt from the 'limited hours of study' ruling, and may study full-time.

"As a graduate, he could have done a one year postgraduate course, but knowing his physical limitations, he preferred to take the full three years for a first degree LLB. I tightened my belt further and looked on it as his 'occupational therapy'. He missed half a term in both the first two years through illness, not to mention those days when he was not well enough to travel, or to study.

"[He was then very ill] and was in hospital for the whole of the first term of his final year. The College advised him to defer his studies for a year, so did the hospital surgeon and specialists. My son is a very stubborn and determined young man. He got back to his studies, sat the final exam and obtained an Upper Second Class degree."

Still at school? Some brief notes

Besides reading the rest of this chapter, and chapter 31 on employment, look at the Family Fund's free booklet *After 16 – What Next?* (from the Joseph Rowntree Memorial Trust). Get the free *Just the Job* (see *Just the Job* in Appendix 2) for information about government-funded training and enterprise schemes, etc. Look too at non-disabled publications like Ann Jones' *The School-Leaver's Handbook*, (National Extension College), full of the sort of advice a good friend would give you. Look too at *Your Choice at 15+* and *Your Choice at 17+* by Michael Smith and Peter March (CRAC/Hobsons Press), the 'Schoolleavers' chapter in *Second Chances* (see page 244); and the DLF information sheet on *Further, Adult and Higher Education*. You'll get advice too from people like Careers Officers/Specialist Careers Officers, teachers, DROs, Skill, Young Arthritis Care, and the Lady Hoare Trust.

When weighing up what to do, get up-to-date advice on how studying will affect your benefits from a social worker, welfare rights adviser or Citizens Advice Bureau. The position's complicated, and varies depending on age, disability, and what you're studying.

For everyone: where to start

The best source of information is a friendly, readable non-disabled goldmine of a book: *Second Chances – A National Guide to Adult Education and Training Opportunities*, published annually by COIC, the Careers and Occupational Information Centre. There's one chapter on disability, but *do* look at the whole book too. Find it in a library, in a bookshop, or from COIC by post (but p&p's expensive). COIC also publish a cheaper, shorter guide *It's Your Chance*, chattier than *Second Chances*, but with far less in the way of specific information. It aims to help you sort out what would be best for you, how best to fit it into your life, and how to tackle any doubts you might have. *Second Choices* is much more detailed. It's in four parts:

– Part 1: The practicalities. Where to get help, advice, money, etc.
– Part 2: Users. Different reasons for wanting education and training, and some facilities for people with special needs (eg people with children, unemployed people, people with disabilities, people with children and other dependents).
– Part 3: Providers. Main types (eg university, adult and further education, training schemes, open learning, returning to study, basic reading, writing, maths, learning by post, teach yourself systems, self-employment).
– Part 4: General reference. The range of qualifications and subjects, and a gazetteer of places to study (includes all the local education authorities in the country, their further education colleges, and arrangements for adult education).

By using *Second Chances* you can do a lot of research from your armchair or library chair. If you need to search further, then try your local library, CAB, and local education authority guidance service. Try your local polytechnic/university/college library, if there's one nearby. Look at *Just the Job* (page 243) for information about government-funded training services. Don't forget Skill (page 241) and EGSA (page 241), both wonderfully helpful. A brief, cheap guide focusing on the disability angle is DLF's *Further, Adult and Higher Education – Assessment and Training for the Physically Disabled*.

If you're studying with a career in mind one or more of the following publications might also help you make sure the studies are going to get you where you want to go:

– The *Skills for...*, *Choice of Careers*, and *Working in...* series of booklets, covering different professions, industries and jobs, recruitment, training and prospects, etc (published by COIC: write or phone for the COIC publications list).
– CRAC publications (Careers Research and Advisory Centre, a registered educational charity). Write to CRAC for a list. Three examples:
  – *Careers and Jobs Without O Levels*, by Thelma Barber
  – *Your Choice at 17 +*, by Michael Smith and Peter March
  – *Jobs and Careers after A levels*, by Mary Munro
– *Careers Encyclopaedia*, edited by Audrey Segal, (Cassell)
– *It's Never Too Late* by Joan Perkin (Impact), who took A levels at a college of further education when in her 40s, and then went on to do a degree.
– *Returning to Work: Education and Training for Women* (Longman). A directory of over 1400 courses for women returning to work.
– Look too at chapter 31 on employment.

Some of the many qualifications you could study for

Basic skills   Many adults have never really learnt to read or write or do simple maths (or all three). Maybe you were in manual work until the arthritis appeared on the scene? And now want to brush up on the basics before retraining? There are courses specially for you. More information from the Adult Literacy and Basic Skills Unit or ask at your local library for information. Some YPAs are themselves adult literacy tutors.

GCSEs Don't worry if you didn't get manage to get your GCSEs at school. There's a special GCSE (mature) syllabus, designed for one year courses. They can be studied in various ways – day, evening, full-time, part-time, adult education, correspondence college, or totally on your own (using the 'external' syllabus). For details contact your nearest examinations board (ask the DES for the address).

BTEC (Business and Technician Education Council) qualifications These include business and finance, computing and information systems, public administration, plus some pre-vocational and continuing education courses. They can be studied at further education colleges, polys, and some by distance learning. Get the free booklet *Opportunities for Adults*, available from BTEC (from SCOTVEC for Scotland).

RSA (Royal Society of Arts) qualifications These cover office, secretarial, and business studies, computers and information technology, counselling, languages, and general training for work. Also the Certificate of Continuing Education, for adults with little academic background who want to increase their confidence before returning to work or going on to further education. More details from RSA.

City and Guilds certificates Cover over 400 subjects, mainly industrial and commercial. For a free publications list write to City and Guilds of London Institute.

Teaching qualifications Mainly studied at HE colleges. Mature entrants are welcomed. For *A Career in Teaching* and more information contact the Teaching as a Career Unit (TASC) at the DES in London, or the Scottish Education Department, or Department of Education for Northern Ireland.

Second Chances has excellent chapters on qualifications and subjects to study, which include where to find out more about those I've mentioned, plus many others. The National Extension College (NEC) publishes a range of books to help people brush up on their academic study skills, eg *How to Study Effectively*, *How to Write Essays*, *Clear Thinking* and *Answer the Question*. Get a full list from NEC.

Further education (FE)

FE colleges have various names (eg College of Technology, Tertiary College), and are run by local education authorities (LEAs) in England and Wales, Regional or Islands Councils in Scotland, and Education and Library Boards in Northern Ireland. They offer a wide range of courses, usually below degree level, to anyone over 16 who's left school. Courses may be full- or part-time, day or evening, or day release. Specially interesting for us are their open learning courses, their courses for updating basic skills, and their special arrangements for mature students. Some courses help you start studying again after a break, or prepare for a return to work; some have specially helpful hours (eg 10 till 3, once a week, with childcare facilities). Many colleges run 'access courses' (or higher education preparatory courses), alternatives to school exams as an entry qualification for some degree courses (*Second Chances* has a list).

Open learning courses may also be called 'Flexistudy', 'Learning by Appointment', 'distance learning'. You do your studying at times to suit yourself. The courses often use correspondence materials and new technology (computers, audio-visual aids) but you also get help and support from a tutor. Subjects include GCSEs and A levels, BTEC courses, or vocational studies for a specific job. Your local library or jobcentre should have a copy of the *Open Learning Directory*, with more information. More information in *Second Chances*, too, and from the Open College. Ask the National Extension College (NEC) for a list of centres running NEC 'Flexistudy' courses. In your library you should find the *CRAC Directory of Further Education*, which lists all FE (and HE) colleges, polys, with full course information.

Once you've chosen a likely sounding college, send for its prospectus. Then write asking for an interview with a college adviser to discuss the course which interests you, your special needs, and how any difficulties might be overcome (eg access, avoiding having to queue in person to register). Some colleges have a Coordinator for Disabled Students. If the college seems unhelpful, contact Skill for advice.

Some FE colleges are residential, and specially for students (all ages) with physical disabilities, eg Hereward College, Coventry. Though it's run by Coventry Education Authority, students come from all parts of Britain, sponsored by their own LEA.

Studying for pleasure/adult education (AE)
(may also be known as continuing or community education)

Adult education opens up a vast world of learning for pleasure. Topics range from arts and crafts, family tree researching, flower-arranging, cookery, to languages and creative writing. No exams to pass, it's a good way of meeting other people, and an excellent way of distracting your mind from the arthritis. Evening classes are the best-known form of AE, but if evenings don't suit, look instead at daytime classes, or one-off all-day classes on a Saturday, or short residential weekend or summer courses (some are for the whole family).

Jenny's just one example of what you can get up to. As an active young mum she was shocked to find she had RA. But encouraged by her family she asked about lace-making classes at her local AE centre. She'd been worried about being different from the other class members and slowing down their progress, but found that everyone worked at their own pace on their own project with lots of individual help. Her tutor advised her to work on Torchon lace (a coarser variety than others), to avoid difficulties manipulating smaller bobbins. Jenny said her self-esteem had increased enormously, and to her children she was again *"the mum who can, rather than the mum who can't"* (*Replan Newsletter*).

AE classes are run by all sorts of institutes, eg AE colleges, FE colleges, the WEA, Women's Institutes, Townswomen's Guilds, National Housewives' Register. Many universities, polys and other colleges run special courses, 'extramural studies', for adult 'outsiders'. You don't usually need any previous academic knowledge.

The OU too has lots of short non-degree courses and study packs for home-based use, ranging from *Looking at Paintings*, to *The Handicapped Person in the Community*, or courses for parents like *The Pre-School child*, *Childhood 5 - 10*. Look too at the section on 'Distance Education', on page 247, for other mainly home-based courses.

AE prospectuses are available in libraries, by post, and advertised in the local press. Some mention 'special provision for disabled students', though you'd still need to check out whether your own special needs could be met. Ask about special arrangements for registration, to avoid mad queueing scrambles. Worth asking too whether they can suggest ways of overcoming any difficulties you might have in actually getting to the classes. Or try your social worker or OT or DIAL, or maybe someone else in the class could give you a lift? Transport to her evening class was the big obstacle for YPA and writer Pamela LaFane. She contacted her LEA, who said it was 'something they hadn't come across before', but they'd see what they could do. Amazingly, they solved the problem!

Where to find out more about adult education
- Look at *Second Chances*, especially chapters on further and adult education and leisure classes: part-time, weekends, holidays.
- For OU continuing education courses write for *Open Opportunities* from the Associate Student Central Office, Open University.
- For information on voluntary adult education centres write for the low-cost *Educational Centres Association Directory* to the Educational Centres Association (for England), or Scottish Institute of Adult and Continuing Education.

- The Workers' Educational Association (WEA) runs part-time classes for people who live in deprived areas or who are educationally disadvantaged in some way (single parents, elderly, disabled or unemployed people). Subjects range from social and political education, to local history, art and literature. Classes are day or evening, and free or very cheap. Some have nursery facilities. For information contact WEA.

- Many Women's Institutes organise classes. The WI also has its own residential college, Denman College, Oxfordshire. Contact your local WI, or the National Federation of Women's Institutes.

- Get the low-cost booklet *Time to Learn* packed with a wealth of short residential courses throughout the country, on almost every subject under the sun, from singing to butterflies to poetry or philosophy. You could take the family, or even if you're on your own, it's a great way to have a stimulating weekend or week away, with other people and many of the courses take place in lovely centres in the countryside. A wheelchair symbol indicates centres with access, ground floor bedrooms and lifts. *Time to Learn* is published twice-yearly, in August and January, by the National Institute of Adult Continuing Education (NIACE).

- The Arts Council (send SAE) publishes *The Directory of Arts Centres*.

- The Government's REPLAN programme aims to improve educational opportunities for unemployed adults. To see if there's a REPLAN project near you, contact NIACE.

Distance learning

'Distance learning' means study by correspondence, plus, sometimes, radio and TV programmes and face-to-face tuition. Best-known of the distance learning providers is the Open University (OU), and several of us have benefited from its flexibility. If the idea appeals, why not find out from other Young Arthritis Care members how they got on? One wrote to me *"they are so helpful to people with disabilities. The sense of achievement is so important for one's self-esteem – and the hard work keeps your mind off your aches and pains (most of the time)"*. Besides degree courses, the OU also has a range of shorter, non-degree courses: write for *Open Opportunities*. Distance learning is available through other bodies, too.

Drawbacks of study for OU degree courses are that it's hard-going and you need to be able to study on your own with little feedback from other people. You'd probably need at least 12 hours a week for study, maybe as much as 20, and you'd need to be sure you could fit in with other commitments to family, work, or whatever. Because it's 'part-time' you can't get an LEA grant. However if finance *is* a problem, the OU might be able to help (see page 251). On the other hand, the OU encouragingly points out that the only qualifications are that you should be 18 or over, live in the UK, have a determination to improve your life and are prepared to work hard in order to earn a degree.

OU degrees are 'modular'; you choose your own combination of subjects. There's a choice of over 130, from science and technology to the arts, from maths to social sciences. They can be taken a section at a time over a longer period than a normal degree course. Each section you successfully complete earns you a full or a half credit. Six credits make an ordinary degree, eight an honours degree. Credit exemptions may be awarded for any relevant qualification you already have.

Study's by four different methods: (1) correspondence materials sent at regular intervals; (2) broadcasts; (3) personal contact with tutors, counsellors, study centres; (4) summer schools – one-week residential courses, usually at a university – a chance to meet and work (hard!) with other students and staff.

The OU year starts in February, so you'd need to apply the previous year, no later than October, but the earlier the better as it's first come, first served. Write to the OU Admissions Office for the *Guide for Applicants for BA Degrees*. For specialist information, contact the OU Adviser for Disabled Students. The Adviser may for instance be able to help with financial problems, specialist equipment (eg computer/word processor on loan), etc. Sometimes a helper can be provided for the summer school if you need help and there's no one to go with you.

Here are some personal experiences of studying with the OU, first from YPA Carol J:

"My husband suggested I try the OU to give me some interest. At first I was reluctant as I had left school at 16 and had no higher education and I felt I wouldn't be able to cope with academic study at university level. After preliminary enquiries in which the OU were very helpful, I was accepted and I began my studies...Initially studying was difficult, particularly the essay writing as that had always been a weak point at school. Self-discipline and organisation are key factors when studying at home alone and these I had together with a determination to do my best, pass or fail. The mental challenge was a great stimulus and just what I needed and I began to feel that I had found something worthwhile to aim for. Since the early days with the OU I have gained enormous self-confidence...I certainly think positively now, my maxim being accept what you can't do and do to the full that which you can do!"

In the Open University's booklet *005 – Occupational Information – a Supplement for Students with Disabilities* (1985), disabled graduates explained what studying with the OU meant to them. For instance, a tutor, aged 51, with arthritis:

"...thanks to my degree, I can and do coach eighteen children (in groups of four) for their Common Entrance examinations. One of the reasons for needing such coaching may be that the child missed quite a lot of school because of some illness or other..."

Someone else, aged 43, described as chronically sick:

"Since I have not even got O grade examination passes, I was often turned down when I applied for things. Apart therefore from changing me as a person (I am more self-reliant now), studying with the OU has opened doors that previously were firmly shut. I am now employed as an unqualified nurse tutor and plan to attend a full-time university in October and complete an MSc degree."

A housewife, aged 30, with arthritis:

"I am currently a housewife and have also done a little tutoring. But I would like to become an audiovisual librarian in a university. Since I only obtained one A level at school (and failed three times to get more A levels!) I was not able to be a librarian as this requires two A levels. The OU was an ideal opportunity to get started again..."

For many people, what they found out about themselves was at least as important, if not more so, than their increased academic knowledge. Studying was a morale-booster, and pleasure in itself.

Other distance learning courses

OU degree courses may be too tough-going or too advanced for many people, but luckily other schemes offer education by post, too. One YPA, for instance, did a 'Software Technical Authorship Course' at home, funded through her DRO, using a computer and printer on loan. That was for the City and Guilds (Technical dissertation) exam.

For other ideas send for free prospectuses from the Open College (founded 1987), and the Open College of the Arts (founded 1988), and write for the National Extension College (NEC)'s free *Guide to Courses*. NEC offers home-study courses for adults in subjects including maths, computing, economics, business studies, English, history, languages and science, at introductory, GCSE and A level, plus professional and leisure courses, eg playwriting, playgroups, religions, child development. NEC's a non-profit-making college, governed by an educational trust.

A multitude of other correspondence colleges offer a multitude of courses. Some are more reputable than others, so be wary. There are adverts all over the place. Get prospectuses and compare them, but *don't* part with any money unless you're sure the college is reputable, and promises value for money. Check with the Council for the Accreditation of Correspondence Colleges (CACC) to see if it's accredited by them. CACC operates with the approval of the DES. *Second Chances* includes a CACC list.

Finally, you can also study for University of London external degrees by correspondence. The courses are cheaper than the OU, but you usually need to have A levels, and the courses aren't modular. For *First Degrees and Diplomas for External Students: General Information*, write to The Secretary for External Students, University of London. Waring Bowen, founder of what's now called Arthritis Care, gained an external degree in history and an LLB from the University of London before going on to become a solicitor. He had AS and had to do much of his studying while lying flat on his back in a spinal jacket (quite the opposite of present day treatment).

See also *Second Chances* for more about distance and open learning.

Higher education (HE)

The OU's done wonders in making higher education accessible to people with a disability, but many of us still prefer the idea of immersion in a full-time (or part-time) course at an 'ordinary' centre of higher education. Many universities, polys, and HE colleges now make a special effort to be helpful, for instance through special parking and access arrangements, campus residence, extra time to write exams. Some universities, eg Southampton, York, Sussex and Oxford, provide residential housing for students with disabilities, where 'continuous care' is available if necessary. Polys offer courses similar to university courses, though usually with a stronger bias to training for jobs. Many run part-time courses, and have nursery facilities.

Some HE colleges are flexible about entry requirements, which may be lower than those for universities. For instance, all places offering CNAA degrees have the automatic right to admit unqualified mature students. You might be asked to do an HE preparatory exam, or the college's own entry exam, instead of GCSEs and A levels. Alternatively, work experience or evidence of recent study and an interview might do instead.

Some CNAA degrees are now available in modular form, like OU degrees, where you get credits for individual course modules (eg at Oxford Poly). Hatfield Poly, where YPA Martin E did a social sciences degree course as a mature student, looks sympathetically at any non-standard qualifications or experience, and also runs a wide range of non-standard 'just for interest/pleasure' courses in their continuing education programme and helpfully runs shortened day courses from 10 am to 3 pm.

Some HE colleges offer DipHEs (not in Scotland). Entry requirements are the same as for degree courses, but it takes only two years, qualifies for a mandatory grant, and can be used as credit towards professional bodies' courses or for transfer to a degree course.

Skill may be able to help you negotiate your way through any rules and regulations at your chosen HE institute which don't cater for unconventional education and career patterns. Look at Skill's *Applying to Higher Education: Some Notes for Disabled Students, their Parents and Advisers* (free to students with a disability). Other sources of general (non-disabled) information about HE courses include the following:

- *The School Leaver's Handbook* (National Extension College): Ann Jones offers a friendly guiding hand through the maze of getting into and making the most of higher education (including dealing with money and deciding where to live).
- For a list of most universities, their addresses, courses, and how to apply, get *How to Apply for Admission to a University*, free from UCCA. If you're a mature student ask also for the booklet *University Entrance for Mature Students*.
- For details of CNAA degrees get *Directory of First Degree Courses* and *Opportunities in Higher Education for Mature Students*, free, from the CNAA.
- For details of how to apply to a polytechnic write to PCAS. Look too, in your library, at

Polytechnic Courses, published by Lund Humphries.
- Look in a library at *Which Degree?*, published in five volumes, arranged by subject (eg Arts, Humanities and Languages, Maths, Medicine and Sciences). There's a synopsis of every degree course in the country, at universities, polys, and HE colleges.
- Send for the CRAC publications list and look at *Second Chances*.

You might find helpful too:
- Observer Helpline: free information about higher and some professional education throughout the UK.
- EGSA: see page 241.

Individual prospectuses will tell you lots more. Some places also have 'alternative prospectuses', produced by the students there, which focus on *un*official but enlightening views. The annual *Student Book* (£9.99, 1991, Macmillan) looks at courses and facilities in every HE establishment and includes all-important consumers' views, too.

Ask in your library about HE courses available locally. You might come across something as amazingly useful as Bradford and Ilkley Community College of HE's 'Mature Students' Certificate Course', a drop-in group for mothers and toddlers and anyone else who needs to drop in. It can be done just for fun, or as the first step to a DipHE.

Other helpful bodies

The Disabled Graduates' Careers Information Service and The Association of Disabled Professionals both have lots of information and helpful advice culled from actual experiences of people with a disability. More details on pages 260 and 261.

Financing your studies

Write to the DES for *Loans and Grants to Students: a Brief Guide* (or to the Scottish Education Department or Department of Education for Northern Ireland for similar leaflets. Write too to Skill for *Financial Assistance for Students with Disabilities* (free, but send SAE). The two main grants, applied for through your local education authority, are:

- ***Mandatory grants***   Provided you meet certain conditions, you automatically get the award, for certain designated degree courses or degree-equivalent courses, ie most courses in universities, polys, and colleges (including teacher training, the DipHE, HNDs and BTEC Higher Diplomas). Almost all are full-time, except for a few teacher-training courses. Special conditions and allowances may apply if you're a mature student, and/or have dependants.

- ***Discretionary grants***   *Not* automatic. Only limited funds available. If you plan to do a further education or part-time course, this is the sort of grant you'd normally apply for. Amounts payable vary considerably. You might get as much as a mandatory grant, something very small, something in between – or, alas, nothing.

You could also apply for a 'Disabled Students' Allowance', for extra disability-related costs (other than travel). In 1991/92 it allows for up to £4,240 for non-medical helpers, up to £3,180 for major items of specialist equipment, and up to £1,060 for other costs. If you receive a mandatory or a discretionary grant, you can claim DSA, but it's discretionary and not awarded automatically. You don't have to be registered or severely disabled to apply, but do need to be able to convince your LEA the extra expense is necessary (a) because of your impairment/disability and (b) because of the course. Examples of claims reimbursed have been for typewriters, microcomputers, tape-recorders, and paid help, but not for extra travel costs incurred because of disability. If travel costs are 'necessarily incurred' for a course, apply separately to your LEA for assistance.

If you're turned down for a mandatory or a discretionary grant, or think you've got too little, you can appeal, first to the LEA, then to the Department of Education (or equivalent) if you're still unsuccessful. There's no guarantee of success, but it's worth a try.

You could also talk to local councillors, especially if they're on the education committee, and your MP.

The Student Loans Scheme aims eventually to account for half a student's income. Normally borrowers have to repay loans in 60 monthly instalments, starting from the April following the end of the course. However, disabled borrowers are allowed to negotiate special conditions, for instance the repayment start date may be deferred if your monthly income is low, or repayment over a longer period may be allowed. Income from disability benefits doesn't count as 'monthly income'. For borrowers under 40 an outstanding loan will be cancelled when they reach 50 or if the loan has been outstanding for 25 years or more. For more information on loans get *Loans for Students – a Brief Guide* (free from DES). For information specific to disabled students contact Skill or RADAR.

Because OU courses are regarded as part-time, there are no mandatory grants for them. LEA help varies. If your LEA won't help, write and explain your problem to the OU. They may be able to help you from a special fund for unemployed students. (By the way, beware of a nasty trick where if you get an OU degree and then want to do a 'first degree' somewhere else you forfeit your eligibility to a mandatory grant for that course, even if you paid all OU fees yourself.) If financial dificulties put you off doing an NEC correspondence course, see if the NEC's Student Services Adviser can help.

Fees for adult education classes are often waived or reduced for students in special need. Your DRO can tell you about special training opportunities for disabled people, eg financial assistance with part-time or correspondence courses, like the YPA who did the Software Technical Authorship course (page 248), or help to train for a professional career if you're not able to get a grant. Other sources of limited financial help include:

- Arthritis Care. May be able to help, perhaps from the Waring Bowen Fund, set up in 1980, as a tribute to its founder, Arthur Mainwaring Bowen. The fund aims to help people whose studies are interrupted by a rheumatic disease, eg by giving limited grants to buy computers, books, stationery, calculators.
- The Snowdon Awards Scheme for Disabled Students makes several awards annually to help disabled students with extra expenses incurred because of disability (but can't cover all costs of a full-time course). In 1986, for instance, one student received £1,000 to buy an electronic typewriter and help with other expenses on a secretarial course. Applications have to be in by 31 May each year.
- Skill administers the COMET scheme (Concerned Micros in Education and Training), which helps disabled students who need microcomputing equipment. Skill also has a limited number of bursaries for students unable to pay course fees and living expenses.
- The Electronic Aids Loan Scheme – page 146-147.
- Some universities, polys and colleges have funds to assist students in special need. Apply to the Registrar or Principal.
- EGSA (page 241) may be able to advise on sources of funding.
- Ask your LEA, CAB, library and local clergy about any local trust fund that might be able to help (the amounts are usually small, if any), and look in your library at the *Directory of Grant-Making Trusts*, the *Charities Digest*, the *Educational Grants Directory* (Directory of Social Change) and the *Guide to Grants for Individuals in Need* (also Directory of Social Change).
- Ask the National Union of Students for advice (they publish *Educational Charities*).
- You could look too at COIC's *Sponsorships and Supplementary Awards*

What happens about income support, and other benefits? The position's complicated, and depends on individual circumstances. eg your age, whether the course is full or part-time, whether you're considered 'capable' or 'incapable' of work, your family circumstances, etc. Seek reliable advice, well before you apply for a course, eg from the BEL helpline, CAB, Skill, and sources in chapter 17.

Chapter thirty-one

EMPLOYMENT

Many younger people with arthritis work normally. Some, like me, are in full-time employment outside the home. Others work from home, either in paid employment, or perhaps doing unpaid voluntary work. Some opt instead to be full-time housewives/househusbands (housespouses/housespice?). In this chapter I'm going to concentrate on paid employment.

Not everyone feels up to doing a job. At one extreme many YPAs are so mildly affected that they have few or no problems. Other people simply can't work, or have to work in some form of sheltered employment. Most YPAs are somewhere between the two extremes, sometimes wobbling nearer one than the other, depending on how much we can maximise our abilities (the 'can dos'), minimise our disabilities (the 'can't dos'), *and* overcome the handicaps put in our way by other people and by conditions such as access, mobility, inflexible working hours. Success brings worthwhile rewards: money (and the priceless independence that goes with it), a sense of purpose, self-esteem and self-confidence, social contact and social status.

I hope this chapter gives you encouragement and helpful tips. Getting and keeping a job isn't easy at the best of times. However, with courage, determination, and persistence you're half-way there. The right information helps considerably, too. Alas, even some professionals — even some doctors and Disablement Resettlement Officers (DROs) — suffer from the 'ignorance handicap', so don't assume they necessarily know everything.

Perhaps one day we'll be able to get all the help and information we need by consulting just one wonder-person (complete with wonder-computer). The right job will be identified and any employer will be so well-informed that s/he will be able to ignore the arthritis and judge you, the employee, solely on your abilities and job potential... But back to earth now, with a bump. At present *you're* the person who must (and can) do most for yourself. Not *completely* on your own. There *is* information and help out there for the asking, but it's up to you to do the asking!

What sort of jobs do YPAs already do?

Time for some ideas and encouragement, before you get too downhearted. Here are examples of paid jobs some of us already do/have done, which all go to show that if you *want* to work, and if the arthritis lets you, you shouldn't be discouraged.

Employment agency interviewer (female with RA)
British Petroleum (male, RA)
Cashier in Sainsburys' (female with RA)
Personnel officer in the DSS (female, JCA)
Worker in residential children's home (female, RA)
Clerical assistant in centre for handicapped people (female, RA)
Secretary for local Consumer Council (female with JCA)
Clerk in British Airways Revenue Accounts Department (female with JCA)
Trainee doctor (female with RA)
Staff nurse in a London hospital (female with RA)
Estate agent (male with RA)
Librarian at the National Maritime Museum, Greenwich

Local government manager (male, RA)
Senior manager in firm of auditors (male with RA)
Freelance photographer (male with RA)
Legal executive (female with RA)
Administrator with the British Council (female with JCA)
Stockbroker (female with JCA and partial sight)
'Setter' – setting machines and jigs for 100 people to work on (male with RA)
Foster parent (female with RA)
Member of parliament (Jo Richardson, Labour MP with RA)
Local councillor (female with RA)
Hospital telephone operator (female, with RA)
Central Television office worker (female, AS)
Computer programmer with the RAF (female with RA, and blind)
Equal Opportunities Officer for a County Council (female, psoriatic arthritis)
One 25 year old has set up his own employment agency (male with RA and blind)
Self-employed, male with RA, offering CAD (computer aided draughting) planning and design service to small businesses
Administrative Officer in Disability Resource Centre (female, JCA)

Some people with arthritis have achieved fame through their work – see chapter 29.

Some YPAs who can't manage a full-time job have found the 'Sheltered Placement Scheme' helpful. A sponsor shares financial responsibility with a host employer (details from DROs). One sponsor is the Shaw Trust. Here are some examples of people with rheumatic disorders the Trust has sponsored, the jobs they're in, their 'assessed working ability' (WA), hours of work, and location:

Male, aged 48, with AS: assistant architect; 60% WA, 37½ hours, Cirencester;
Female, 27, with RA/Still's: general office work, 30% WA, 30 hours, Trowbridge;
Male, 53, polyarthritis: technician, 60% WA, 30 hours, Winchester;
Male, 24, RA: admin assistant, 55% WA, 36 hours, Cheam;
Female, 41, RA: clerical assistant, 40% WA, 20 hours, Wrexham;
Female, 18, arthritis: telephonist/receptionist/clerk, 50% WA, 38 hours, Llanelli;
Female, 42, arthritis of spine and hands: telephonist/clerk, 60% WA, Carmarthen;
Female, 23, RA: clerical/lab assistant, 45% WA, 40 hours, Port Talbot;
Male, 39, RA: vehicle mechanic, 50% WA, 40 hours, Hereford;
Female, 37, RA: medical secretary, 60% WA, 18 hours, Norwich;

The scheme means you can work in an ordinary workplace with non-disabled people. Even if your output is lower than your colleagues', you receive the full wage for the job, because costs are shared between the host (who pays only for your actual output) and a sponsor, who could be a local authority, a voluntary organisation, or Remploy. Host firms have included Chappell Music International, Gainsborough Chocolates, Jaguar Cars, Laura Ashley, London Electricity Board, Tesco, F W Woolworth.

Deciding what work you could do

Think 'non-disabled'
First, remind yourself that you're an individual, first and foremost, with a whole lot more to you than just arthritis. Don't be browbeaten by other people (even some DROs or doctors) into accepting *their* limited notions of what 'a disabled person' or 'an arthritic' can – or can't – do. You've already seen examples of what some YPAs have achieved. That doesn't mean they haven't had their problems, but it does mean many, at least, can be overcome. And of course the frontiers of what *anyone* can do are being pushed back all the time, by modern technology, improved social attitudes, etc.

So don't overlook everything that's on offer for people *without* arthritis or a disability!

Otherwise you'll close too many doors, and goodness knows these days *everyone*, disabled or not, needs to keep as many open as possible. To become, say, a secretary, a bookkeeper, a lawyer, an accountant, a banker or a computer programmer, get all the advice available for any non-disabled person:

- Look back at page 244 on finding out about careers.
- Write to organisations that interest you, asking for their advice (eg if you're interested in travel, try firms like Thomas Cook, British Airways).
- Read newspapers and journals, for job ads, and for news of new developments and organisations in your area. Your library should have a good selection.
- Talk to other people. The unlikeliest friends and contacts may tell you about jobs you'd never have thought of or unadvertised vacancies.
- Visit a jobcentre, either locally, or in a more promising area.
- The Careers & Occupational Information Centre (COIC) publishes masses of information on careers, occupations and vocations. Write for their publications list.
- Visit private employment agencies. Reputable agencies charge fees to employers only, so don't go to one that wants *you* to pay.
- Look in the *Yellow Pages* and *Thomson's Directory* for ideas.
- *The Job Book* (CRAC), gives details of over 1,000 employers, hundreds of training and career schemes. Ask in your careers or public library for directories giving details of other companies throughout Britain
- Plus, yes, look too at special information for disabled people (details later)

OK, exclude anything totally unrealistic; there are plenty of non-arthritic reasons for excluding lots of things, anyway. But do first keep the emphasis on your interests and abilities, and on what you'd *like* to do. Only after that think about special needs and problems. Think positive, as obstacles that may seem insurmountable can often be overcome, and if *you* think positive, it'll rub off on other people, including prospective employers, and get *them* thinking positive too.

With physical abilities below par, concentrate on non-physical skills. Use education and training (see chapter 30) to the full, and where possible to give you qualifications that *prove* those abilities to employers. Elizabeth, for instance, did a YTS course in typing, word processing and general office duties. That led to a position with Central Television as a YTS trainee, and she was later taken on to their permanent staff.

Other things, like voluntary work and hobbies, interesting in themselves, can give you useful experience and prove to a potential employer your abilities, commitment and reliability. Karen, for instance, did voluntary work for Women's Aid, and for a community programme dealing with alcoholism. She's now got a full-time paid job as admin officer in a Disability Resource Centre.

You'll get ideas from what other YPAs have done, and how about other possibilities like telephone sales work (for newspapers, airlines, banks etc), employment agency work, estate agency work, word processing, correspondence tutoring, private coaching, book-keeping and accountancy? COIC's *Second Chances* (page 244) is a good source of ideas and information.

The rapidly expanding field of information technology (IT), working with computers, suits many people. The more obvious openings include programming, systems analysis, word processing, computerised book-keeping, hardware research, design, construction and manufacturing, technical support and user training. Some office employment agencies, Alfred Marks, for instance, have set up high street learning centres to introduce people to personal computing and skills such as word processing and spreadsheets. Computer skills may even enable you to work at home (see chapter 32). Look too at page 291.

Find out more by getting COIC's leaflet *Working in Computers*, and by looking at books such as *The Handbook of Information Technology* (CRAC/Hobsons Publishing), which describes the wide variety of jobs available, courses and over 800 employers. You can also get helpful information on training courses and employment using microcomputers from OUTSET, and from the British Computer Society (which has a Disabled Specialist Group). Last, but not least, DROs in jobcentres can help in various ways, even by providing computing equipment for work at home or in an office, and can advise on training, and can sometimes put you in touch with prospective employers.

If you're already trained and well qualified before arthritis strikes, that's often an advantage, though you may still face problems; even, at worst, the threat of redundancy, though employers and employees are now encouraged by the government's *Code of Good Practice* to consider less drastic alternatives first, such as rethinking your current job or maybe retraining you for something else.

Be realistic, too

OK, so you have got arthritis. OK, so it does have to be taken into account. What can you do to minimise its effects? Are there any jobs you'd do better to avoid?

Make sure, first, you're getting good medical care. Change your GP if necessary and ask to see a rheumatologist if you haven't already seen one. Though there's no cure yet, there's so much that *can* be done and you need to be sure it's being done, so that the 'bad' or 'worse' times are minimised and so that as much of your energy as possible can be diverted away from battling with the arthritis and back to other things like work. A good job in turn will help keep your morale up and Arthur Itis firmly in his place.

Remember that types of inflammatory arthritis like RA or AS, are 'up and down' disorders, with bad or variable times, but, thank goodness, with good or better times too. Remissions may last months or years or for ever, and even in persistent disorders modern medicine can minimise problems, so that many YPAs are potentially capable of working once the bad episode is over or once medical treatment has brought the rheumatic disorder's activity under control.

Find out through your doctor whether any special work guidelines apply to your particular sort of arthritis and you. Keep in mind any advice on joint care given to you by your healthcare team, so you don't choose a totally unsuitable job. Some **general guidelines** now to be going on with. First, from consultant rheumatologist, Professor J M H Moll:

"Certain occupations are particularly liable to put an extra strain on your rheumaticky parts – especially your back...mining, farm labouring, and working in the docks. Jobs involving forceful manoeuvres and repetitive work may aggravate or trigger rheumatic problems in your hands and arms. Working in cold, damp surroundings may increase rheumatic pains, but contrary to general opinion, these factors do not cause rheumatic ailments." (*Arthritis and Rheumatism*, Churchill Livingstone's Patient Handbook).

Melvyn Kettle and Bert Massie's *Employers' Guide to Disabilities* (Woodhead-Faulkner in association with RADAR), writing on **rheumatoid arthritis**:

"Where the wrists and fingers are painful and swollen there will be difficulty in gripping small objects, grasping, using manual typewriters, picking up heavy objects and applying sustained pressure on small pieces of equipment."

Though it's amazing what arthriticky hands *can* do, given the right equipment (eg word processor) and the absence of a flare-up.

Ankylosing Spondylitis. A Guidebook for Patients, published by NASS (National Anky-losing Spondylitis Society), advises:

"Pay special attention to the position of your back when at work, so that you do not have to stoop. If you sit at a desk or bench, see that your seat is at the proper height and do not sit in one position too long without moving your back. A job that gives a variety of sitting, standing and walking is ideal. The most unsuitable work is one in which you stoop or crouch over a bench for hours at a time. If you have a heavy or tiring job do not tackle other activities at home or elsewhere until you have had a break, if necessary, resting flat for a time. It may also help if you can rest flat for twenty minutes at mid-day.

*At such times try to lie for part of the time facing downwards. If your job is entirely
unsuitable and involves much stooping or back pain, talk this over with your doctor. He,
or a doctor from the Employment Medical Service* [see page 260], *may be able to advise
you on how you may change to more suitable work.*"

For people with **Raynaud's phenomenon,** the Raynaud's Society advises avoiding
situations where you're exposed to cold. Sometimes Raynaud's develops in someone who
works with vibrating tools (eg chain saws, floor polishers). The Raynaud's is then known as
'Vibration White Finger' (an industrial disease eligible for compensation). Workers with
polyvinyl chloride may similarly develop ulcerations of the fingers due to spasm of the
arteries.

J Edmonds and G Hughes wrote encouragingly about **juvenile chronic arthritis:**

*"Overall, 70 − 80% of children make a satisfactory recovery without serious functional
impairment. At 15 year follow-up, more than 80% of a group of children with JCA were
able to work."* (In *Lecture Notes on Rheumatology,* Blackwell Scientific, 1985)

Remember − problems are for solving − though the arthritis itself can't be removed,
plenty of the problems caused by it or by the environment *can* be. One of the best people
to help is a good OT. More about OTs on pages 38, 142 and in chapter 6.

Think 'disabled' − are there any advantages?

Now you're going to think I'm barmy, having earlier told you to 'think non-disabled'. But
bear with me and let's turn things upside-down. Employment *is* an area where there are
sometimes advantages in accepting the label 'disabled', even if you simply don't consider
yourself disabled. Some people wear the label in an official sense, by becoming 'registered
disabled' (page 126); others in an unofficial sense, just by acknowledging they have a
disability.

What advantages? Even if you're not badly affected, 'wearing the label' can sometimes
give you access to that extra bit of financial or practical help through a jobcentre, or extra
flexibility in an employer which could make all the difference to your working, and
working enjoyably and successfully too.

Unfortunately there can also be disadvantages, especially if you're dealing with a
prejudiced, ignorant, or misinformed employer. Twenty years ago 'the label' was a big
hindrance. I believed it would reinforce other people's prejudices against me, and even
without it I did have a very difficult time, first getting a job, and then getting satisfactory
terms of employment from my employer.

Nowadays I do wear the label, with fewer misgivings, and do see advantages to myself or
to other people (the 'stand-up-and-be-counted advantage' for instance). By working *and*
being registered I hope too I'm making my own tiny contribution to showing society that
disability doesn't mean 'inability'. I decided to become officially registered six years ago,
which coincided with my employer becoming an Equal Opportunities Employer. I confess
however that the main reason was because I wanted to learn to fly, and had applied for a
Sir Douglas Bader Flying Scholarship (page 291), open only to registered disabled people!
Other advantages?

● Though there's still a long way to go, public awareness of, and provision for, the special
needs of people with a disability have improved in recent years. The Employment
Service's *Code of Good Practice on the Employment of Disabled People* (HMSO), is
written for employers, but well worth reading by employees, too. It urges employers not
to miss out 'on the contribution of potentially valuable employees', with 'proven skills,
abilities and commitment', and gives examples of good employment practice.

● The *Code of Good Practice,* and another booklet, *Employing People with Disabilities:
Sources of Help,* explain financial and practical help available. For instance grants of up
to several thousand pounds can be made to adapt premises or equipment; financial

assistance to encourage an employer to employ a disabled person for a trial period, or for fares to work; free long-term loan of special tools or equipment, eg computer. Not all employers are aware of these schemes, but if *you* know about them you could use them as a reassurance to an employer that problems can be overcome, and as an incentive to take or keep you on.

● Have you heard about the Quota System? In theory, employers with 20 or more workers are expected to employ a quota of registered disabled people (RDPs). The standard quota is 3% of an employer's total workforce. An employer below quota is not supposed to engage anyone other than an RDP without first obtaining a permit to do so. And an employer must not discharge an RDP on medical grounds 'without reasonable cause' if s/he is or would then be below quota. In practice, unfortunately, the Quota System has often proved ineffective, and is under review.

● At present, only people on the Employment Service's Register of Disabled People (page 126) count towards the Quota, though this may change. Registration's voluntary. If you're accepted you get a 'Green Card' (useful for proving entitlement to other concessions). Some jobcentre Employment Service schemes are restricted to RDPs, though many aren't, so don't be put off applying for them if you haven't registered.

● Rules applying to some goverment training schemes (and benefits) for unemployed people may be more flexible if you're disabled. If you discuss these with, say, a Welfare Rights Officer, make sure that person knows about this flexibility, and doesn't put you off applying by giving you advice meant only for *non*-disabled unemployed people. Cross-check with someone who *does* compile specialist advice for disabled people, eg the Disability Alliance. And make sure any adviser you consult knows about your type of arthritis, eg if it's an 'intermittent disability' special regulations may apply.

● Several organisations (eg Opportunities for People with Disabilities, the Association of Disabled Professionals) have done a lot to increase opportunities and public awareness. More about them, and how they might help you, on page 260 onwards.

It's to the benefit of all of us to take advantage of progress already made and to build on it for the sake of other people with disabilities and special needs.

Getting or keeping work: who can help you

Doctor/social worker/occupational therapist
Your doctor might help by giving you letters of support, eg to get working hours changed, so you can avoid the rush hour, work a flexitime system, or have a rest at lunchtime; or help you get a special parking space; or to help testify to your wonderful perseverance and self-motivation; or perhaps to support a request for your job to be kept open during extended sick leave, for instance if you're trying a second-line drug, like gold, a doctor might be prepared to testify that it's likely to take 10 to 20 weeks to show results, and could ask for you to be given an appropriately long period of grace.

A social worker could help you sort out practical and financial difficulties, eg transport, benefits. If you receive income support, or other benefits, seeking paid employment will affect them. The position's complicated, so get early advice.

An OT can give lots of practical help, especially with joint care and overcoming functional problems, eg hand problems using a phone, writing, typing; seating difficulties, can help you organise your life to make the most of limited energy rations, suggest ways of getting working conditions adapted, eg special equipment, hours of work, fitting in rest periods. Ask for an assessment by an OT. Later, if your condition changes or you come across new or different problems, ask for another. More about OTs in chapter 6.

Other people with arthritis

Find out how they've overcome difficulties. Often simple adjustments can make all the difference. I now work happily full time, with difficulties overcome by, for instance, keeping a folding longreach gadget in my drawer, having files shelved beside me at the right height, sitting on a higher than normal chair, access to a word processor (though I dictate most letters on an audio-typing system), and, best of all, the joy of flexitime which lets me harmonise my ups and downs with the job's, to our mutual advantage. Carol J's had RA since she was 18 months old. She described her work with the Civil Service:

> *"My work mainly consists of sitting at a desk answering telephone enquiries and writing letters. Sometimes I have to carry books etc from one desk to another but if it's too heavy or if I can't cope then I tell them and someone will lift the items for me. Something I do find difficult is getting things from a high shelf because I'm only 4'6" but again I ask and someone lifts it down for me. I drive to and from work and am lucky enough to have a place reserved in the car park."* (*In Contact*)

Another YPA works in British Airways Revenue Accounts Department:

> *"I do find work tiring but can cope providing I don't have too many late nights. I have a desk job, so there is not too much walking around. I work in a multi-storey building, with the car park directly below. Ideal in bad weather, no walking on snow or ice, and a lift straight to the offices. Only disadvantage is the building is large, and there is a bit of a walk from the lift to my place of work. It keeps me fit though!"* (writing in *In Contact*)

See if your self-help group can give you any helpful information. NASS, for instance, makes a special point of helping people with AS and employment queries.

Citizen's Advice Bureau (CAB)

Independent general advice and information. If they can't help they'll usually know someone who can. And in the tricky area of benefits and officialdom you can try out questions at the CAB that you might hesitate to put directly to an 'official' (eg how would doing a particular job affect your benefits?). Try CAB for help too if you face legal difficulties in your employment, eg job dismissal. (More about CAB on page 118)

Jobcentres, DROs and government training and employment schemes

Jobcentres provide a job-finding and advisory service. They used to be part of the Manpower Services Commission (MSC) but are now run by the Employment Service (ES), an agency in the Employment Department Group. If you can't find the address of your local jobcentre in an old phone book, try looking under 'Manpower Services Commission'.

An excellent introduction to the many ways jobcentres can help is the free booklet *Just the Job*, available by post (see *Just the Job* in Appendix 2). Jobcentres are run on a self-service basis. Disabled or not, you can apply for any of the jobs advertised. You'll find useful leaflets too, eg the *Jobhunting Pack*. Although there are specialist services for disabled people, don't restrict yourself to those. Make sure you're told about what's available to anyone, disabled or not.

DROs (Disablement Resettlement Officers) are jobcentre staff who specialise in helping people with a disability (whether registered disabled or not). DROs also liaise with employers and should know about job openings locally. A home visit can usually be arranged if you're physically not able to get to the jobcentre.

The sort of help you'd get from a DRO varies in practice. Some DROs know more than others. You'll probably get more help if you go in with some clear ideas yourself, about what you'd like to do, and what might be realistic, eg rather than saying 'What can you do for me?', try something like:

"I'd really like to apply for a job in 'Browns' on the industrial estate, working in their data processing department, but I think I'd need some special gadgets to help me, and I'm worried about the travelling involved. 'Browns' might look at my hands and my stick, and think I can't cope, but maybe a trial period of employment would convince them I could."

Try not to get too disheartened by the effort *you* might have to put into getting the right sort of help: as Martin Ellingford said, in *In Contact*:

"Professional advice from a doctor, or DRO in my experience, is only useful once you have come to an initial decision about your future. Often comments are made by people who know too little about the nature of arthritis to give any intelligent advice."

DROs can tell you about special training and emploment services for disabled people, and they're explained, too, in various helpful leaflets (eg leaflet PWD 16, *Jobhunting for People with Disabilities*) available from DROs/your jobcentre. If you can't get to the jobcentre easily, phone and ask if they'll post them to you. Many are also available by post from RADAR (send a second-class stamp for the publications leaflet which lists them all).

Take note, too, of what's available to encourage *employers* to employ people with a disability. It might make all the difference to your getting (or keeping) a job if you can tell an unknowing (many are) employer that s/he could be paid to give you a trial period, or the DRO could provide adaptations to premises or special equipment considered essential to help you, etc. Employers' leaflets are also available through RADAR and these include the *Code of Good Practice on the Employment of Disabled People*.

Examples of special schemes and leaflets available (shown in brackets) as I write include:

- *Job Introduction Scheme* You could dangle this carrot in front of a prospective employer, to encourage him/her to give you a trial, usually six weeks. (Leaflet EPWD 7)
- *Aids and adaptations* Aids are issued on free loan, ranging from simple reading or writing devices, to typewriters, special chairs, or sophisticated computer equipment. Worth remembering that the DRO might be persuaded to provide a powered wheel chair for work, whereas DSA will not. A solicitor with MS even got a nifty stair-climbing one, so she could get in and out of the courts. Some powered wheelchairs can 'stand up' to overcome reaching difficulties. Capital grants (up to several thousand pounds) can be given to employers who need to adapt premises or equipment for you, even for something like a stair-lift, provided the DRO agrees it's essential. (See leaflets PWD 3 *Special Aids to Employment* and PWD 4, *Adaptations to Premises and Equipment*, and, for employers, EPWD 9 and EPWD 10.)
- *Assistance with fares to work* If you can't use public transport. (Leaflet PWD 1)
- *Assessment of newly disabled employees* The Training Agency runs centres where disabled employees can be assessed (free) in industrial, commercial, and clerical tasks, and helped to regain confidence and skills. (EPL 201, *We Can Help You*)
- *Sheltered employment* For very disabled people the DRO can arrange employment in sheltered workshops. There's also the Sheltered Placement Scheme, where you work in an ordinary job. (Leaflet SPSL 1, and see page 253)
- *Personal reader service* For blind or partially sighted employees. Full details from the RNIB's Employment Department, and in leaflet PWD 2.
- *Working at home with technology* If your disability prevents you travelling to work regularly, your DRO may be able to provide computer equipment to help you work from home. (Leaflet PWD 6)

Non-disabled schemes may also be relevant. Eligibility rules are often made easier for people with a disability, so don't let the ordinary rules put you off applying, through your jobcentre. The schemes are outlined in *Just the Job*. For example:

- *Restart programme* For anyone who's been unemployed for over six months; the

qualifying period's shorter if you're disabled) (Leaflet RESTL 2)
- *Travel to interview scheme*   Financial help with travelling to job interviews further than normal daily travelling distance from home.
- *Training and enterprise services*   Training for unemployed people, with special arrangements for people with disabilities (eg waiver of the qualifying period, and the possibility of part-, rather than full-time training). Help, too, if you want to become self-employed or to set up your own business.
- *Jobclubs*   These can coach you in job-hunting techniques, and provide stamps, telephones, newspapers, etc, free of charge. Unemployed disabled people can join at any time, other people have to have been out of work for at least six months.

The Disablement Advisory Service (DAS)
Part of the Employment Service. Knowing about DAS might help you point an employer in the right direction to get help to help you. Many employers don't realise they can contact DAS for advice on improving job opportunities for existing or prospective employees, eg advice on practical and financial help, on job restructuring, career development and retention. Why not hand an unknowing employer the leaflet *Disablement Advisory Service (EPWD 12)*? DAS can be contacted through jobcentres or the Employment Service Head Office.

The Employment Medical Advisory Service (EMAS)
Can be contacted through local offices of the Health and Safety Executive or EMAS Head Office. Nationwide organisation of doctors and nurses (Employment Medical Advisers), who can advise disabled people on any aspect of their fitness for work, and advise employers on any health and safety aspect of the employment of disabled people. They also advise doctors, trade unions, DROs, etc, on medical aspects of employment and training. Maybe if you're having trouble at work you could try them as a sort of 'third party' (like a marriage guidance counsellor), sometimes a helpful way of resolving difficulties, especially if the 'third party' can bring in fresh ideas and specialist knowledge.

EMAS also advise on fire safety procedures, so if these worry you or your employer, get on to the experts. Getting you out in a fire needn't mean adaptations to premises; EMAS may suggest simple alternatives, such as a carrying sling or transi-seat, kept handy to carry you downstairs in an emergency.

Opportunities for People with Disabilities
Like an employment agency. Any disabled person in the areas covered by its offices can seek advice on getting a job, retraining, or career development. It's funded by enlightened employers and has charitable status. It was founded in 1980 by the Chairmen of the Bank of England, BP, CEGB, IBM, Midland Bank, P & O, Price Waterhouse, Sedgwick Group, Stock Exchange, and Unilever. All its senior staff are on secondment from industry or commerce, eg big banks, Marks and Spencer, IBM, ICI, Access, so they have practical experience of the working world. There are offices in several parts of Britain. *Opportunities Annual Report 1985* mentioned a young man with heart trouble and arthritis, who was found work as a plant engineer in a small precision toolroom machining firm. Opportunities also works to educate and advise employers.

Disabled Graduates Careers Information Service (DGCIS)
Helpful careers and information service for people with a disability, and for careers advisers and employers. Databank of graduates in open employment. Unemployed disabled graduates can join the job vacancy list for details of openings with employers keen to take on disabled people.

Association of Disabled Professionals (ADP)

Charity, founded 1971. Useful source of information and advice based on real experiences of professionals with various disabilities. Members' professions include law, engineering, medicine, accounting, teaching, management. ADP works to improve opportunities for all disabled people. Publishes regular, informative bulletin.

Local schemes

Find out what special schemes may be operating in your area. Ask your town hall inform-ation service, social services, CAB, local DIAL/disability advice centre. As I write, for instance, Suffolk County Council has announced that any disabled person who applies for a job will automatically get an interview. Elsewhere, local authorities are funding schemes to put disabled employees in touch with employers.

Careers advice

The right careers advice may help you find the job you want. Look back at page 254 and 244.

Getting a job: some tips

Read the advice given in the publications on page 268. RADAR's *Into Work* is a particularly good guide (free!) to the process of applying for a job, the interview, your rights, etc.

Job-seeking techniques

Brush up on the basic techniques which anyone needs, arthritis or no arthritis. From a jobcentre, get *Jobhunting for People with Disabilities* (PWD 16) and the pack on *Jobhunting* (both free). Look at something like the Consumer Association's *Getting a New Job*. Ask at your jobcentre about jobclubs (page 260), where you can get useful tips and practical help. Write for CRAC's publications list, which includes *Decide for Yourself*, to help you choose your career, *Write Your Own CV*, and *Surviving Interviews*.

Increasing your chances

Apply for jobs where you can make the most of your skills and interests. Don't just wait for vacancies to appear: an amazing number of jobs (*You and Yours* TV programme in March 1987 estimated about 70%) are filled without advertising. Write to firms that interest you, mention to anyone you know that you're looking for work, watch for news of new firms opening, contact Opportunities for People with Disabilities, etc.

Go for a firm which says it's an Equal Opportunity Employer or 'welcomes applic-ations from disabled people'; it's likely to have a fairer and more informed attitude. Large organisations (eg local government, civil service, banks) usually have more flexible practices (eg flexitime), more financial resources, better facilities and more generous sick leave provision. They may also have more experience of employing people with disabilities. Keep in mind practicalities like commuting time and methods.

Apply with as much thoroughness as you intend to put into a job when you get it. And meanwhile occupy your unemployment in ways you can use to impress a potential employer, eg with a demanding hobby, or community work. A temporary spell working in a Citizen's Advice Bureau, for instance, looked good on my application forms.

Details count

Aim to create a good impression from the start, from the first application form or first letter and CV. Think of everything as your own personal advertisement and ensure you're advertising a well-organised person who's serious enough about getting a job to take time and trouble over it. Write clearly and legibly, or type (unless they specify handwriting). Letters on A4 paper look businesslike and are less likely to get lost on the employer's file. Be informative but keep to the point. Tailor your application to the job you're looking for. Keep a dated copy for reference. If you're writing on the off-chance of a vacancy, say you'd welcome any advice or information if there isn't a vacancy currently available.

Accentuate the positive

All the time, stress your *abilities*. That's what the employer's looking for: relevant skills and abilities, evidence of commitment and enthusiasm, and someone who's going to fit in well. Focus attention on just how right you'll be for the job and company. *Don't* go into a lot of detail about arthritis and 'problems'!

Formal qualifications help tremendously, so do what you can to increase them. But non-formal skills and personal qualities can also prove a lot, if you write or talk about them the right way. Hobbies, voluntary work, household management skills, etc, can all be used to demonstrate qualities sought by an employer. For instance, family tree researching as a hobby can demonstrate attention to detail, an enquiring mind, perseverance and commitment to a long-term task. Interest in penfriends shows that you can write/communicate, and are interested in other people. 'Playing' with a home computer can demonstrate no end of skills − mental, yes, but manual dexterity too, to someone who may have doubts about your hands. Even mention of travelling on holiday, driving a car, etc, can all help reinforce the idea of you as an active, doing, person.

Don't be put off by the fancy terms employers use, for instance, communication skills, administrative ability, interpersonal skills (relating to other people), management of resources (managing time, money, other people), delegating and supervising skills, financial planning. Most are as as necessary for running a home as they are for running a business successfully, and you're probably already skilled in many, if not most of them.

How much should you say about the arthritis, and when?

(1) At the application stage   Only you can really decide. If an application form specifically asks about disability, then best to mention it, but keep what you say short, and in your favour. If it doesn't ask, then you might choose to wait till later, till you're offered an interview. Whatever you decide, don't make it seem the main feature of your application, and *don't* go on about 'problems'. No employer wants to take on a 'Problem'! Whatever you say, make it a *positive*, encouraging statement, eg something like this, if true:

−   RA: Diagnosed in 1980. Now well controlled with medication/in remission.
−   JCA: Diagnosed when aged 10. Studies show that 70 − 80% of children with JCA make a satisfactory recovery without serious functional impairment. My medical history strongly indicates that I am among that 70%.
−   RA: Diagnosed in 1975. Medically under control. Some limitation of joint movement, but this has no effect on my efficiency at work.
−   Ankylosing spondylitis: No effect on my work. (In one review, 80% of people with AS were in full-time work.)

Put yourself in the employer's shoes − what questions may come to mind as s/he reads your application for a job that involves typing, for instance? S/he may think 'RA equals crippled hands − how can crippled hands type?' You could write something like:

−   Rheumatoid arthritis: Am proficient on electronic typewriter, which could be supplied by Disablement Resettlement Officer. (Check that first with the DRO)
−   RA: Typing speed with electronic typewriter is 'x' words a minute.
−   RA: My referee, Mr X, can testify to my typing/car-driving/whatever ability.

You might want to include among your referees a professional who knows about your disorder (eg DRO, doctor or OT) *provided* you trust them to give a fair *and* positive picture of your abilities, including, if relevant, how you've overcome any problems.

Discuss in advance what they might say. Even the most well-intentioned referee can inadvertently write something an employer might misinterpret negatively. You don't have to wait to be asked to name a referee; if you think it would be to your advantage, offer a name or send a reference anyway.

(2) How much should you say at an interview? Even if you say little or nothing about the arthritis at the application stage, do be prepared to say more if the application gets taken further. Evading the issue might cause problems later. At worst, whether you win or lose a claim on unfair dismissal against an employer could depend on whether or not you'd disclosed your arthritis. Instead, better to take the initiative yourself, anticipate questions about your arthritis, and *be prepared.*

Practice for the interview with a friend playing the employer's part. Be ready with calm, straightforward answers, which illustrate how brilliantly you manage yourself and the arthritis. Don't ramble on about difficulties (eg with shopping or cooking or dressing or washing) which have nothing to do with the job you're applying for. Handling tricky questions the right way can do as much as anything to convince an employer of your efficiency and aptitude for doing a job well. Being evasive or fearful or unprepared or emotional will make him/her uncomfortable and won't help you sell yourself.

Impress the employer that you have the right attitude. For instance, s/he asks 'how will you cope with...?'. You, with a convincing, reassuring smile, say 'There's always a way around a problem..', 'My arthritis has made me very skilled at problem-solving' or 'Luckily, I'm very resourceful. I usually know or can find out *where* to go for a solution to a problem even if I can't immediately think of a solution myself.' *Don't* begin with something negative, like agreeing 'Yes, I do have dreadful trouble with my legs...' (even if that's true).

What skills have you learned (even unwillingly) through your illness? Ability to adjust to change, flexibility, problem-solving skills, organisational skills, ingenuity, resilience, patience, self-motivation? What about psychology too – eg how people relate to each other, especially in a difficult situation? One YPA felt her arthritis experiences helped a lot in her job as customer services liaison officer with one of the big banks:

> *"I have time to listen, I know how other people feel when faced with a system which they can't understand (eg the NHS), where everyone seems so big and important and busy that you're afraid to ask questions, because they sound so silly." (In Contact)*

Have answers ready for specific problem areas too. Research beforehand possible solutions. Be ready with evidence of how you've overcome problems in the past. I, for instance, know that my hands look fairly useless. To look at them no one would believe I can write, type, grip, etc, magnificently. But I can prove that by referring to achievements such as cooking skills (winner of best fruit flan several times running!) and articles I've written and had published. I do hate being asked about my hands, but to be fair, I guess I'd ask (or certainly think) the same questions if roles were reversed. At least once the problem's aired and talked about, unfair and wrong assumptions can be dealt with. Be alert to *un*spoken questions. You might be better off coaxing them into the open, difficult though that may be.

Here's a checklist of some arthriticky difficulties. Pick out those relevant to you, and using information in this book, work out how best to deal with questions about them.

- Mobility – eg getting to work, getting about at work
- Stiffness and functional limitations – eg reaching up, down, standing, sitting, lifting things, moving things (would a trolley help? helping hand? lower shelves? higher seat?)
- Manual dexterity – eg gripping, grasping, exerting pressure, working a machine, writing, typing, telephoning. If, like me, you can still cope perfectly well despite hand problems, quote examples as proof, or another approach might be to quote to a doubtful employer the *Code of Good Practice*:

"A physical disability, such as a damaged hand or fingers, does not mean that a disabled person cannot be considered for a job which involves manipulating objects or which is highly skilled and calls for dexterity. Disabled people often find ways of minimising the effects of such disabilities – one engineering company employs a man to make miniature wax moulds; he is a quick worker yet he has only three fingers and one thumb. Where a disabled person does have difficulties concerning dexterity, special aids can often be supplied which will help."

- Fatigue, pain, and time-keeping – might it be worth looking out for part-time jobs, jobsharing, or flexitime? Might a nap in the first-aid room at lunchtime help? Or ten minutes 'counting the breath' meditation (page 108) at your desk help?

- Standards of attendance, likelihood of having to take time off. Difficult to generalise, but if you're reasonably confident that your attendance record will be good, try going armed with authoritative quotations such as another from the *Code of Good Practice*:

"Disabled people are not necessarily more likely to lose days through sickness and absences, and indeed research has shown that many disabled people are more conscientious than other workers. For instance, in one branch of a leading chainstore which employs a number of disabled people, the average length of service of its disabled employees is ten years and their average loss of time through sickness and absence is one and a half days per year, well below the national average."

- Safety aspects. Again the *Code of Good Practice* advises employers:

"There is nothing to show that disabled workers are any less safe than others, either in terms of safety aspects relating to particular types of work or safety matters generally, for example coping with an emergency such as a fire alert...In certain cases you [the employer] may need to ensure that specific precautions are taken so that a disabled worker can do a particular job safely or that he or she will be safe in the case of an emergency, such as a fire. Given such precautions, however, the disabled worker will be as safe as others. If you are not sure about some aspects of safety concerning a prospective disabled employee, then the Employment Medical Advisory Service...will be able to give advice."

Being aware of the need to protect our joints and bodies, we may even be *more* careful than *non*-disabled people.

- An encouraging note in Kettle and Massie's *Employers' Guide to Disabilities* might be worth quoting to an undecided prospective employer:

"Neither arthritis nor rheumatism are likely to lead to an undue increase in sickness absence and, provided sensible note is taken of the physical limitations associated with the conditions, there is no reason to fear an increased accident rate. Similarly, with appropriate attention given to the demands of the job and the use of aids where necessary, there is no reason why the worker with arthritis or rheumatism should not be as productive as any other worker." (Woodhead-Faulkner in association with RADAR)

Finally, although it's wise to prepare for the awkward questions, don't get so carried away that you forget to prepare for the old chestnuts *everyone* gets asked, like 'What relevant experience do you have?' 'Tell me why you think I should give this job to *you*?' Avoid saying you need the money, or couldn't find anything better!

Going for interview

Boost your self-confidence by preparing yourself thoroughly beforehand. Do your homework about the company, the job, and how you're going to handle questions. Make sure you can get to the interview on time and in good shape. If necessary, phone beforehand to ask about lifts, to ask whether a chair of 'dining-chair' height can be provided, etc. Allow time to pull yourself together and to show yourself at your best. Don't agree to an early appointment if travelling's awkward or if morning's not your best time. No need to give reasons; just ask politely if a later appointment would be possible.

Dress smartly, show an informed, enthusiastic interest in the job and company, give good reasons why you should have the job, and don't make salary seem your first priority. Don't dwell on the arthritis, but give honest, to the point, answers, which demonstrate how sensible and positive you are, even if you don't feel it. Try to see the interview not as an ordeal, even if it is, but as an *opportunity to sell yourself and your good points.*.

Some employers may be too embarrassed or just plain useless at asking sensible questions about your arthritis. You may need to help things along; the important thing is to get doubts into the open and cleared up, while stressing that the most important thing about you is not the arthritis, but your excellent skills for the job. Try not to get angry at absurd assumptions about what you can or can't do, but try consciously to slow yourself down, and take things calmly. Take a deep breath, smile, and produce the 'trump card' you've prepared beforehand (eg 'you might like to see this photo of me abseiling/sailing at Kielder Adventure Centre; if I can do that....!'). A sense of humour or a smile can help things along.

A naughty employer might try to draw you into talking about problems that simply aren't relevant to your ability to do the job, eg 'How do you manage to do the shopping?' Just say something like 'No problem there', or 'I've got that well organised'. If you start going into detail about irrelevant problems you'll only reinforce the employer's picture of you as a 'Problem'. Steer the talk back to your *abilities* and their relevance to the job.

If an employer seems to like you, but still has some doubts because of the arthritis, be bold and suggest a trial period, or be ready with such comments as 'If you'd like more information about me perhaps you'd like to talk to my DRO, Miss X' or 'I've brought this booklet along to show you what help's available to overcome any difficulties' or 'perhaps you'd like to have a word with EMAS about how other employers/employees with my particular sort of arthritis have got on?' I had to agree to a trial contract of a year when I joined my organisation. During that time I managed to take not one day's sick leave, and was able to prove my ability to do the job. On review after that year my good record helped get me a confirmed contract with full pension rights.

YPA and secretary Janet Flower is an old-hand at interviews:

"At the interview the interviewer may/may not put you at ease. Some do not appear at all friendly but try not to let this worry you. Probably after everything else has been gone into, then will come the questions about RA. Remember the interviewer probably has no idea what it is, or what to ask, so don't let it put you off, if their questions seem stupid. It is easy to say too much, going into your whole medical background, which they don't need to know. Just relate everything to the job you're applying for. For instance, if the person asks how it affects you and what things you can't do, don't feel you have to mention that you can't get in the bath, or do your shoes up. Merely mention that, say, you can't lift heavy things, or stand for too long, or whatever. In other words, be honest about your abilities concerning the job, but leave out what doesn't matter.

"If you are asked about time off for hospital visits, be truthful about it. Even if you'll need a lot of time off, if they are impressed with you in every other respect, this may be acceptable to them. Perhaps a compromise of less holiday entitlement can be agreed in lieu of time off for hospital visits. If they do seem unhappy about the time off you'll need, perhaps mentioning this may allay their fears and you will be showing that you are willing to be helpful and are not going to take liberties. Mention your good attendance at school/work. This is simply adopting an attitude that emphasises what talents, abilities, qualities you personally have for the job, while playing down what you can't do. After all, the things you can't manage probably aren't important in the job you are after. Things that are a problem will probably be slight or easily overcome. If you try to overcome the nerves, and give a positive impression, then even if there are going to be problems, the firm will probably be willing to accept them." (In Contact)

Even embarrassing happenings at the interview needn't mean disaster:

"One interview room had low chairs. To have said I'd sit elsewhere might have been okay, but it would have meant me feeling awkward from the start. So, I sat down, and went through the interview, giving as good an impression as possible, while trying not to worry about how I was going to get up! I got the job, and I'm sure it's because, having proved I had the necessary qualities for the job, the fact that I had to be helped up was irrelevant. If you can make RA seem unimportant compared with your other qualities/ abilities, your chances of success are much greater, no matter how bad your disability."

Successful – or not?

No? – Put it down to experience and try not to get too disheartened. Tell yourself the loss is theirs. Plenty of other people get rejected too, arthritis or no arthritis. If it's a job or a company you're really keen on, no harm in writing to them saying you'd still be interested in being considered for future openings. Keep beavering away at the job applications and make full use of any support services available, eg jobclubs. The struggle will eventually prove worthwhile.

Already in a job when arthritis strikes?

Time and information are crucial. Don't be panicked into making hasty decisions. You'll need time to see how the arthritis develops, time for treatment to show its effect, time to think what to do for the best, and information to help you make the right decisions. It takes time to adapt to any new situation, especially something like RA, AS or lupus. To reassure you and your employer, listen to Kettle and Massie:

"There are many effective medicines to diminish pain and stiffness and several long-acting drugs which, after a few months, have more than an even chance of bringing the condition under control. In severe cases surgery or physiotherapy can help although it should be emphasised that often arthritis or rheumatism need cause little or no interference with work." (In *Employers' Guide to Disabilities*)

You and your employer may be able to make adjustments that can keep you in your present job, or perhaps in another job in the same firm. Keeping a job is probably in your interests financially, socially and psychologically, and in your employer's interests too.

So, with your GP's and rheumatologist's support, try to get your job kept open as long as possible. Even if the employer stops paying you, see if you can be 'kept on the books' until you can return to work or until there's a suitable vacancy.

Find out who to contact, at work and outside work, to help with particular difficulties (eg look back at page 257 onwards). Consult your personnel/welfare officer/union for help and advice. Make sure your employer knows about the *Code of Good Practice* – there's a section on 'Assisting employees who become disabled' (eg who to consult for advice, changes that could be made, legal obligations). Look too at the publications mentioned elsewhere in this chapter, and at the *Disability Rights Handbook* (page 127).

Be wary of anyone making wrong assumptions too early on about what you can or can't do. Arthritis and rheumatic disorders are notoriously misunderstood, *even* by professionals. Do everything you can to ensure that what happens to you is based on professional advice given by a professional with reliable, up-to-date, and *specialist* knowledge of *your* particular type of arthritis, preferably a rheumatologist. You might find it useful to know that Professor Anne Chamberlain, holder of the Charterhouse Clinic Chair of Rheumatological Rehabilitation at Leeds University, specialises in the socio-economic effects of arthritis, including employment implications.

Keeping a job you're already in

You might be able to continue in the same job
–   with no changes

- for a trial period, to assess whether you can cope with your old (or a new) job if you or your employer have doubts (financial help is available through DROs)
- with a gradual return to full-time hours, starting first with shorter hours, as you work out ways of coping and regaining confidence
- with OT and DRO advice on adjustments
- with changes to the job specification to eliminate difficulties (eg some of the physical aspects, replacing them with more non-physical aspects)
- with changes in hours of work, eg allowing for a rest period in the middle of the day, using a flexitime arrangement, or starting later and finishing earlier/later, or working part-time, or job-splitting (grants are available to employers to assist) or job-sharing (information from *New Ways to Work*), or a Sheltered Placement arrangement.
- by working at home, temporarily or possibly permanently (see chapter 32).
- modern technology may help, depending on the type of work.

Or maybe you could return to alternative work in the same company? Retraining might be necessary. If your employer can't arrange it, your DRO should be able to help.

You and your employer may need to consider the implications for pay and conditions if your hours of work are changed. The *Code of Good Practice* advises the employer: *"Any changes to terms and conditions of employment which become necessary should be based, as far as possible, on agreement between your company and the employee. If you have any queries about terms and conditions of employment, then the Advisory Conciliation and Arbitration Service (ACAS) may be able to help."*

Make sure you know your firms's sick leave regulations, and keep your own record of time off in case of any disagreement. Sometimes it's worth using a day or so's annual leave for a short rest if the arthritis is playing up, rather than taking frequent periods of sick leave. And as YPA Anne Ryman wisely advises:

"Employers and work mates will be helpful if you don't use your disability as an excuse. Try to do as much as you can for yourself without asking for help. Always be punctual and reliable."

If you lose your job

Try not to, if at all possible: the longer you can keep it open the better the chances of improvements in medical treatment and in you. However, if you *are*, sadly, faced with the prospect, contact the DRO at once, your union (if you're a member), and your doctor. Talk too to Arthritis Care/Young Arthritis Care or other relevant patient support group.

A disabled person, like all employees, is covered by employment protection legislation. You can get legal advice from a Citizens Advice Bureau and/or local law centre or Network (page 122). Jobcentres have leaflets on employment protection legislation. Free advice is available too from ACAS or a trade union. There's a helpful chapter in the *Disability Rights Handbook* (see for instance the section on 'Sickness and Unfair Dismissal'). Note particularly that any claim for unfair dismissal *must* reach a central office of the Industrial Tribunals within three months of the effective date of termination of your employment (leaflet IT1 from jobcentres tells you more). It's worth knowing that if you're registered disabled (a Green Card holder):

"Your employer would have to prove that special consideration had been given to your case, and that the needs of business made your sacking absolutely necessary. If your employer failed to do this then a tribunal would probably say that your dismissal was unfair." (*Disability Rights Handbook*, 16th edition).

Finally, remember again what I said earlier. Rheumatic disorders are notoriously misunderstood, *even* by professionals and people you'd expect to know better, so do your best to insist that any decisions about you are based on advice given by a professional with reliable, up-to-date and specialist knowledge of *your* particular type of rheumatic disorder, preferably a rheumatologist.

Points of law and disabled employees

Although discrimination against employees on grounds of race and sex is outlawed, discrimination against people because of disability is, alas, not illegal. However that needn't stop you seeking advice from the Equal Opportunities Commission (EOC) or RADAR, and ACAS or your trade union can advise on employment law.

All people with disabilities have the same employment rights as fit employees, and since the Wages Act 1986, the law no longer allows a disabled person to be employed on less favourable terms than someone who is not disabled.

Under the Health and Safety at Work Act 1974, which covers all employees, an employer can refuse work to a disabled person on health and safety grounds *only* if that person's overall condition means s/he can't perform the job effectively and/or safely.

Under Section 7 of the Act an employee has certain obligations which mean s/he should disclose to the employer any medical condition likely to affect safety at work. If it isn't disclosed and the disability caused an accident or injury you might be held responsible, which could mean dismissal.

Employment and benefits

A horribly complicated area, dealt with in more detail on page 133. Do get advice, and cross-check it from different sources. Try CAB, social worker, rights officer, DSS BEL freephone (page 127), DRO, jobcentre Claimant Adviser. Though the *Disability Rights Handbook* takes some ploughing through, it does give you a good start in unravelling the complexities of benefits and employment/unemployment.

Helpful publications

Even if you don't consider yourself disabled these are well worth looking at:

–   RADAR's free *Into Work* (send a stamp), a particularly good step-by-step guide (free!) through the process of applying for a job, the interview, your rights, etc.

–   Employment Service and Training booklets (see page 259), especially the *Code of Good Practice on the Employment of Disabled People*, *Jobhunting for People with Disabilities* (PWD 16), *Employing People with Disabilities. Sources of Help* (EPWD 11). From jobcentres or by post from RADAR (for the cost of postage.)

–   Mary Thompson's paperback *Employment for Disabled People* (Kogan Page). She looks at the whole field of employment, not just areas or schemes exclusively for disabled people. Unfortunately my edition appeared before the changes in the social security/income support system and the Employment Service, so needs to be read with care and you'd need to check more up-to-date information elsewhere.

–   Expensive, and aimed at employers rather than employees, but worth looking at in a library is *Employer's Guide to Disabilities* by Melvyn Kettle and Bert Massie (Woodhead-Faulkner Ltd, in association with RADAR).

–   *Disability Rights Handbook*. Details on page 127.

Look at non-disabled publications, especially *Just the Job* (page 258) and anything aimed at other people with special needs, eg working mothers, women returning to work after time off, unemployed people, information from the organisation New Ways to Work, and:

–   *Working Mother – A Practical Handbook* by Sarah Litvinoff and Marianne Velmans (Corgi), guide to combining motherhood and work successfully.

–   *The Working Mothers' Handbook* available from the Working Mothers' Association.

Chapter thirty-two

WORKING AT HOME, AND
STARTING YOUR OWN BUSINESS

Working at home has its attractions. You can be your own boss, and arrange working hours and surroundings just as you like. But there are pitfalls. The right sort of work's not always easy to come by, pay may be poor for very long hours, and legal and financial regulations or family and domestic demands may cause complications. Bear in mind that benefits may be affected if you start earning money, so take advice first (see page 133). It's helpful, though not essential, if you've already got particular skills and experience which can be adapted to homeworking, such as computer skills or accountancy, or an employer who wants to keep your skills and is enlightened enough to see the advantages of 'teleworking'.

What sort of work could you do?
Homeworking possibilities include book-keeping, giving private lessons, coaching, or correspondence course tutoring, typing/word processing, telephone answering service for small businesses, writing, indexing, proof-reading, data preparation, design work, crossword and quiz compiling, writing technical publications. Don't fall for adverts that ask you to send money in return for directories of homeworking or lists of employers. Most are useless and some simply out to make money for nothing.

Unless you're working for an existing employer, you'll have to find customers yourself, through local contacts, firms, newpapers, etc. Some work such as typing, word processing, addressing envelopes, is done on an agency basis and you could try approaching local agencies listed in *Yellow Pages* or *Thomson's Directory*. Or if you can offer services such as computerised mailing lists, sorting programmes for catalogues or prospectuses, or database, spreadsheet and book-keeping services, even programming or systems analysis, you could approach small firms direct.

The Market Research Society can provide a list of firms which may need outside help with data preparation (preparing information on returned questionnaires ready for computer processing). Contact the Society of Indexers for advice on becoming an indexer. For information on writing, see page 281.

Teleworking in computers/information technology (IT), is a rapidly expanding area. Firms such as Rank Xerox, ICI, Barclay's Bank, British Airways, and British Telecom use homeworkers with programming or other appropriate skills. With IT, everything's in front of you on one keyboard and without having to move you can communicate with other computers and businesses through special telephone and fax links.

Look back at page 259 and talk to your DRO, who may be able to help with advice, finance and equipment. From jobcentres or RADAR, get leaflet PWD 6 *Working at Home with Technology*. One YPA was lent a computer and funded, in conjunction with a technical publications company, to do a Software Technical Authorship course at home, leading to the City & Guilds exam in Technical Communications Techniques. This qualified her to work at home writing manuals for computer packages. For information on careers and courses in technical writing try the Institute of Scientific and Technical Communicators.

Getting relevant experience in IT isn't always easy, but there are special projects which may help (ask your DRO) such as OUTSET and ITeC projects, which include experience of working life, basic computer and electronic skills, software training, word processing.

You don't need to be particularly good at maths. Being able to think clearly and communicate effectively is more important. Clerical skills may be a good starting-point.

General information for people working at home

The Consumers' Association's very readable *Earning Money at Home* covers all aspects, from deciding what to do and selling your work to practicalities such as insurance, keeping accounts, tax and VAT. Marianne Gray's *Working from Home. 200 Ways to Earn Money* (Piatkus) is amusing and full of tips and information. Mary Thompson's *Employment for Disabled People* (Kogan Page) has chapters on 'Running your own business' (including self-employment at home) and 'Information technology'. Andrew Bibby's *Home is Where the Office is* (Hodder and Stoughton Headway) is a practical handbook on teleworking.

OwnBase is a nationwide mutual support organisation of home-based workers. Its informative newsletter appears every two months, and there are local groups, a members' contact list, and a mail-order service of books on homeworking.

A Citizens' Advice Bureau may be able to tell you if there's a homeworking association in your area which could offer general advice and help, though not jobs. You could also try the National Homeworking Unit or the Guild of Disabled Homeworkers.

Specially for disabled people, RADAR produces a cheap employment factsheet *Working from Home*. Remember that your DRO can tell you about special financial and practical assistance available.

For information on legal rights and employment protection legislation for home-based workers, contact the Advisory Conciliation and Arbitration Service (ACAS).

Starting your own business

If you're interested in starting your own business, much of chapter 31 will still apply. Other business and enterprise services specially geared to potential self-employers are on offer through your jobcentre. You can also get free advice from the Small Firms Service (Freephone 0800 222 999). They issue several really helpful free information booklets, eg *Starting and Running your own Business*, *Your Guide to Government Help for Small Firms*, *Accounting for a Small Firm*, *The Secret of Business Success*, *Marketing*, *Selling to Large Firms*, *Franchising*. Local Enterprise Agencies can also help with free advice (071 253 3716 for your nearest agency).

There's a whole chapter on 'Training for Self-Employment' in the excellent book *Second Chances* (page 244), packed with information and addresses, including correspondence courses in starting a business, book-keeping, marketing, etc. The Consumers' Association's book *Starting Your Own Business* is another very helpful, clearly written guide to all aspects of self-employment. You might also like to look at *The Woman's Guide to Starting Your Own Business* by Deborah Fowler (Thorsons). A good introduction to the thorny areas of tax and accounting are three leaflets *Starting in Business* (IR 28), *Thinking of Working for Yourself?* (IR 57) and *Simple Tax Accounts* (IR 104), free from your local Tax Enquiry Centre (in the phone book under Inland Revenue).

Specifically to help disabled people set up their own businesses is the 'Business On Your Own Account Scheme' (details from DROs). The Prince's Youth Business Trust is also keen to help disadvantaged people aged between 18 and 25 who opt for self-employment. The Trust can provide grants and low interest loans, plus professional advice and training for at least one year after the business is established.

When YPA Martin* was made redundant after working for 16 years he studied for the City and Guilds Computer Aided Draughting (CAD) course, and passed with credits. He then took the plunge and started his own business in CAD, offering a planning and design service to small businesses, working from an office in a local business centre. The Enterprise Allowance Scheme gave him professional guidance and back-up, and the Disablement Advisory Service (page 260) provided computer equipment.

Chapter thirty-three

VOLUNTARY WORK

Many YPAs are involved in voluntary work of some sort, and find it a very fulfilling way of making the most of their talents within any limitations imposed by their arthritis. Volunteering can give you a purpose in life, and the great feeling that you're doing something worthwhile. Sometimes voluntary work can lead to a paid job, too, and it's a good way of showing a prospective employer that you have valuable skills and commitment.

What sort of things do YPAs do? Someone from ARC came to talk at a WI meeting that Pamela Waterhouse went to, and she found things snowballed:

"Don't be too disheartened by the effort you have to put into getting the right sort of help: Out of the 100 or so women there, our WI president pounced on me to give the vote of thanks. Well, those few words changed the course of my life! The speaker approached me afterwards and asked if I could start a group locally. I wrote an appeal for help in our parish magazine and was overwhelmed by the response. The group was officially formed in July. The Mayor-elect is our Chairman and I'm the secretary which keeps me extremely busy. It's a wonderful feeling to be doing something positive at last...We now have over 60 members. Last month we held a committee dinner to celebrate raising £1,200 for research in just seven months."

Jacqueline Senior spent many years living with the ups and downs of RA. She and her doctor recently tried out a new drug. – After a shaky start they found the right dose, and *"hey presto!"* she felt so well she

"rejoined the WRVS and joined a team who go to the local prison to serve tea and coffee etc to the prison visitors. Then in October I was asked to go to a local day centre to help out in the shop. It was lovely to feel useful again and to get out and about to meet people."

Barry Hayward volunteered to work on his local hospital radio:

"I became a ward visitor at first but due to a lack of presenters I soon got the chance to appear on one of the programmes. This was a 'magazine' type programme where I read the news and featured a recipe of the week. I pretended to make the recipes 'on the air', whilst all I was actually doing was banging a saucepan and spoon together now and then. It sounded quite good though, and the studio stayed clean!...I now host my own programme called 'All in a Week' in which I look at the news of the previous week and play both old and new records..." (*In Contact*)

Some YPAs get involved with local action groups or with the local church. Doing voluntary work doesn't necessarily mean you have to be physically energetic. One YPA, more or less confined to a wheelchair, was able to use her skills as an active founder member of the local Dial-a-Ride and Crossroads Care Attendant Schemes: *"The Lord really made sure I was in the right place at the right time."* Another wheelchair-using YPA teaches creative writing to adults with learning difficulties. Some YPAs work for their local DIAL information service (mainly on the phone). Others work for the Samaritans, or in the local Citizens' Advice Bureau (CAB). I enjoyed helping at the local CAB at one time, all sitting-down and phone work. Relate (formerly the Marriage Guidance Council), needs not only volunteer counsellors, but also volunteers to staff the telephone and reception points, so too does the WRVS. Or how about offering to record newspaper and magazine articles on cassette for the Talking Newspapers Association? Or become an adult literacy tutor, teaching basic reading, writing and arithmetic to mature people in your home? (See Adult Literacy in Appendix 2).

If your arthritis is too unpredictable you might find it more sensible to avoid committing yourself to any specific task, but there's still lots you can do. If nothing else, do make 'educating' other people about arthritis your cause! Goodness knows they do *need* educating. Just sitting here with my ankle in plaster I managed to have a go at that – taking part in a radio phone-in, writing letters to newspapers, etc.

Far from being a barrier to doing voluntary work, your arthritis or disability could be a positive *asset*. Peter Stubbings, in a paper produced for The Volunteer Centre UK, *New Resources for Old Tasks: Disabled People as Volunteers* (now out of print), pointed out how some apparent disadvantages of disablement can be turned into advantages:

"Apart from any individual attributes, disabled people in general may have these among their assets:

– *immobility, which can be translated into the capacity to be in the same place for fixed periods*
– *time itself, a crushing burden for many disabled people when there is nothing to fill it, but a scarce commodity in modern life*
– *patience, very often stemming from experience of having to be patient*
– *motivation to work to escape the routine of inactivity*
– *experience of being dependent on someone else, all too rare among people who give care or service*
– *sensitivity stemming from experience of one's own or other people's suffering*
– *often, a high development of unimpaired faculties, such as...hearing or speech*
– *highly organised routine, making for reliability."*

A wheelchair-user with MS described in *MS Bulletin* what she does:

"In the corner where I sit by the window where I can keep an eye on the world passing by, there is a digital telephone on one side and an entryphone on the other. Here, I am able to act as a co-ordinator for my local community care group, receiving calls and passing them on for action by volunteers. I also act as an answerphone for a friend who is a professional photographer out a lot on assignments wanting someone to take his incoming calls."

If you want more ideas, try your local Council for Voluntary Service or Volunteer Bureau. If there isn't one in the phone book, ask your CAB, or contact the National Association of Volunteer Bureaux or the National Association of Councils for Voluntary Service.

Chapter thirty-four

HOLIDAYS

Nowadays there are all sorts of holidays to choose from, even if you *have* got arthritis dogging your steps. A good holiday will refresh you inside and out, recharging your batteries, so you return to everyday humdrum with renewed mental and physical vigour, and with plenty to chat about to anyone who'll listen! It's also something to look forward to, and back on – with pleasure, ideally!

Arthritis-problems can usually be overcome, be they great or be they small; it's a question of gathering plenty of information, being realistic, and forward planning. I'll give you a few ideas; up to you then to work out what's best for you. Cans and can't-dos vary so much from person to person.

A favourite with under-45 YPAs are the Young Arthritis Care holidays. Because they're specially for YPAs (friends/family too) you can more or less ignore the arthritis and get on gleefully with other things. *"We just didn't have time to feel arthritic, there was so much to do"*, enthused one YPA after an action-packed holiday in Blackpool. Young Arthritis Care's regular holidays at the Kielder Adventure Centre in Northumberland certainly don't give anyone the chance to blame arthritis for not being able to do something they've always yearned to do. Janet Flower raved about her stay at Kielder:

"Where to begin?...The exciting choice of activities? The idyllic scenery? The terrific instructors, friendly companions, the outings? ...An unforgettable week... Each day there's a choice of activities – eg sailing, horse-riding, archery, fishing, canoeing, abseiling, orienteering, swimming – from which you can usually choose two each day, with a break between for lunch. Or if you prefer you can potter around and relax – there's no compulsion to do any unless you want to.

"...I found it a good idea to do something active in the mornings and then a gentler activity in the afternoons. One of the most exhilarating activities was sailing...We spent the whole day sailing, and it was a real sense of achievement – just the elements and us, working together.

"As with all the activities, once we were helped into the boat, Dave the instructor involved us totally in handling it, telling us what things were for and some elementary principles of sailing. That's what made it so enjoyable – rather than if he did all the work. Similarly with horse-riding, you are shown how to guide and instruct the horse, and with canoeing how to stop or turn the canoe. It's fascinating learning, and gives you a real sense of achievement. It's terribly impressive when you get home too, to casually drop into conversations something about abseiling techniques, or maybe a nautical phrase you've learnt.

"...Also enjoyable...swimming in the heated pool (carpeted inside *so you can't slip), archery and riding in the horse and cart. Some of the others did fishing, abseiling and shooting. Also available was bird-watching, and believe it or not, specially adapted water-skiing!*

"...Even if, like me, you haven't much self-confidence, at a place like Kielder anything's possible! The staff do their utmost to help you with any of the activities you want to try and if you find it difficult or uncomfortable they come up with ideas to make things easier.

"In the evenings there was plenty to do too...pool, table-tennis, a TV/video/piano room. One night a hilarious indoor hockey match took place, on another some of us had

great fun with a TV quiz game. Another night there was a party...another a meal out. One crazy evening we all set off on a Treasure Hunt in two mini-buses – it was a maniac Anneka Rice-type competition... We even found time for outings too...and just about saved enough energy for a disco on Friday night..

"...although in our group we had arthritis in common, our mobility and conditions varied considerably – some of us with artificial hips and/or knees, some using crutches, some unable to walk more than a few yards. And yet by the end of the week we'd all managed to have a go at almost all the activities on offer. Where necessary, some of us stayed in wheelchairs for some of the activities, eg abseiling, in order to ensure both safety and as little strain on grotty painful joints as possible. But much to our amazement, we did it, we really did it!" (In *In Contact*)

Kielder's purpose-built for anyone with a disability – you can go alone, in a group, or with your family. The building's all on one level, and each room has private access to the lovely countryside outside. Beds have been specially made to cater for different disabilities, and washbasins are at different heights too. Besides the main dining-room and small licensed bar, there are small kitchens for self-catering and laundry. To go in a group, write to Young Arthritis Care, or if you prefer to go independently contact Kielder direct. The services at Kielder, and at nine other adventure centres for disabled people, are described in the Stackpole Trust Support Group's leaflet (free, but send SAE) *Adventure for All*.

Other holidays for not-too-disabled YPAs

Some of us have been fit enough and foolhardy enough at times to travel, on our own, to exotic foreign parts like Norway, Canada, or even Czechoslovakia. We've had to plan ahead carefully, but managed with fairly straightforward modifications to otherwise 'ordinary' holidays, for instance by ensuring hotel bedroom and main public rooms are accessible by lift, by getting extra help from an airline, and by getting manageable luggage, eg shoulder bag, suitcase on wheels – some have built-in wheels, others are strap-on, or luggage trolleys/carriers (eg from Norland Gazelle Travel Goods).

Don't overlook 'disabled' publications just because you don't feel disabled: they contain many useful tips for making ordinary holidays easier. More about those later. Look back too at chapter 24 'Out and about' for ways of overcoming mobility problems, and page 174 on getting-to-the-loo problems. Ask, too, the Holiday Care Service (page 277) and Tripscope (page 184) for information specific to your needs.

More and more ordinary publications and travel agents are anxious to help people with special needs too, so don't be afraid to mention yours. Be wary though that 'special facilities' may not be as wonderful as they sound, or might not suit your own particular needs. Don't take bland reassurances for granted, but cross-check facts, eg ask how many steps there are, don't just accept that 'there aren't many'. Be specific about what *you* need, rather than accepting what *they* think you need.

Difficulties may be overcome just by choosing your holiday cannily, like Peter Nightingale, who maximised scene changes and minimised leg-work by taking a boat trip one Easter: 11 nights at sea travelling the length of the Norwegian coast. Or how about a weekend or longer on a 'residential course' in a lovely old country home or university, meeting other people and dabbling in anything from singing or crafts or English literature to astronomy or computing? (In *Time to Learn*, page 247). Seek inspiration too in the English Tourist Board's *Activity and Hobby Holidays*, which includes special interest breaks, and residential activity centres for children to go off on their own. If you're wanting simply to travel in Britain, it's worth remembering that hotel chains such as Travelodge, Granada Lodge and Travel Inns usually have ground floor rooms. Every Travelodge has at least one room designed for disabled people.

For a quieter break, how about going on a retreat, a period of time set aside for meditation, rest and spiritual reflection? These take place in houses, convents, or monasteries. The Macleod Centre for instance, on the island of Iona, was specifically designed to be accessible to people with disabilities. In some centres you spend the time in your own way; in others guidance is offered. Some offer 'theme retreats', where you're helped to develop inner stillness and reflection through painting or music. For details send an SAE to the National Retreat Centre.

Or how about a holiday centre, where each member of the family can be as active or as lazy as s/he likes, like Center Parcs, for instance? There are several abroad and two in Britain, one in Sherwood Forest and one in Norfolk. There's a huge central tropically heated dome with swimming pool, wild water rapids, whirlpools, water slides, sunbeds, saunas, etc, and plenty to do outside the dome too. Some of the self-catering villas have special features for disabled people, and there's a choice of restaurants. No cars are allowed: you get around by bike or on foot, so you might want to take a wheelchair or electric 'scoota'. Full details from Center Parcs.

If warm sunny Tenerife tempts you, there's a purpose-built, wheelchair-accessible holiday centre there, called Mar y Sol, with swimming pools (one heated with a hoist), poolside bar, sports and health facilities, etc (see Mar y Sol in Appendix 2).

One YPA, who'd brought up her family singlehanded, on state benefits, unexpectedly found *her* holiday dream came true thanks to her local council:

"I approached my local council (holidays section). The ladies were particularly helpful and friendly. I told them that my two young sons were going on a camping holiday, could they consider me for a holiday on a health farm? ...A little later, one of the ladies telephoned to say that the council had agreed to funding, and that they would organise everything! They also said that my request was the first time that anyone had asked for such an unusual holiday, and that I had to promise to tell them all about it when I got back! (I think they were as excited as I was). So, as you see, because a thing hasn't been tried before − it doesn't mean that it can't be done!

"Contrary to popular belief, health farms aren't full of the 'idle rich' either. I made friends with a headmistress, a mother and daughter, a Welsh policeman and a journalist − 'The Gang of Six'! Of course, you 'rub shoulders' with some monied people, but spending all day in dressing-gowns is a great leveller! (By the way, my dressing-gown was much admired by an actress, and I took immense pleasure telling her it cost £4.99, 'down the market').

"The staff were very efficient and helpful, and guests were treated equally − and a nice touch, I thought, was on departure day. On checking out, people paid by cheque or cash, but my bill was being paid by the London Borough of Greenwich. I presented myself at the desk, and the receptionist said 'Hello, Mrs P−, we do hope you've enjoyed your stay, your bill has been taken care of by your company!' Great eh? I swanned out of reception like 'Lady Dunnabit'..." (In Contact)

Local social services departments are required to assess the need of a disabled person for a holiday, if asked to do so, but their reaction in practice to a request for help is unpredictable. Still, worth a try if a holiday any other way seems out of the question.

Holidays for more disabled YPAs

Besides considering Young Arthritis Care or PHAB holidays, others of us who are older, or more limited in what we can do might prefer something like one of Arthritis Care's hotels, or self-catering holiday units, where you and your family do your own thing. Ask Arthritis Care for their *Holiday Centres* leaflet. Other organisations too have hotels or centres with special facilities (addresses in Appendix 2), for instance:

−   Ashwellthorpe Hall Holiday Hotel, Norfolk. Beautiful moated Elizabethan mansion, in lovely grounds, owned by the Disabled Drivers' Association. Whether disabled or not, you can have an ordinary holiday there, or book for one of their speciality weekends, eg fishing, bridge, history, Scrabble, or gourmet!

- John Groom's Association for the Disabled has hotels in Minehead, Somerset, and Llandudno, Gwynedd, and runs the Visitors' Club, which offers reduced rates in specially converted rooms (eg electric hoists, automatic toilets, handrails) at the London Tara Hotel. Also has mobile holiday homes and self-catering accommodation.
- The Winged Fellowship Trust has purpose-built holiday centres in Surrey, Essex, Nottingham and Southport which offer activities and outings and cater for disabled people who don't have a helper to bring with them. Volunteer able-bods help out. The Trust also organises holidays abroad.
- Park House, on the Sandringham Royal Estate, is where Princess Diana grew up. It was presented to The Leonard Cheshire Foundation by the Queen in 1984, and is now a modernised country house hotel specially equipped for people with disabilities, with qualified staff able to provide 24 hour care. There's room for 25 guests in single and twin bedrooms, a leisure hall with bowls, snooker, and table tennis, and also a spa bath, hairdressing salon, and heated swimming pool.
- The National Trust has some specially adapted cottages which can be rented. Details from Valerie Wenham, National Trust.

One mother (with very bad RA) and her family decided to pool their holiday money to buy a caravan, so they could take advantage of it the instant she had a period of good health.

Several tour operators now specialise in organising group or individual holidays for disabled people, taking all the worry out of the whole business. Some holidays are in Britain, others abroad in exotic places like Florida or Majorca. The Holiday Care Service and publications mentioned in this chapter will tell you more.

Holidays on the ocean wave

How about an adventurous sailing holiday, perhaps off Britain, or even the Bahamas, helping to crew a square-rigged boat, the Lord Nelson? It's been specially built to be crewed by a mixed team of physically handicapped and able-bodied people. Details on page 290, where you'll find other information to inspire holiday ideas.

Visiting London

Some sources of information to help you plan your visit in advance:
- Nicholson's *Access in London*, by G Couch, W Forrester and P Mayhew-Smith (by post from Pauline Hephaistos Survey Projects). Really excellent.
- The London Tourist Board's guide for people with mobility problems, *London Made Easy*, includes sights, entertainments, restaurants, and transport (available by post).
- London Regional Transport, Unit for Disabled Passengers: can give information on transport, including lift-equipped buses linking Paddington, Euston, King's Cross, Waterloo and Victoria, and others linking Heathrow with Victoria/Euston. They publish *Access Around London for Disabled People* (free), and *Access to the Underground* (cheap).
- Artsline: Information for disabled people on arts and entertainment in Greater London: what's on, ticket prices, concessions, access. Artsline can help too with making a booking and sorting out venue and transport arrangements. Produces free magazine *Disability Arts in London*.
- The Visitors' Club can provide information about London hotel facilities for disabled people.
- GLAD (Greater London Association for the Disabled): information service.
- See also Tripscope, on page 184.

Single-parent family holidays

A divorced mum (with RA) wanted a holiday she and her sons could go on together:

"In the past, my sons and I have been on holidays for the elderly and mentally handicapped. That wasn't too successful. A week at Butlin's, absolutely great for the children, but awkward for me, as the holidaymakers were in groups, or two parent families. Gingerbread (single parent group), fine, you would think − not so! The common denominator is the one parent but not a disabled *one parent!*

"I thought I'd cracked it − our last holiday, two years ago, was a caravan, parked almost on the water's edge, in a quiet seaside resort. I imagined spending all day on the beach together − only one snag! It was sandy beach but you had to scale a mountain of shingle to get on to it. The boys spent all day on the beach all right, but alone − without me. I was back at the caravan relaxing. (Trying to, that is) hoping they hadn't been swept out to sea, or savaged by crabs on the almost deserted beach." (*In Contact*)

The solution was to go to Kielder (page 273) with Young Arthritis Care, where they had a wonderful time, *together.* An alternative might be to go somewhere like Center Parcs or Ashwellthorpe (page 275) or to an Arthritis Care self-catering unit or hotel, or to a National Trust adapted cottage (page 276), and to persuade friends and other people from a self-help group to go along too (an local Young Arthritis Care Contact might help put you in touch).

Another option, though not cheap, is to send the children away on their own to special activity camps. Some have swimming pools, gyms and playing fields. Some are multi-activity, others specialise in anything from computing to football coaching. The British Activity Holidays Association (BAHA) operates a code of practice and makes safety inspections of camps. Write to BAHA for a list of members.

Gingerbread (page 236) publishes a *Holiday Guide for One Parent Families*

Further general information (look back at chapter 24 too)

The Holiday Care Service Have you ever wished you could just say to a specially understanding travel agent 'I'd like to go to Tenerife − but I've no idea how to do it or how on earth I'd manage to get over the arthritis/mobility difficulties' − and receive the reply 'Here's just the information to help you'? Or maybe you fancy birdwatching? Or wonder how you could travel by air with a wheelchair? Or whether there's an accessible hotel in the resort of your dreams? Well, the Holiday Care Service could be the answer.

It's a charity, partly funded by the English Tourist Board, which provides free information and advice on holidays for people with special needs. It *doesn't* actually make bookings, but gives you the information to help you make your own choice of holiday, whether it's an 'ordinary, independent holiday' or one specially geared to disabled people.

There's a wide range of factsheets, including a list of accessible hotels in the Mediterranean. They also operate a free service, Holiday Helpers, to introduce experienced volunteers to disabled people who can't go on an independent holiday without someone to help. One of these was Sheena, with Still's disease, who thanks to Holiday-Helpers was able to tour the Scottish Highlands in a specially adapted vehicle. HCS only make the introductions; it's then up to the holiday-maker and helper to sort out details, including finance.

You can write or phone for information. You'll need to give full details of your needs, explain what kind of holiday you're looking for, where you'd like to go, what sort of budget you're working to, and what your arthritis limitations are.

Tripscope See page 184. Information by phone, to help you plan your travelling, wherever and whatever it's for. To keep your phone bill low, they'll phone you back if you want.

Travel Companions   If you're fit enough to travel on your own, without help, but would prefer someone else along for company (and to avoid single room supplements), Travel Companions, for an annual membership fee, offer three introductions to possible holiday partners (age range 35 – 75). They stress they're *not* a dating agency!

Department of Transport   DoT's free *Door to Door* guide is packed with travel information, including rail, coach, air and sea travel, with all sorts of gems tucked away, for instance a ferry from Aberdeen to Lerwick with a specially designed cabin for disabled people, cross-Channel ferries with lift access. The guide's well worth a browse.

RADAR publications   Various prices, all available by post from RADAR. Books first:
–   *Holidays in the British Isles* is published annually each December, and includes holiday homes, camps, guest houses, hotels and private houses with accessible accommodation. Also covers activity holidays and transport.
–   *Holidays and Travel Abroad – A Guide for Disabled People*. Similar, but this time outside Great Britain. Includes travel by sea and air, as well as coach or escort services. Provides useful contact addresses in countries as varied as Barbados and Yugoslavia. Not only country by country information on accommodation, but also useful hints such as where to hire and repair wheelchairs.
RADAR Holiday Factsheets include:
–   *Useful addresses and publications for the disabled holidaymaker*
–   *Sport and outdoor activity holidays/courses*
–   *Holiday insurance cover*
–   *Holiday finance*
–   *Planning and booking a holiday*
–   *Escort, taxi and private ambulance services*
–   *Red Cross portable equipment loan*
–   *Holiday accommodation with nursing care*
–   *Holiday accommodation for children and young people*
Send SAE for RADAR's full publications list, which includes leaflets and books published by other bodies, for instance *Travelling with British Rail – A Guide for Disabled People*, *Disabled Traveller's International Phrase Book*, a full range of *Access* guides (eg in different towns in Britain, also *Access in Paris*, *Access in Brittany*, *Access in Israel*, *Access at the Channel Ports*).

Disabled Living Foundation   Will send, for a small payment:
–   *Holidays information* – includes specialist travel agents
–   *Accommodation for handicapped people of all ages*

Automobile Association (AA)
–   *Travellers' Guide for the Disabled*, updated each year, free to members, few pounds to non-members. Excellent guide, includes 'Where to stay', 'Where to eat', 'Places to visit', 'Getting around', 'Travelling abroad', motorway service areas and their suitability for disabled motorists

Other possibly helpful publications :
–   *Holidays and Courses for Disabled People*, 258 pages, free (!) from Countrywide Publications
–   *The World Wheelchair Traveller*, by Susan Abbott and Mary Ann Tyrell (Spinal Injuries Association)
–   *Nothing Ventured – Disabled People Travel the World*, edited by Alison Walsh,

who has RA (Harrap Rough Guide)
– *Access in Paris*, from the Pauline Hephaistos Survey Project

Financial help

Arthritis Care will sometimes consider applications for financial assistance. RADAR produces a holiday finance factsheet. The Holiday Care Service may be able to advise on sources of help, and it's worth trying your local social services, and any local charity too.

Special needs while away

Don't forget to take your medication, and any portable gadgets you'll need. Make a 'Holiday Checklist' well in advance – a great sanity-saver! List all the clothes and whatnots you might need. Choose a limited number of coordinating clothes and colours, which can be dressed up or down. Don't load yourself down with clutter you won't use. Put the list away for a while then go through it again and ruthlessly prune it.

The sort of gadgets I take include a folding longreach gadget, a long-handled bathbrush (for feet), stocking puller-up, small non-slip bathmat, plus my National Key Scheme key (for 'disabled' loos – page 174). You might want to include a tap-turner. The nearest thing to a portable raised toilet seat is a collapsible 4" high seat which fits most standard toilets. It's made of polypropylene, and folds flat into its own carrying bag. Details from Aremco. Remember, some items can be hired from the British Red Cross, for instance a wheelchair or commode, useful where there's no downstairs loo. Some can be folded for travelling. See RADAR's *Red Cross portable equipment loan* factsheet or contact the British Red Cross direct. Or take a discreet 'portable urinal' (page 144).

Include your drugs in your checklist. Take with you a separate note of drug types, dosage, etc, in case they get lost. If flying, pack the drugs in your hand luggage, not your suitcase, in case that goes astray.

If, horror of horrors, you forget to take your tablets with you, and you're in Britain, you can visit a GP in your holiday area, under the NHS, as a 'temporary resident'. The GP will ask you to sign a form. If you can't get to a GP, visit a pharmacist. Provided the drug's not on a controlled list, and the pharmacist is convinced your need's genuine, s/he can give you an emergency supply (usually three or five days' worth). You may have to pay. If you normally use a 'season ticket' for your prescription payments but have forgotten it, ask the pharmacist for a receipt so you can claim the money back later.

If you're going abroad, Britain has reciprocal health care arrangements with some other countries. Some are complicated. Well before you travel ask at any local social security office or post office for a copy of leaflet SA30: it includes a form you'll need to send off for the certificate of entitlement (form E111) which you'll need with you in EEC countries. Take out health insurance, especially if you're visiting countries without reciprocal agreements (see the section on holiday insurance on page 139).

Find out whether there are any special health precautions you need to take. Get leaflet SA35 *Notice to Travellers: Health Protection*. Both leaflets SA30 and SA35 are also available by post from DSS Overseas Branch.

In some countries overseas (eg Pakistan, India, Middle East) injections or anti-malarials are necessary which may upset RA or SLE/lupus in some people (though in a few, anti-malarials have instead helped the RA). Beware anti-cholera and anti-typhoid which can cause unpleasant reactions in RA and SLE/lupus. Check with your rheumatologist.

Chapter thirty-five

PASTIMES AND CLUBS

I hope here to inspire you with tales of what other YPAs get up to, plus information on specialist groups, gadgets and mail-order sources, to spur you on to overcome any hurdles the arthritis puts in your way. Only enough room here to tickle your fancy, but no matter! As Pamela Waterhouse says *"The biggest tip is to keep yourself busy – mentally and physically."* An absorbing hobby will help keep your mind off pain and frustrations, give you a sense of achievement, put you in touch with new friends, and help keep the old by giving you something wonderfully *non*-arthritic to share with them. So – get cracking!

For other ideas, browse in a library, bookshop (including the children's section), hobby magazines and TV programmes (especially children's). For armchair browsing, try the Search Press's colourful mail-order catalogue of arts, crafts, cookery and organic gardening books. Readicut's crafts catalogue (page 283) includes books and Reader's Union even has a Craft Book Club. Short residential courses (on anything from singing or painting to obscure fungi) are a good way of meeting other people and indulging a hobby without long-term commitment or recurring transport problems – send for NIACE's *Time to Learn* (page 247). For heaps more ideas and addresses, you could try too the Disabled Living Foundation's low-cost leaflet on leisure activities, and maybe the *Disability Arts Magazine*. Look too at studying for pleasure in chapter 30.

Try saying 'I wonder *how* I could do x/y/z' rather than 'I don't think I can do x/y/z'. Find out *how* by consulting RADAR, DLF, SHAPE or Artsline, (both work for access to all aspects of the arts), by talking to other YPAs, or put your problem to a relevant 'non-disabled' organisation and ask if they can help; eg write for information about a residential painting weekend, and explain your accommodation needs. The reply might be a pleasant surprise saying they've a ground floor bedroom and shower. Or contact your local WI or photography club, say, and explain you're too shy to come along on your own – perhaps one or two members could visit you first so you'd know someone to go along with?

Even if you're not very disabled, just the right bit of equipment might make all the difference to keeping up or abandoning a favourite hobby. If you can't find one mentioned here, or commercially available, why not see if Technical Aids for Disabled People (formerly REMAP – page 146) might be able to make something?

Art
Did you know many of Auguste Renoir's masterpieces were painted when he had severe RA? When his hands got really bad he had to have the brush tied into his hand. Fortunately most of us can manage without having to go that far. Haydn Martin (who has RA) paints watercolours:

> *"I fortunately don't have any problems with holding my brushes. Now and again the tendons in my wrists seem to get crossed and make me jump a bit, but it's not too bad. I find it most absorbing and am hoping to hold a one man exhibition sometime in the future."*

Art's an area where you really can forget can't dos and concentrate instead on can-dos. Very therapeutic. If you're the competitive type you can compete on equal terms with anyone else, like Sue Gunn (she has RA):

> *"I have been learning calligraphy for about 18 months and have entered an exhibition. No one in the exhibition knows that I have arthritis so I will be judged along with*

everyone else." (*In Contact*)

Sue now teaches calligraphy at evening classes, and has her own small business too.

Painting and drawing courses are a lovely way of getting out and meeting people. NIACE's *Time to Learn* (page 247) lists a variety (short residential), in really beautiful places, some of which I know are happy to cater for someone with special needs, if you write and explain. For information on other facilities around the country, see RADAR's *Guide to Arts Centres and Creative Opportunities for Disabled People*. The Search mail-order catalogue includes lots of low-price art books (eg watercolours, oils, calligraphy).

Reading for Pleasure

There are now more than a quarter of a million books in print! Make the most of your local library – if you're housebound ask about the visiting library service, which may be run by the local authority or the WRVS. If like me you can't easily get out to buy books in the shops, buy by post instead (see page 114).

Scan magazines and TV and radio programmes for news of new books and keep a note in your Infokit of any that take your fancy. Ask in your library to see *The Bookseller* new book lists; ask someone to pick up a copy for you of W H Smith's free *Bookcase* magazine; or think about subscribing to *The Good Book Guide*, a bi-monthly magazine of reviews with a bookpost service. I enjoy browsing through the publishers' catalogues which my wonderful paperback supplier (J Barnicoat – see page 115) sends back with my order.

Another armchair browser's guide is Waterstone's regular newsy *Guide to Books: an Ordering Service for Readers*. You get a year's account facility enabling you to order books from the guide by post or phone. You have to pay postal charges.

Book clubs abound, widely advertised in magazines and newspapers (eg ask Readers Union for their list). Some are general interest, others specialise in anything from military matters to romance. One drawback is that you usually have to agree to buy a specific number of books, to start with, anyway. That apart, their leaflets are usually inspirational, and they're a good source of presents.

Reading doesn't have to be a solitary occupation. Why not start a reading group, with, say, four or more members, meeting once a month in each other's homes to discuss a chosen 'book of the month'? It needn't be terribly intellectual, just people who want to do something easy but different, other mainly housebound people, maybe mums with young children?

For tips on overcoming physical difficulties in holding books, look back at page 149. Your OT can advise you on book rests or DIY solutions. Or plump for tapes and cassettes instead. Many libraries stock a good range. Travellers Tales specialise in lending out books on cassette by post and have a wide range, ideal for car, kitchen, or while you're languishing in bed. The service isn't specifically for disabled people, so not cheap, but worth finding out about nonetheless. ISIS also run a mail-order library of audio books, again with subscription and loan charges.

Cheaper, and sometimes free, are several specialist taped books (fiction and non-fiction) organisations, catering not only for blind people but also for people who can't hold books, provided you send a doctor's certificate describing the disability. Some, like the National Listening Library, hire out special tape/cassette players, manageable by people with arthritis. Other tape-lending charities are Calibre and the Muriel Braddick Foundation. DLF's *Communication* list gives details of these and others.

Ask DLF for information about special cassette players. Clarke & Smith Manufacturing Co Ltd, for instance, make the Easiplay Audio Cassette Player. Clever, though not cheap, it includes remote control on-off, automatic side change and light action controls.

Writing for pleasure or profit

Popular, despite dodgy hands. Two well-known authors, Rosemary Sutcliff and Marie

Joseph, are fellow YPAs. Rosemary has juvenile chronic arthritis, and Marie RA, which developed in her 20s. More about them in chapter 29. Many others of us enjoy writing prose or poetry for pleasure, and dream of fame even if we never achieve it!

The Writers' and Artists' Yearbook (A & C Black), updated each year, is the key reference book to look at, packed with names and addresses of publishers, information about writing for radio and TV, literary prizes, copyright laws, desktop publishing, self-publishing, etc. (Also greeting card producers.) *Don't*, as they stress, be tempted by 'vanity publishers', who get you to foot the bill for publishing your work. It could turn out very expensive.

The inspirational monthly *Writers' News*, available on subscription, is packed with information, advice, and news of competitions and helpful publications.

Where else to get tips on how best to write? Widely advertised summer writing schools (some included in the NIACE's *Time to Learn*) and correspondence courses might help, but make sure you're you mean to complete the course before parting with any money. One way of meeting writers and learning from them is to join a local Writers' Circle. Ask your library for information or see Jill Dick's *Directory of Writers' Circles*.

There are various 'how to' books available, for instance *Write a Successful Novel* by F E Smith and M Sherrard-Smith (Escreet), author and former publishing editor Michael Legat's *An Author's Guide to Publishing* (Robert Hale) and *Writing for Pleasure and Profit* (Robert Hale), Jill Dick's *Freelance Writing for Newspapers* (A&C Black), John Braine's *Writing a Novel*, Patricia Highsmith's *Plotting and Writing Suspense Fiction*, or *How to Publish Your Poetry* by Peter Finch, himself a poet. Mary Wibberley's written a book on writing romantic novels *To Writers With Love* (Buchan and Enright). Mills and Boon will send guidance notes to would-be romantic novelists, along with a cassette *And Then He Kissed Her...*, (£7.50, 1991).

A booklet *Writing for Radio* is available free from Radio Drama, Broadcasting House, and *Writing for the BBC* by Norman Longmate (BBC Books) explains how to approach appropriate sections of the BBC. Rosemary Horstmann's *Writing for Radio* (A&C Black) or the *Writers' and Artists' Yearbook* will tell you more, too.

Word processing and desktop publishing make it much easier these days to publish your work yourself, though costs and quality vary tremendously. You'll need to do a lot of homework first before committing yourself. I've only a basic (but much loved) Amstrad 8512 PCW, not even IBM compatible, but was delighted to find two firms (Daisywheel and Inspiration) who could produce laser-printed, camera-ready copy direct from my disks, and by return of post. That did away with expensive typesetting costs, and the hassle of translating disks first into ASCII.

To find out more about desktop/self-publishing, look at Charlie Bell's low-cost *The Writer's Guide to Self-Publishing* (Dragonfly Press), Susan Quilliam and Ian Grove-Stephensen's *Into Print* (BBC Books), Peter Finch's *How to Publish Yourself* (Allison & Busby). *Publish! An Author's Guide to Doing it Yourself Using Desktop Publishing*, by Nicholas Saunders refers in particular to Neal's Yard in London, where you can do DIY typesetting and graphic design yourself, using all manner of hardware, including Apple Macs, and software including PageMaker, Illustrator 3, Quark Xpress, WordPerfect. Write too, to the Small Press Group.

Family tree researching/genealogy

I've been hooked for years! It's a fascinating detective story that can turn up all sorts of discoveries, about your family and social history in general. I learned several generations of one side of the family were mole-catchers, and even found the very plot of land where my great great great great molecatching grandfather lived. Even better, discovered distant cousins in America and Canada, who we never knew existed. One, in particular, in his 80s, writes wonderfully entertaining letters, and we hope to meet up very soon.

Start by collecting together everything you and other relatives know. Birth and marriage certificates from St Catherine's House, in London, will help take you further back (from General Register Office (Scotland) for Scotland. Two of the best sources of cheap, often free information are the census records and the microfiche records of the International Genealogical Index. A lot can be done by post, though nothing beats tackling the hunt in person, if you can. Your local Family History Society (address from the Federation of Family History Societies) can give you information about local sources, and there are lots of helpful publications, eg George Pelling's *Beginning Your Family History*, Willis and Tatchell's *Genealogy for Beginners*, P Palgrave Moore's *Tracing Ancestors*, Jean Cole's *Tracing Your Family History*. Your library should have some. *Family Tree Magazine* is an inspiring read, too, and many useful books are available through its postal book service. There's even one called *No Time for Family History?* by Eve McLaughlin, which focuses on what can be done by post (one of several guides available by post from her).

Crafts including sewing and knitting

"I am very happily married and at present entering my third year as an OU student...I have recently rediscovered the pleasures of embroidery although weak and stiffened fingers prevent me attempting anything too ambitious." (Carol J, who has RA)

DLF's *Leisure Activities* information sheet lists gadgets (plus suppliers' addresses) to make sewing, knitting, pottery, scraperwork, woodwork, etc, easier; for instance needle threaders, self-threading needles, electric sewing machines with special features, even a tapestry kit with larger holes to make life easier for arthritic hands. Battery-operated scissors are useful for cutting cloth, if you've weak or limited hand movement, like me.

Bear in mind that OTs advise against keeping a joint in one position for long periods, especially if you're trying to grip tightly, as you might with fine sewing. That could exacerbate RA hand deformity. If you must sew by hand, try tacking, cross-stitch or blanket-stitch. Anchor your material firmly to a stand, your knee, or your chair arm, so you've a firm surface and don't need to grip.

Machine sewing may be better, though more expensive to start with. Once you've mastered it, you can make your own clothes, or adapt bought clothes. You can make toys, children's clothes, and gifts, too. I use a portable lightweight machine with foot control. Some machines have helpful built-in features, eg needle-threader, bobbin extractor, thread cutter. Other adaptations can be made too. Take a good look at what's available before buying, try out different machines, and if you come across any particular difficulty, contact various manufacturers (or DLF) to see if they can suggest a solution.

Most of the major pattern houses (eg Vogue, Simplicity, Style, Butterick) have regular magazines you can study at home and even buy patterns from by post. Some publish guides to basic techniques. Or try a book like Ann Ladbury's *Making the Most of Your Sewing Machine* (B T Batsford). Small ads in the magazines are useful sources of mail-order fabrics and accessories like belts and buttons. *The* place for buttons by post is Button Box (send SAE for leaflet). Two mail-order suppliers of haberdashery (eg fastenings, tape, ribbons, elastic, zips, shoulder pads, facings) are Myra Coles and Couture Haberdashery.

Knitting and needlework I know several YPAs who enjoy knitting, though it's something OTs aren't usually too keen on for dodgy finger joints. For mail-order supplies, both Readicut and Falcon by Post produce wonderful catalogues with designs, well-known yarns, books, plus useful accessories (Readicut's includes a set of bamboo and birch needles which they say are ideal for people with arthritis). Other suppliers of wool by post are the Direct Wool Group, St John's Wools, Yorkshire Mohair Mill and Brockwell Wools (both do a wide range: from acrylic or wool or cotton, to mohair or even silk or alpaca). Needlework kit suppliers include Readicut (their crafts catalogue includes 210 shades of Paterna pure wool yarn), Needlework Kits by post (all sorts, plus special Christmas and

Easter designs), the Royal School of Needlework, St John's Wools. All produce wonderfully inspirational catalogues.

Other crafts   Endless possibilities! Seek inspiration in magazines, your local library and bookshop, the Search catalogue, catalogues below and Women's Institute publications. Mail-order firms can supply everything from patchwork templates, dolls' house fittings, soft toy fillings and patterns, to teddy bear eyes and growlers! There's usually a small cost for the catalogue, so check by phone or SAE first. Suppliers include:

- Fred Aldous, Manchester: jam-packed catalogue includes candle, cracker and paper flower making, crochet and leather work, raffia, embroidery tapestries, dolls' kits, faces, toy stuffings, fur fabrics. (Send two first-class stamps for the catalogue.)
- Beckfoot Mill: vast range, like Fred Aldous. Includes soft toy kits, patchwork templates, handicraft kits, craft books.
- Marsland Textiles: patchwork pieces, remnants and materials, from gent's suiting to lurex lamé and gingham, and zips, vilene, etc.
- Midas Mail Order Ltd: catalogue includes craft fabrics and toy making materials
- Craftkit: hobbies from calligraphy to quilling.
- Janet Coles Bead Ltd: very attractive colour catalogue (£2.75, 1991) of ready-made and do-it-yourself earrings and other jewellery.
- Creative Beadcraft Ltd: sequins, stones, iron-on diamanté and beads for embroidery, knitting and trimming. Also earring wires and necklace clasps, shoe and hair clips to decorate.
- Hobby Horse Ltd: everything for costume jewellery.

Singing and Music

Pamela Waterhouse found it very frustrating when RA stopped her doing her favourite keep-fit, yoga, and disco dancing:

> *"Luckily, I also have a small singing talent and have always been in a choir or singing group. I was always too nervous to sing solo but in the last four years I am quite in demand locally! I'm making this sound quite grand but I have sung to an audience of 200 and often sing to a group of about 100 ladies in WI. I can't believe it's me sometimes."*

Maybe, like me, you aren't sure you share Pamela's talent? Despite grave doubts about hitting the right note, I was fired with enthusiasm by my keen singing friend Gwen (also with RA), and found some Saturday afternoon classes for beginners. Nerve-racking at first, but we were all in the same wobbly boat. I still can't sing brilliantly, but I felt really exhilarated after the classes. Wonderful to do something with my body which I could (more or less) control, unlike most of the time when it does its own thing regardless.

A good starting point might be a local choir which doesn't take things too seriously. Your local library could help you find one. Many already have members with a disability, and should be helpful if you explain any arthritis difficulties. An alternative to a regular commitment would be to go on a residential singing weekend. Gwen and I sampled some. Great fun. Details in NIACE's *Time to Learn*. A couple of helpful books are Graham Hewitt's *How to Sing* (Elm Tree Books) and Howard Shanet's *Learn to Read Music* (Faber). Even if you can't get out to classes or a choir, practice at home, learn a few songs, and lead the festivities at the next get-together of friends or family!

Some YPAs have made records. *Frost at Midnight* is a cassette of songs by Alan and Denise Whittle (available by post from them). Many are 'country' songs, but some are about Denise's arthritis, eg *Cure for Arthritis Rag* and one about other people's reactions to her *"What do you find to do all day...sitting in that chair?"*. Young Arthritis Care Contact Julia-Ann Kerner wrote and recorded *Christmas All Over the World* (copies available from her). Another Contact, Kata Kolbert, is a singer/songwriter whose records include *Live Your Life* (Nevermore) and *By Word of Mouth*. She's happy to give advice to anyone wanting to know more about making records or selling songs. She's an enthusiastic member of the London Disability Arts Forum (LDAF), which has:

"registers of disabled performers in all areas of the arts and and organises 'workhouse' cabaret evenings all over the capital on a regular basis, where disabled artists perform (for a fee) in accessible venues...Even if like myself, someone wishes to perform for disabled and non-disabled people alike, getting on to the disability arts circuit is a must. Not only is it very active and vibrant, growing all the time, but it offers a good grounding in the art of performing...One important point: the views of many performers of this scene are considered radical and 'anti-establishment': we're not talking about 'art therapy' or 'charity' peforming – in fact charity is a dirty word in these circles and if these views make you feel uncomfortable then you may not fit in!"

Playing music, rather than singing, may be difficult, but Janice Simons found she could manage a small electronic keyboard (weighing 1.5 kg/3.3 lb):

"Soon I was able to play quite acceptable tunes from the large lettered music..The sounds that can be made with the 44 small keys and nine instrument voices sound really quite professional, anything from string, flute, piano, guitar, to vibraphone, together with the rhythm box of waltz, swing, rock, and latin, make some really up-to-date music. Accompanying the melody with the left hand [is] less of a problem than on a piano where you need to be able to span the keys. These keyboards have a one-finger chord button which when depressed turns the keys at the left-hand side of the keyboard into automatic chords, thereby making one key sound like a three-finger chord." (*In Contact*)

Artsline can supply general information to help with musical projects both amateur and professional. Besides giving information about access to the arts for people with disabilities it actively encourages participation in the arts and can tell you what exists in different parts of the country.

Photography

Many of us enjoy taking and showing photographs. There are courses and clubs for anyone who wants to take it more seriously; ask your local library for information. The Disabled Photographers' Society can advise on overcoming disability problems, publishes a newsletter with equipment, tips, sales, small ads, and also runs an annual competition.

Glyn Barney, who developed RA at 15, works as a freelance photographer, and has worked for *Homes and Gardens*, the publishers EMAP (particularly on custom car magazines), and for Shell. He took a three year diploma course in photography at West Surrey College of Art and Design. The photographs on the cover of this book were all taken by Glyn.

Penfriends

If your legs won't take you to meet other people and to see other countries, this is certainly one way of overcoming the frustration. Great fun, anyway, even if that's *not* a problem. One YPA, who's in her 20s and has had RA since she was 16, has 70 or so penfriends!

Some penfriend clubs cater specially for people with disabilities, some are mixed, and others are general, for anyone. If you have difficulty writing, you might prefer a club where correspondence is by tape or cassette. Send an SAE always, when writing to a club for information. Specially for disabled people:

- For people under 35, contact Carolyne Lees, c/o Young Arthritis Care. If you're over 45, contact Arthritis Care for details of the 'Caring Friends Pen Club'
- *Wider Horizons* is a magazine by people of all ages, plus correspondence groups.
- *Contact* is a monthly postal tape magazine, which includes stories, poems, interviews, music and news. Recorders available on loan to members. Details from Birmingham Tapes for the Handicapped Association.

– Correspondence club specially for disabled and housebound people uses letter, tape or telephone. Details from Lisa Rowe.

Two special interest correspondence clubs (for anyone, not just people with a disability):

– The Postal Scrabble Club (PSC) has over 200 members around the country who play Scrabble by correspondence

– The Hardy Plant Society has a correspondents' group of people interested in hardy perennials, bulbs, and other border plants.

You could ask if your library knows of others, connected with your own special interests. Other 'non-disabled' general groups (don't forget to send an SAE) include:

– Safari, which runs correspondence groups, each of six to eight people. Letters are generally chatty or on a specific topic, eg animal lovers, housework haters, gardeners.

– The International Friendship League (IFL) aims to promote a spirit of mutual respect and friendship among peoples of the world. As part of its work, it runs two pen-friend schemes: IFL Pen-Friend Service to link people of all ages in the UK and Ireland with pen-friends overseas; and IFL Pen-Friend Service UK to link people in one part of the British Isles with pen-friends in other parts. Vice-Presidents of the League include Terry Waite, Sir David Steel, and Katie Boyle.

Citizens' Band Radio

"I discovered CB radio and soon made lots of friends. Even now eight years on I don't know what I'd do without it. I joined clubs and went on 'eyeballs' and to meetings. Even my Mam used to go to the discos. Even romance has blossomed a few times although nothing permanent as yet! It's great company for me." (Janet Mason, JCA)

To join in, you'd need a CB transceiver, not cheap (cheaper second-hand) plus small transformer, but after that it's cheaper than the phone because there's no charge for 'calls'. There's a special magazine and many areas have local CB clubs with social evenings and talks. Some members volunteer to run the emergency channel on which people can call for help. For information send for *CB Citizens' Band magazine.*

The countryside and birdwatching

The Royal Society for the Protection of Birds (RSPB) produces leaflets on birdwatching, including *RSPB Reserves for the Disabled* which describes reserves with wide surfaced pathways and nature trails, special boardwalks, rest benches, toilet facilities, birdwatching hides and information centres. There are also leaflets for armchair birdwatchers! The Suffolk Ornithologists' Group has produced the excellent low-cost *Easy Birdwatching*: a guide, with maps and photos, to access and facilities at 60 sites mainly in Suffolk. In Court Associates do a gadget, Threshold A Frame, which makes supporting binoculars easier for people with stiff shoulders.

The Countryside and Wildlife for Disabled People (RADAR, in association with the Country Landowners' Charitable Trust) lists over 950 accessible sites throughout the UK, and includes birdwatching, beauty spots, fishing, farm and nature trails, and bed and breakfast places. I visited two sites recently, Pensthorpe Waterfowl Park (near Fakenham, Norfolk) and Peakirk Wildfowl Trust, Cambridgeshire – both fascinating, and wheel-chair/electric scooter accessible.

The AA *Travellers' Guide for the Disabled* includes a section on countryside parks and picnic sites with special toilet facilities. Several water authorities publish helpful leaflets, eg Welsh Water's free booklet *Reservoir Recreation with Special Interest to the Disabled* (fishing, birdwatching, accessible Visitors' Centres and car parks with good views). Ask your own local water authority if they produce anything similar.

Besides historic houses, the National Trust owns more than 100 beautiful gardens, 465 miles of breathtaking coastline, 530,000 acres of open countryside and entire villages. The Trust produces a booklet *Facilities for Disabled and Visually Handicapped Visitors* (free for SAE). It includes NT properties where you can borrow a wheelchair, just for your visit; phone beforehand to check availability.

Even some of the NT's countryside facilities are more accessible than you might imagine. Wicken Fen, for instance, is a nature reserve where the Trust has built a circular 1km long boardwalk route that gives wheelchair users the chance to see unusual wetland. There's also a disabled toilet and exhibition centre with ramped entrance.

Gardening

One compensation for being forced to slow down by the arthritis is finding more time to enjoy nature and the changing seasons. And a garden, provided it doesn't become a burden, can be a real tonic, and incentive to 'keep going' as you wait eagerly to see what each season unfolds.

"At the moment I'm sitting in a small conservatory which we had built on to the back of our house. It's so peaceful, as I watch the birds come and go, with the sound of light rain hitting the glass. The garden isn't huge, by any means, but it's full of various shrubs and flowers. Hubby curses the job of looking after the garden but when it's done and tidy it really is lovely." (Marilyn S, who has psoriatic arthritis.)

You might still manage all or some of the gardening yourself. Make things easier by changing the layout and plant types. Find the right tools to overcome bending, reaching and gripping problems. Sit instead of standing, and ration carefully what you do and don't do. Or copy one YPA's particular talent: *"although only able to participate in a limited way I am however very good at supervising and nagging my husband in the garden!"*

I concentrate on perennials, ground cover plants and on allowing nature to do its own thing (partly, anyway), and have actually won local flower show prizes for my apples and roses! I sit on a high stool to garden and use long-handled lightweight tools, which include a long-handled weeder and long-handled flower-picker which cuts the flower then holds it (from suppliers on page 144), and a lightweight range of garden tools which fit interchangeably on to a long extension handle. Mine are by Gardena; Wolf Tools make others, and Griffin tools have variable telescopic handles, adjustable for individual height and reach. One of my best finds is a ratchet pruner, which cuts easily through anything from a flower stem to a thickish branch with next to no strain on the fingers (Ceka Works).

Look for problem-solvers in the excellent *Gardening* (in the Disability Information Trust's *Equipment for Disabled People* series). It includes garden design, garden tools, choice of plants, tackling weeds, hanging baskets, indoor gardening, buying wisely, clubs for disabled gardeners, other sources of information. Superb ideas for any gardener.

DLF's *Leisure Activities* sheet lists other books with a specifically disabled slant. Look too at the vast range of garden books aimed at making life easier for *any* gardener, like Judith Berrisford's *The Weekend Garden* (Faber), Laurence Fleming's *The One Hour Garden* (Ward Lock). Learning about weed control techniques, mulching, ground cover plants, etc, all helps cut down on the work.

Plenty of enjoyable gardening can be done simply sitting in an armchair, looking through the window, or browsing through gardening books and magazines and catalogues for hours on end. For inspirational books look out for writers like Christopher Lloyd, Rosemary Verey, Robin Lane Fox, Peggy Cole, Alan Titchmarsh, and Dorothy Hammond-Innes (Her *My Home is My Garden* is just the read when confined miserably to bed).

Seeds and seed catalogues (eg Suttons, Thompsons, Hilliers, Mr Fothergill's), and plants (eg Highfield Nurseries) are available by post; these and others are advertised widely in newspapers and gardening magazines. Try some unusual ones too, for instance:

–   Suffolk Herbs: fascinating list of seeds for herbs, wild flowers, unusual vegetables, salads, even oriental vegetables. Includes tips, eg how to grow and use the plants, pennyroyal is a great ant repellent, nasturtiums are edible and high in vitamin C.

–   Chiltern Seeds: no pictures, but entrancing descriptions of seeds from all over the world. You can buy exotic seeds, plus the dreams that go with them, quite cheaply.

- Carnivorous Plants speaks for itself! Easy to grow as house plants, need little attention, and fascinating to watch as they devour nasty house-flies and other insects.
- Unusual Plants (Beth Chatto): Specialises in interesting plants for difficult areas.
- Growing Carpets specialises in ground cover plants, useful for keeping weeds down.
- The Country Garden sells by post gadgets and garden aids which would otherwise take ages to discover trundling round garden centre after centre. What joy to order from your armchair such delights as slug pubs, a long-handled 'touch' weedkiller, potato barrels, long-arm fruit pickers, or even a brass sundial or croquet set.

Even without a garden you can enjoy window boxes and house plants and growing things from pips. For ideas dip into *The Pip Book* by Keith Mossman (Penguin) or *How to Grow Weird and Wonderful Plants* by Paul Temple (Beaver Books). Hazel Evans' *The City Garden* (Futura) explains how to grow almost anything even if you've only got a window-box. Or how about some plants, or even a whole real garden in miniature (tiny trees, eg willow, mountain ash; fuchsia just 2″ high, even a tiny thatched cottage and miniature lawn mower!). – Get the catalogue *Nursery of Miniatures* from George Thrasher, in Devon. Borrow from somewhere Anne Ashberry's *Miniature Gardens* (David and Charles, 1977, now out of print) or J Constable's *Landscapes in Miniature* (Butterworth, 1984).

You could specialise in a particular type of house plant, for instance:

- *African violets* Send for Tony Clements' catalogue (African Violets Centre).
- *Bonsai* Herons Bonsai sell trees, seeds, books, and special equipment.
- *Cacti* For a mass of cacti and succulents by post, try Abbey Brook Cactus Nursery. More information, too, from the British Cactus and Succulent Society (BCSS).
- *Geraniums* For hundreds (yes) of geranium varieties by post try Redvale Nurseries or the Vernon Geranium Nursery (catalogue includes over 80 miniature varieties). You could contact the British Pelargonium and Geranium Society, too.

The Good Gardener's Guide (Consumers' Association/Hodder & Stoughton) lists many more specialists. Local flower shows are enjoyable, but not if you've got to fight your way through a crush of people. The Ipswich Flower Show thoughtfully opens an hour early on one day, just for disabled visitors. Something worth suggesting in your area?

I've mentioned two specialist clubs above. Another, the Hardy Plant Society, has several specialist groups within it, including a Correspondents' Group. The Group's for anyone who wants to keep in touch, solely through the post, with other people, worldwide, who share an interest in plants. There's a chatty, informative quarterly newsletter. Two clubs now specially for people with disabilities:

- Horticultural Therapy, which publishes a quarterly magazine *Growth Point*, for disabled gardeners. HT has set up centres where gardening tools can be tried out (eg at Battersea Park and Islington, London; Sheffield and Manchester). HT operates through groups of volunteers with skills in horticulture, and through Voluntary Garden Advisers, who help disabled and elderly gardeners.
- The Gardens for the Disabled Trust runs a Garden Club to exchange information, plants, and seeds, and produces a regular magazine. Grants are sometimes available for members to help them adapt a garden.

Sports and physical recreation

You may have to give up very energetic sports like tennis, squash, badminton and football, but you don't have to give up everything. There are other activities you could try, like swimming, pétanque, croquet, horse driving. With the right equipment and help, YPAs at the Kielder Adventure Centure (page 274) have even found themselves riding, canoeing, orienteering, shooting, sailing, abseiling, and doing archery! Try Technical Aids for Disabled People (page 146) for help if a special piece of equipment or modification might make all the difference to your doing or not doing something. Take heart from an *In*

Contact article by Chris Wood (has RA):

"Two years ago, after constant nagging from friends, that swimming (as we all know), would do me the world of good, I learnt to swim. It took me just two lessons to get up the nerve to take both feet off the floor of the pool and from then on there was no stopping me.

"Of course it didn't stop there. Once the lessons were over, I joined a disabled people's sports group at the local recreation centre. And, as I said, there was no stopping me. I have now added darts, skittles and table tennis to my repertoire, although I can't own to be an expert in any of them.

"...I always had a desire to try archery. No doubt you're thinking it's a strange sport to want to try, since it requires strength in the arms and hands. But, with help from an expert to choose suitably weighted equipment, I was able to have a fair crack at it. And surprisingly enough there were no serious after-effects. Mind you, I can't claim to be ready for the Olympics, I haven't even hit the target! But it has made me a lot more open-minded about trying new ventures, instead of being so sure I'd be no good..."

Whatever you decide to try, get your doctor's blessing first, and do it only if you and your body enjoy it and feel some benefit. Don't see it as a challenge match between you and a disobedient body. If it causes pain and strains your joints, stop.

You could also participate by becoming, say, a cricket scorer, a tennis umpire, or simply a keen spectator. You might find helpful Peter Lawton's *Spectators' Access Guide for Disabled People* (RADAR). It includes all sorts of sports and over 250 venues, with information on viewing facilities, car parking, access to toilets.

The DLF produces a long list of sport and recreational facilities for disabled people plus useful publications. The major national co-ordinating body for sport – the Sports Council – can put you in touch with the national organisation for any particular sport. Even if it doesn't specifically cater for people with a disability it may be able to offer advice. Try the British Sports Association for Disabled People too, and your local DIAL.

Swimming Swimming's the A1 sport for grotty joints, allowing us to exercise muscles without straining joints or fighting against gravity. There are sometimes off-putting problems like public sessions monopolised by Incredible Hulks or Over-Active Brats.. One YPA solved the problem by getting a special session set up on Saturday evenings. Another decided the fact she couldn't swim was irrelevant:

"I was in one of my bulldozing moods in which I don't even contemplate defeat. I would buy three pairs of armbands for myself and the kids and we would all splash about merrily together in the learners' pool, and I wouldn't care a damn if people wondered who on earth was the misshapen 30 year old woman with armbands. So before all my good intentions came unstuck and before my knees turned back to jelly I phoned the Olympic pool, explained my difficulties to one of the managers and was kindly informed that we (me, hubby and kids) could use one of the school changing rooms any Sunday. In that way, hubby would be there to help dry and dress me." (PB)

Find out if there are special sessions locally, eg for adults only, ladies only, or specifically for disabled people (sometimes warmer than usual). Some pools may have a hoist, or special steps to help you get in and out. Ask your local authority's Leisure Department, or the Association of Swimming Therapy. AST has over 50 clubs in Britain, and runs special sessions, with trained instructors and helpers if needed, so you could go along even if you've no one to go with you. Some clubs can even help out with transport. The AST has published a book *Swimming for the Disabled*. Glenda Baum's *Aquarobics* (Arrow Books) is 'non-disabled', but might give you ideas for adding interest to water sessions: check which are OK first with your doctor or physio. One YPA who tried them out enjoyed the slow warm-up and wind-down sections, but very sensibly avoided the fast middle section.

Exercise supervised by physios/hydrotherapists in very warm water, hydrotherapy, is prescribed for some people with arthritis. Pools are specially equipped to ease getting in and out, and some have sessions open to the public, eg the Worcestershire Clinic & Brine Bath in Droitwich, and the pool in Nairn, Scotland, managed by the Nairn Hydrotherapy Trust, a charity. Members of Arthritis Care can use the hydrotherapy pool at the Horder Centre for Arthritis, Crowborough, East Sussex, at a reduced cost. Ask your local DIAL or rheumatologist if there's anything similar near you.

Pétanque   The French equivalent of bowls, pétanque (or 'boules') is something Haydn Martin (RA diagnosed at 44) enjoys:

"Having played most sports myself to a fairly high standard and eventually having to give them up and as a result, inevitably losing contact with various circles of friends, I can truthfully say that the people who play pétanque are the most friendly and without exception wherever I have played have made me most welcome."

You can play pétanque purely for pleasure, or take it up competitively. Haydn takes part in international competitions. His team has represented Britain in the World Pétanque Championships. His other talents – artistic – have led to him selling caricatures of pétanque players and giving the proceeds to arthritis research. For the name of your nearest club contact the British Pétanque Association. By the way, there's a natty gadget for avoiding problems bending to pick up the boule – a magnetic boule lifter, available from OBUT Boule (UK), who sell a range of boules accessories.

Boating and sailing   Specially designed dinghies at places like the Kielder Adventure Centre allow people even very disabled by arthritis to have a go. Find out about other opportunities through Water Authority leaflets. Some inland waterways narrowboats are now specially modified to take disabled people. The British Waterways Board publishes a list of operators.

On a larger scale, how about crewing a square-rigged sailing vessel at sea? The sailing ship Lord Nelson is purpose-built to be crewed by a team of able-bodied and physically-handicapped people working together. There are lifts between all decks, which are all flush with no steps, the main mast has a lift seat, there's an audio compass for blind people, and a bright track radar screen for partially sighted people, etc. Each cruise lasts an average of 11 days. Most of the volunteer team is sponsored (maybe a self-help group or charity might help sponsor you?). Details from the Jubilee Sailing Trust.

Angling   'Wheelyboats' are wheelchair-accessible boats for fishing on inland waters, and there are now over 20 dotted around the country, from Craigavon Lake, Northern Ireland and Alaw Reservoir, Gwynedd to Elsham Park, Yorkshire and Ardleigh Reservoir, Essex. Individual water managers have information on hire charges and availability – contact your water authority, or the Handicapped Anglers' Trust for information. Gadgets like the 'Rodmaster' may help some people – it transfers the weight of a rod from wrist to upper arm (from Hawton Ltd).

Horse riding and horse driving   *"Before arriving at the Kielder Adventure Centre my last ride on a horse had been 19 years back when I was 12. A bad experience at that time, and the difficulty of getting on to a horse ever since, had convinced me that I would never ever ride a horse again...With the help of some of the Centre's staff we were able to get on our mounts. The same staff led us on our walk, each one leading one of the horses on a length of rope...It was a great experience. Life seemed different from the pony's saddle, slower, but with more to see."* (Peter Nightingale, writing in *In Contact*)

If Peter could do it, how about you? Contact the Riding for the Disabled Association for the address of your nearest branch. As an alternative to sitting on a horse, how about driving one, comfortably seated on a specially converted buggy, accompanied by a trained attendant? Contact Riding for the Disabled, and ask about 'Driving for the Disabled', or contact the British Driving Society.

Cycling Some YPAs manage on ordinary bikes or trikes; one Irish friend (with RA and 15-year old knee replacement) enjoys cycling holidays in France. Another, Babette, 'enjoys' the occasional sponsored bike ride: *"it feels good to be able to join in"*. Others, like Pamela Waterhouse, use an adapted bike now and again (page 184).

Ask your local DIAL if there's anything locally like the Cycling for Disabled People cycle hire scheme, operated by the Macclesfield Groundwork Trust. They hire out tandems and tricycles at Tatton Park, Cheshire.

Flying Have you ever dreamed of learning to fly? *And* at someone else's expense? In memory of Sir Douglas Bader the Royal Air Force Benevolent Fund annually awards several 'Flying Scholarships for Disabled People'. Each is for a flying course of about a month at an approved flying school. Candidates must be between 17 and 40 years old, and registered disabled. Apply in October to Flying Scholarships for Disabled People.

Shortlisted candidates attend a residential selection board at RAF Biggin Hill in April. It's the same as prospective jet fighter pilots undergo, and therefore pretty strenuous and demanding. I speak from personal experience! The Board was stimulating and fun, and the other candidates were great company. (Hot tip: brush up on your maths.) Alas I didn't win a scholarship, but received a consolation prize of complimentary tickets for the fabulous International Air Tattoo at RAF Fairford the following July.

The Duke of Edinburgh's Award Scheme

The booklet *A Challenge to the Individual* describes how a young person with a disability can take part. Details from Duke of Edinburgh's Award Office. The scheme's in four sections – service, expedition, skills and physical recreation.

Competitions

A good way of passing the time *and* giving yourself something to look forward to: the day you win! There are two newspapers for keen competitors – the *Competitors' Journal* (CJ), fortnightly, which dates from 1913, and the more recent *Competitors' Companion* (CC), monthly. Both list current competitions with closing dates, and give helpful tips.

Computers

For a total novice's introduction, look at books in the children's section of your library or bookshop, something like *The Beginner's Computer Handbook* (Usborne), and go on from there! Or L R Carter and E Huzan's *Computers and Their Use* (Teach Yourself Books, Hodder & Stoughton). Computing magazines and user groups (eg Amstrad User Group, Lotus User Group) are treasure-troves of information. You can enjoy computing at so many different levels, and who knows, a computing hobby might lead to a computing career. (See also pages 254 and 269.) Roger Jefcoate (page 146) can give specialised advice on using and obtaining computers, and tell you about any special discounts. For instance, as I write, IBM is offering a 40% discount on all PC and PS/2 products to disabled people who would 'gain therapeutic or rehabilitative benefits through using the products'. The British Computer Society has a special Disability Programme, with a quarterly journal and an advice helpline. The DLF publishes *Computers and Accessories for Disabled People*.

Clubs

Joining a club or society connected with your hobby or other interests, eg environment or politics, is an excellent way of making friends and taking your mind off the arthritis. Ask at your local library or church for information on local clubs (some have nursery or 'baby-watching' facilities, if needed). One YPA got back into church life, where she found herself *"part of a lively, caring church"*, joined two choirs, and *"all in all I rarely seem to have an evening in. I wonder how I found the time to go to work."*

Don't overlook clubs like Young Arthritis Care/Arthritis Care, other self-help groups, or PHAB (Physically Handicapped and Able Bodied, page 122). Just because they're geared to people with a disability or arthritis doesn't mean that you won't find a lively group of people with a kaleidoscope of interests there too. (*And* you'll be accepted for what you are, rather than a curiosity-that-must-be-cross-examined.) PHAB has more than 450 clubs where physically handicapped and able-bodied people meet and mix. Or channel your energy into your local ARC group, DIAL, or Access group. It's good to feel you can make something positive out of your unwanted acquaintance with the arthritis.

Several general (non-disabled) social clubs operate throughout Britain including:

−   Nexus (founded 1974): local groups countrywide of men and women (single, divorced, widowed), who meet for friendship and social events and mutual support (given through the 'Skill bank', everything from shifting wardrobes to baking cakes or hanging curtains). Members receive regular bulletins, a Leisure Interest Directory, and the Folio, a collection of open letters ('ice-breakers') from members writing about their interests. Through the Tape Service you can dial a special number and hear members talking about themselves.

−   National Federation of Solo Clubs: less expensive, local clubs for single, divorced, widowed, separated people aged between 25 and 65. Arranges holidays.

There are plenty of groups, too, linked to particular hobbies and interests, many dotted around this book, for instance gardening/plant clubs (page 288), fishing (page 290), pétanque and other sports (page 288 onwards), for homeworkers (OwnBase, page 270). Also, for anyone, married or single, with a spice-loving palate, there's even the Curry Club!

Women's clubs

Many people with arthritis are young mums or middle-aged housewives, who can feel isolated and miserable, stuck at home. Besides making contacts through Arthritis Care or NCT (page 234), other groups are worth trying too, as Pamela Waterhouse (with RA) found:

"I joined WI 18 months ago. It was one of my better decisions. It has given me a lot of enjoyment and fun. I even persuaded my mother to join. I was honoured to be voted on to the committee in November and am now 'Press and Publicity Officer' which keeps me quite busy."

The National Federation of Women's Institutes can tell you where your nearest WI is. Branches hold monthly meetings with talks. The Federation also has its own Adult Education College, Denman College, in Berkshire. Here are some other (also non-disabled) women's groups to choose from:

−   National Union of Townswomen's Guilds: offers women the chance to exchange ideas, learn new skills, lobby on women's issues and make new friends.

−   National Women's Register: local groups meet in members' homes for discussions on anything, from green issues to crime prevention, alternative medicine to running a business, ie anything *except* home and babies.

−   National Association of Women's Clubs: aimed at women who want to meet others for friendship, recreation, education, and social service.

−   National Council of Women of Great Britain: a pressure group, working for the establishment of human rights, particularly the rights of women.

The Women's National Commission (WNC) publishes a free booklet − *Women's Organisations in Great Britain*, which lists more than 160 groups.

SELECT BIBLIOGRAPHY
for doctors and other healthcare professionals
(please look at publications mentioned elsewhere in the book too!)

– *Rehabilitation in Rheumatology. The Team Approach*, by Anthony Clarke, Louise Allard, Bridget Braybrooks (Martin Dunitz, 1987). Overview of the long-term management of the rheumatic patient, aimed at the rheumatology rehabilitation team, including physio, OT, GP, nurse, consultant, surgeon and counsellor.

Anthony Clarke is Consultant in Rheumatology and Rehabilitation at the Royal National Hospital for Rheumatic Diseases in Bath (RNHRD). Louise Allard, formerly RNHRD Deputy Superintendant Physiotherapist, went on to read medicine at Bristol University. Bridget Braybrooks, former RNHRD OT, went on to work at the Lee Abbey Fellowship, Lynton, Devon.

– *Practical Problems in Rheumatology*, by Dr F Dudley Hart, Consultant Rheumatologist (Martin Dunitz, 1983). Comprehensive and very readable. Aims 'to help the baffled diagnostician and assist the confused therapist with some of the more common rheumatic problems'.

– *Manual of Rheumatology*, by J M H Moll (Churchill Livingstone, 1987). Professor Moll is Head of the Sheffield Centre for Rheumatic Diseases. A succinct and convenient manual 'for busy junior clinicians'.

– *Essentials of Rheumatology*, by H L F Currey (Churchill Livingstone, 1983). Written by the Emeritus Professor of Rheumatology, The Royal London Hospital Medical College and Consultant Rheumatologist, The Royal London Hospital. Intended for clinical medical students, but useful for other people wanting a succinct account.

– *The Image of Rheumatic Disease*, by Jan Maycock, a chapter in *Altered Body Image. The Nurse's Role*, edited by Mave Salter (John Wiley, Chichester, 1988). Jan Maycock RGN RM is Nurse Practitioner, Rheumatology, Waltham Forest Health Authority. Excellent analysis of the psychological impact and management of rheumatic disease.

– *Disability and Disadvantage. The Consequences of Chronic Illness*, by David Locker (Tavistock, 1983). Study by Professor Locker and the Department of Community Medicine of St Thomas' Hospital Medical School of the disadvantage and deprivation experienced by a group of individuals with RA. Should be required reading for all doctors, healthcare professionals, and anyone who needs to understand the far-reaching impact RA can have on people's lives.

– *Meanings at Risk: The Experience of Arthritis* by Michael Bury, a chapter in *Living with Chronic Illness* (Unwin Hyman, 1988), edited by Robert Anderson (Institute for Social Studies in Medical Care, London) and Michael Bury (Royal Holloway and Bedford New College, University of London). Explains that something like RA can't be viewed in terms of physical functioning alone: patients also have to live with what the illness means, its impact on daily life and an altered future. Analysis and implications for 'service providers'.

Professionals may also find of interest the bibliographies in these two books:

– *Alternative Therapies. A Guide to Complementary Medicine for the Health Professional* edited by G T Lewith (Heinemann Medical, London, 1985). Dr Lewith MA MRCP MRCGP is Co-Director, Centre for the Study of Complementary Medicine, Southampton.

– *Controlling Chronic Pain*, by Connie Peck (HarperCollins Publishers Ltd). Foreword by Professor Patrick D Wall, MD FRCP. Connie Peck is Senior Lecturer in the Department of Psychology at La Trobe University, Australia, and member of the International Association for the Study of Pain.

Papers

– *Psychological Factors in Patients with Chronic Rheumatoid Arthritis*, review by B Oberai and J R Kirwan, Bristol Royal Infirmary Rheumatology Unit, (in *Annals of the Rheumatic Diseases, 1988, 47*, 969 – 971, British Medical Association). *"Although there are clear anatomical and physiological changes in patients with chronic rheumatoid arthritis (RA), evidence is accumulating for the importance of psycho-*

logical factors as determinants of disease development and of patients' ability to adapt to their condition. There is also an increasing awareness that arthritis treatment and education programmes can be improved by paying more attention to the problems patients face in adapting to a chronic disease both physically and psychologically."

– *The Burden of Rheumatoid Arthritis: Tolerating the Uncertainty*, by C L Wiener, Dept of Behavioral Science, University of California, USA. (*Social Science & Medicine*, 9, 97 – 104). Clear analysis of the often poorly understood socio-psychological implications of living with a fluctuating, intermittent chronic disorder, where uncertainty is exaggerated beyond the usual levels of toleration.

– *Managing a Life with Chronic Disease*, L Reif (*American Journal of Nursing, 1973.* 73, 262 – 265, Pergamon Press plc). Looks specifically at ulcerative colitis, but the basic argument is relevant to chronic rheumatic disorders: "*The conventional perspective defines the medical problems as central, the goal as managing illness, the central managers as the medical personnel, and the central activity as medical intervention.*" Instead, Reif identifies the consequences of illness – "*social and occupational, as well as medical – as central; the goal as managing life in the face of chronic illness; the central actor-manager as the sick person and the central actions as redesign of life style coupled with medical intervention.*"

– *Effects of Psychological Therapy on Pain Behavior of Rheumatoid Arthritis Patients*, by L A Bradley, L D Young, K O Anderson, and others in the Bowman Gray School of Medicine of Wake Forest University, Winston-Salem, North Carolina, USA (*Arthritis and Rheumatism*, 30, 10, Oct 1987, 1105 – 1114). Report of a randomized clinical trial demonstrating reduced pain behaviour, disease activity, and trait anxiety following psychological treatment, of which relaxation training may have been the most important component.

– *Determinants of Disability in Rheumatoid Arthritis*, by A C McFarlane and P M Brooks, Dept of Psychiatry, School of Medicine, Flinders University of South Australia, and Dept of Rheumatology, Royal North Shore Hospital, St Leonards, NSW, Australia (*British Journal of Rheumatology*, 1988; 27: 7 – 14). Longitudinal study of 30 patients with RA over three year period. Psychological factors consistently predicted more of the variance of disability than disease activity, and required specific attention in rehabilitation programmes.

– *Outcomes of Self-Help Education for Patients with Arthritis*, by K Lorig, D Lubeck, R G Kraines, and others, Dept of Medicine, Stanford University, Stanford, California (in *Arthritis and Rheumatism*, 28, 6 June 1985, 680 – 685, J B Lippincott Co). "*Behavioral and health status outcomes of an unreinforced, self-help education program for arthritis patients taught by lay persons were examined in two ways: a four-month randomized experiment and a 20-month longitudinal study. At four months, experimental subjects significantly exceeded control subjects in knowledge, recommended behaviors, and in lessened pain. These changes remained significant at 20 months. The course was inexpensive and well-accepted by patients, physicians, and other health professionals.*"

– *The Impact of Chronic Disease. A Sociomedical Profile of Rheumatoid Arthritis* by R F Meenan, E H Yelin, M Nevitt and W V Epstein, from the Multipurpose Arthritis Center, Boston University and elsewhere (*Arthritis and Rheumatism*, 24, 3, March 1981, 544 – 549). Survey of 245 people with RA, and its impact in the areas of work, finances, and family structure, raising questions of emphasis and approach for physicians involved in the clinical care of chronic rheumatic disease patients.

AA RADAR Group: see Automobile Association

Abbey Brook Cactus Nursery 288
The Desert Life Plant Centre, Bakewell Rd,
Matlock, Derbyshire DE4 2QJ. 0629 580306

Able-Label 112, 176
Steepleprint Ltd, Earls Barton, Northampton
NN6 0LS. 0604 810781

**ACAS (Advisory Conciliation and Arbitration
Service) 267, 270**
83 Euston Rd, London NW1. 071 388 5100

Access Committee 117
35 Great Smith St, London SW1P 3BJ.
071 233 2566

Adams & Jones 156
White Cottage Courtyard, Magdalene St,
Glastonbury, Somerset BA6 9EH. 0458 34356

**Adult Literacy & Basic Skills Unit 244-245,
271-272**
229 - 231 High Holborn, London WC1V 7DA.
071 405 4017

African Violets Centre 288
Terrington St Clements, Kings Lynn, Norfolk
PE3 4PL. 0553 828374

Age Concern England 118, 174
Astral House, 1268 London Rd, London
SU16 4ER. 081 679 8000

Aid Vehicle Supplies (AVS) 187
Hockley Industrial Estate, Hooley Lane, P O
Box 26, Redhill, RH1 6JF. 0737 770030

Allergy Shop 178
P O Box 196, Haywards Heath, West Sussex,
RH16 3YF. 0444 414290

Amstrad User Group 291
PRE Complex, Pallian Ind Estate,
Sunderland, Tyne and Wear SR4 6SN.
091 5108787

Aremco 279
Grove House, Lenham, Kent ME17 2PX.
0622 858502

**Arthritis and Rheumatism Council (ARC) 113,
118, 6, 17, 25, 144**
Copeman House, St Mary's Court, St Mary's
Gate, Chesterfield, Derbyshire S41 7TD.
0246 558033

ARC Cards Ltd 177
Brunel Drive, Northern Rd Industrial Estate,
Newark, Notts NG24 2DE. 0636 73054

**Arthritis Care 113, 118, 16, 17, 22, 25, 144,
249, 251, 275, 279, 285**
18 - 20 Stephenson Way, London NW1 2HD.
071 916 1500. Wyeth Helpline: Freephone
0800 289 170

Arthritis Homecare 140
Leslie and Godwin, Freepost (RCC 1687),
Horley, Surrey, RH6 7ZA. 0293 820888

Arts Council 247
14 Great Peter St, London SW1P 3NQ.
071 333 0100

Artsline Ltd 276
5 Crowndale Rd, London NW1 1TU.
071 388 2227

Ashdown Smokers 178
Skellerah Farm, Corney, Cumbria LA19 5TW.
065 78 324

Ashwellthorpe Hall Holiday Hotel 275
Ashwellthorpe, Norwich, Norfolk NR16 1EX.
050 841 324

Association of Disabled Professionals 138, *261*
Hon Sec Miss S J Maynard, 170 Benton Hill,
Horbury, West Yks WF4 5HW.

Association of Swimming Therapy 289
Hon Sec T Cowen, 4 Oak St, Shrewsbury,
Salop SY3 7RH. 0743 4393

Attends Advisory Service 175
Procter & Gamble Ltd. 091 279 2279

**Autohome, Disabled Travellers' Motoring Club
139**
0604 232334

Automobile Association (AA) 139, 186, 278
Farnum House, Basing View, Basingstoke,
Hants RG21 2EA. AA RADAR: 0800 262050

Avon 179
Nunn Mills Rd, Northampton, NN1 5PA.
0604 232425

Back to School catalogue 236
Freephone 0800 269 396

Banstead Mobility Centre 186
Damson Way, Orchard Hill, Queen Mary's Ave,
Carshalton, Surrey SM5 4NR. 081 770 1151

J Barnicoat (Falmouth) Ltd 115
P O Box 11, Falmouth, Cornwall TR10 9EN.
0326 372628

BBC Radio 114, 282
Broadcasting House, Portland Place, London
W1A 1AA. 071 580 4468

BBC TV and Books
Woodlands, 80 Wood Lane, London W12 0TT.
081 576 2000

Beacon Associates 185
65a Sheen Lane, East Sheen, London
SW14 8AD. 081 878 7060

Beckfoot Mill 284
Clock Mill, Denholme BD13 4DN.
0274 830063

Benefits Enquiry Line (BEL) 112, 127
Freephone 0800 882200

Birch Products Ltd 185
37 Homewood Ave, Cuffley, Potters Bar, Herts
EN6 4QQ. 0707 873075

**Birmingham Tapes for the Handicapped
Association 285**
20 Middleton Hall Rd, Kings Norton,
Birmingham B30 1BY. 021 459 4874.

Body Shop International plc 178
Hawthorn Rd, Littlehampton, West Sussex
BN17 7LR. 0903 717107

BON (British Organisation of Non-Parents) 227
BM Box 5866, London WC1N 3XX

Books for Children 236
P O Box 70, Cirencester, LL7 7AZ.
0793 420000

Books for Keeps 236
6 Brightfield Rd, London SE12 8QF.
081 852 4953

Boots Customer Services 145
1 Thane Rd West, Nottingham NG2 3AA.
0602 592537

Braun Electric (UK) Ltd 152
Dolphin Estate, Windmill Rd, Sunbury on
Thames, Middlesex TW16 7EJ. 0932 785611

Brenda Redmile 154
32 Cherry Tree Ave, Leicester Forest East,
Leics LE3 3HN. 0533 392079

Britannia Home Video 178
Freepost, Ilford, Essex IG1 2JP.

British Activity Holidays Association 277
Rock Park Centre, Llandrindod Wells, Powys
LD1 6AE. 0597 822021

**British Agencies for Adoption and Fostering
(BAAF)** 230
11 Southwark St, London SE1 1RQ.
071 407 8800.

British Airports Authority Head Office 185
Gatwick Airport, Gatwick, W Sussex RH6 0HZ.

British Assn for Counselling 111
37a Sheep St, Rugby, Warwicks CV21 3BX.
0788 78328/9

British Assn of Wheelchair Distributors 183
Grove Cottage, Packwood Rd, Lapworth,
Solihull, West Midlands B94 6AS.
0564 77384

British Cactus and Succulent Society 288
(Hon Sec T E Jenkins), St Catherine's Lodge,
Cranesgate Rd, Whaplode St Catherine,
Spalding, Lincs PE12 6SR.

British Computer Society 147, 291
13 Mansfield St, London W1M 0FH.
071 637 0471. Disability Programme: Tom
Mangan, c/o City University, Dept CCS,
Walmsley Building, 214 St John St, London
EC1V 2PA.

British Driving Society 291
(Jenny Dillon), 27 Dugard Place, Barford,
Warwickshire CV35 8DX. 0926 624420

British Footwear Manufacturers' Fed 156
Royalty House, 72 Dean St, London
W1V 5HB. 071 437 5573/5

British Gas (Home Services Dept) 134, 163
326 High Holborn, London WC1V 7PT.
071 242 0789

British Holistic Medical Assn 71, 89, 107, 109,
114, 206, 217
179 Gloucester Place, London NW1 6DX.
071 262 5299

British Homeopathic Assn 74
27A Devonshire St, London W1N 1RJ.
071 935 2163

British Library Medical Information Service 116
Medical Library Document Supply Centre,
Boston Spa, Wetherby, W Yorkshire,
LS23 7BQ. 0937 546039

British Medical Acupuncture Society 72
c/o Mrs Marcus, New Ton House, New Ton
Lane, Lower Whitley, Warrington, Cheshire
WA4 4JA. 0925 730727

British Medical Assn 49, 68, 114, 225
BMA House, Tavistock Square, London
WC1H 9JP. 071 387 4499

British Pelargonium and Geranium Society 288
R Clifton, 7 Crabble Rd, Dover, Kent
CT17 0QD.

British Pétanque Assn 290
18 Ensign Business Centre, Westwood Park,
Coventry CV4 8JA. 0203 421408

British Psychological Society 111, 217
St Andrews House, 48 Princess Rd East,
Leicester LE1 7DR. 0533 549568

British Red Cross Society 22, 118, 136, 144,
146, 183, 279
9 Grosvenor Crescent, London SW1X 7EJ. 071
235 5454

British Sjøgren's Syndrome Assn 26
16 Jubilee Close, Cove, Farnborough, Hants,
GU14 9TD.

British Society for Nutritional Medicine 65, 68
Stone House, 9 Weymouth St, London
W1N 3FF. 071 436 8532

British Sports Assn for the Disabled 289
34 Osnaburgh St, London NW1 3ND.
071 383 7277

British Waterways Board 290
Canal Off, Delamere Ter, London W2 6ND.

Brockwell Wools 283
Stansfield Mill, Triangle, Sowerby Bridge
HX6 3LZ. 0422 834343

Brook Advisory Centres 225
Central Office, 153a East Street, London
SE17 2SD. 071 708 1234.

BT 147
Dial 150 (free) for general information.

BT Action for Disabled Customers 147
Room B4036, BT Centre, 81 Newgate St,
London EC1A 7AJ. 0800 919195

Building Research Estab (BRESCU) 134
Garston, Watford WD2 7SR. 0923 664428

Bus and Coach Council 184
Sardinia House, 52 Lincoln's Inn Fields,
London WC2A 3LZ. 071 831 7546

**Business and Technician Education Council
(BTEC)** 245
Central House, Upper Woburn Place, London
WC1H 0HH. 071 388 3288

Button Box 283
44 Bedford Street, Covent Garden, London
WC2E 9HA. 071 240 2716

Buyona (Health and Bodycare) 155
PO Box 13, Unit 5, Lealand Way, Boston,
Lincs, PE21 7SW. 0205 362742

Bymail 179
Freepost, 100 Liberty St, London SW9 0YX.
Freephone 0800 246424

Calibre 281
New Rd, Aylesbury, Bucks HP22 5XQ.
0296 432339/81211

Camp Ltd 155
Staple Gardens, Northgate House, Winchester
SO23 8ST. 0962 55248

Care and Repair 118
22a The Ropewalk, Nottingham NG1 5DT.
0602 799091

**CARE Trust (Christian Action Research and
Education)** 212, 218
21A Down Street, London W1Y 7DN.
071 233 0455

Carita House   179
Stapeley, Nantwich, Cheshire CW5 7LJ.
0270 627722

Carnivorous Plants   288
Marston Exotics, Lawnsdown Nursery,
Brampton Lane, Madeley, Hereford HR2 9LX.
0981 251140

Catholic Marriage Advisory Council (CMAC)
212, 218
23 Kensington Sq, London W8 5HN.
071 937 3781

CB Citizens' Band Magazine   203, 258, 286
Argus House, Boundary Way, Hemel
Hempstead HP2 7ST. 0442 66551

Ceka Works Ltd   287
Caernarvon Rd, Pwllheli, Gwynedd
LL53 5LH. 0758 701070

Center Parcs   275
P O Box 200, Nottingham NG1 6JY.
071 200 0088

Centre for Accessible Environments   118
35 Great Smith St, London SW1P 3BY.
071 222 7980

Centre for Independent Living   118
Mark Walsh, 31 Churchfield, Headley,
Bordon, Hants GU35 8PF.

Centre for the Study of Complementary
Medicine   71
51 Bedford Place, Southampton, Hampshire
SO1 2DG. 0703 334752

Centromed Leg Lifter   164
Stafford Close, Fairwood Industrial Park,
Ashford, Kent TN23 2TT. 0233 628018

Charities Aid Foundation   134
48 Pembury Road, Tonbridge, Kent TN9 2JD.
0732 771333

Chester-Care: see Homecraft Supplies

Children's Society   218
Edward Rudolf House, Margery St, London
WC1X 0JL. 071 837 4299

Chiltern Seeds   287
Bortree Stile, Ulverston, Cumbria LA12 7PB.

Citizens' Advice Bureaux (Headquarters)   118,
112, 138, 218, 271
115/123 Pentonville Rd, London N1 9LZ.
071 833 2181

Citizens' Band: see CB Citizens' Band Magazine

City and Guilds of London Institute   245,
269, 270
76 Portland Place, London W1N 4AA.
071 278 2468

Civil Aviation Authority (CAA)   185
071 379 7311

Clarke & Smith Ltd   281
Melbourne House, Melbourne Rd,
Wallington, Surrey SM6 8SD. 081 669 4411

Clayton Socks   155
17 Oakleigh Ave, Clayton, Bradford
BD14 8QE.

Clifford James   155, 179
High St, Ripley, Woking, Surrey GU23 6AF.
0483 211381

Clothkits   179
P O Box 2500, Lewes, Sussex BN7 3ZB.
081 679 6200

CNAA   249
344 Grays Inn Rd, London WC1X 8BP.
071 278 4411

COIC (Careers and Occupational Information
Centre)   244
Moorfoot, Sheffield S1 4PQ. 0742 594563/4/9

College of Health   117, 119, 56, 98, 116
St Margaret's House, Old Ford Rd, London E2
9PL. 081 983 1225.

Community Health Councils   119
Association of Community Health Councils for
England and Wales, 30 Drayton Park, London
N5 1PB. 071 609 8405

Community Service Volunteers (CSV)   118
237 Pentonville Rd, London N1 9NG.
071 278 6601

Competitors' Companion   291
14 Willow St, London EC2A 4BH.
071 638 4937

Competitors' Journal   291
411 Upper Richmond Rd, London SW15.
081 876 8432

Confederation of Healing Organisations   74
113 Hampstead Way, London NW11 7JN.
081 455 2638

Consumers' Association   119, 270
2 Marylebone Rd, London NW1 4DF.
071 486 5544

Coopers   144
Wormley, Godalming, Surrey GU8 5SY.
0428 682251

Cordless Door Entryphones   162
Eureka House, 7 Highwold, Coulsdon, Surrey,
CR5 3LG. 0737 554824

Cosmetics To Go   178
29 High St, Poole, Dorset BH15 1AB.
Freephone 0800 373366

Cotswold Woollens Ltd   179
2 Queens Circus, Cheltenham, Glos
GL50 1RX. 0242 226262

Cotton On   155
29 North Clifton St, Lytham FY8 5HW.
0253 736611

Council for the Accreditation of Correspondence
Colleges (CACC)   249
27 Marylebone Road,
London NW1 5JS. 071 935 5391

Council for Acupuncture   72
10 Panther House, 38 Mount Pleasant, London
WC1X 0AN. 071 837 8026

Council for National Academic Awards: see CNAA

Country Garden   178, 288
53 Dale St, Manchester M1 2HH.
061 228 7471

Countrywide Publications   278
8 Bretton Green Village, Rightwell, Bretton,
Peterborough PE3 8DY. 0733 334433

Couture Haberdashery   283
19 Park Avenue, Bush Hill Park, Enfield,
Middlesex EN1 1HJ.

Cox, Moore & Co Ltd   156
Milner Road, Long Eaton, Nottingham
NG10 1LD

Crabtree Electrical Industries Ltd   162
    Lincoln Works, Walsall, WS1 2DN.
    0922 721202
CRAC/Hobsons Press   245
    Hobsons Publishing plc, Bateman St,
    Cambridge CB2 1LZ. 0223 354551
Craft Book Club: see Readers Union
Craftkit   284
    Freepost, Bewdley, Worcs DY12 2BR.
    0299 404702
Creative Beadcraft Ltd   284
    Denmark Works, Sheepcote Dell Rd,
    Beamond End, Nr Amersham, Bucks
    HP7 0RX. 0494 715606.
Crossroads Care Attendant Schemes Ltd   216, 271
    10 Regent Place, Rugby, Warwickshire CV21
    2PN. 0788 73653.
Culpeper Ltd   178
    Hadstock Road, Linton, Cambridge CB1 6NJ.
    0223 894054
Curry Club   178, 292
    P O Box 7, Haslemere, Surrey GU27 1EP.
    0428 645256

Daisywheel   282
    98 Bell Rd, Wallasey, Merseyside L44 8DP.
    051 630 2457
Damart   154, 179
    Bingley X, West Yorkshire BD97 1AD
Dateline   203
    23 Abingdon Rd, London W8 6AL.
    071 938 1011
DIAL UK   120, 112, 138
    Park Lodge, St Catherines Hospital, Tickhill
    Rd, Balby, Doncaster DN4 8QN.
    0302 310123
Jill Dick   282
    Oldacre, Horderns Park Rd, Chapel en le
    Frith, Derbyshire SK12 6SY.
Direct Wool Group   283
    P O Box 46, Wheatley Works, Ilkley, West
    Yorkshire LS29 8PY. 0943 609896
Disability Alliance   120, 127, 138
    Universal House, 88 - 94 Wentworth St,
    London E1 7SA. 071 247 8776
Disability Arts Magazine (DAM)   280
    10 Woad Lane, Great Coates, Grimsby,
    DN37 9NH. 0472 280031
Disability Information Trust   142, 147, 161, 287
    Nuffield Orthopaedic Centre, Headington,
    Oxford OX3 7LD. 0865 227591
Disability Now   114
    12 Park Crescent, London W1E 3HU.
    071 636 5020
Disabled Advisory Service (DAS)   270
    219 Clapham Rd, London SW9 9BE.
    071 737 6823
Disabled Drivers' Association   185, 187, 275
    Ashwellthorpe, Norwich NR16 1EX.
    050 841 449
Disabled Drivers' Motor Club Ltd   185, 187, 275
    Cottingham Way, Bridge Street, Thrapston,
    Northants NN14 4PL. 08012 4724

Disabled Graduates' Careers Information Service (DGCIS)   260
    Room B10 Bulmershe Court, University of
    Reading, Woodlands Avenue, Reading
    RG6 1MY. 0734 318659
Disabled Living Foundation   121, 144, 278
    380/384 Harrow Road, London W9 2HU.
    071 289 6111
Disabled Photographers' Society   285
    P O Box 130, Richmond, Surrey TW10 6XQ.
Disablement Income Group   121
    Millmead Business Centre, Millmead Rd,
    London N17 9QU. 081 801 8013
Disablement Services Authority   260
    Ground Floor, Government Buildings,
    Bromyard Ave, London W3 7BA. 081 740 1235
Dogs for the Disabled   101
    Edmondscote Manor, Warwick New Rd,
    Leamington Spa, Warwicks CV32 6AH.
    0926 889102
Dragonfly Press   282
    2 Charlton Cottages, Barden Rd, Speldhurst,
    Tunbridge Wells, Kent TN3 0LH.
Driver and Vehicle Licensing Agency (DVLA)   139, 186, 189
    7 Long View Rd, Swansea SA6 7JL.
    0792 782341, or 42091 or 72134
DSS: see Social Security, Dept of
Duke of Edinburgh's Award Scheme   291
    5 Prince of Wales Terrace, Kensington,
    London W8 5PG. 071 937 5205

Early Learning   236
    South Marston Industrial Estate, Swindon
    SN3 4TJ. 0793 831300
Ease-E-Load Trolleys Ltd   168
    Crown Works, Baltimore Rd, Birmingham
    B42 1DP. 021 356 7411/2/3
Easiaids   162
    51A St Anne's Ave, Middlewich, Cheshire.
    060684 4641
Easy-on Designs (Celia Hart)   153
    59 Butlers Grove, Great Linford, Milton
    Keynes, Bucks MK14 5DT. 0908 605573
Ebury Press   172
    Random Century House, 20 Vauxhall Bridge
    Rd, London SW1V 2SA. 071 973 9680
Education for Northern Ireland, Dept of   245
    Rathgael House, Balloo Road, Bangor, Co
    Down BT19 2PR. 0247 466311
Education and Science, Dept of (DES)   245
    Room 2/11, Elizabeth House, York Rd, London
    SE1 7PH. 071 934 9000
Educational Centres Association   246
    Chequer Centre, Chequer St, London
    EC1V 8PL. 071 251 4158
Educational Grants and Advisory Service   135
    c/o Family Welfare Association (FWA), 501
    Kingsland Rd, London E8 4AU.
Educational Guidance Service for Adults   241
    Mrs E Kelly, Room 208, Bryson House, 28
    Bedford St, Belfast BT2 7FE. 0232 244274
Efamol Ltd   178
    Woodbridge Meadows, Guildford, Surrey
    GU1 1BA. 0483 578060

Electricity Association   134, 162
  30 Millbank, London SW1P 4RD.
  071 834 2333

Electronic Equipment Loan Service for Disabled
People   146-147, 291
  Willowbrook, Swanbourne Rd, Mursley,
  Milton Keynes, Bucks MK17 0JA.
  029672 533

EMAS (Employment Medical Advisory Service)
260
  Health and Safety Executive, The Triad,
  Stanley Rd, Bootle L20 3PG. 051 922 7211

Employment Service Head Office   256, 258-260
  Rockingham House, 123 West St, Sheffield
  S1 4ER. 0742 596330/739190

Energy Management and Information Unit   134
  Scottish Life House, 2/10 Archbold Terrace,
  Newcastle-upon-Tyne NE1 1BZ.
  091 281 1303

English Tourist Board   274, 277
  Thames Tower, Black's Rd, London W6 9EL.

Enterprise Agencies Head Office   270
  071 253 3716

Equal Opportunities Commission   268
  Overseas House, Quay St, Manchester
  M3 3HN. 061 833 9244

Equipment for Disabled People: see Disability
Information Trust

Eurospan Group   220, 225
  3 Henrietta St, Covent Garden, London
  WC2E 8LU. 071 240 0856

Exley Publications Ltd   160
  16 Chalk Hill, Watford WD1 4BN. 0923 50505

Factory Shop Guides   178
  G Cutress, 34 Park Hill, London SW4 9PB.

Falcon by Post   283
  Freepost, Westfield Rd, Horbury, Wakefield,
  West Yorkshire WF5 9BR

Families Need Fathers   218
  BM Families, London WC1N 3XX.
  081 886 0970

Family Fund: see Joseph Rowntree Foundation

Family Planning Association   121, 114, 224-225
  27 - 35 Mortimer St, London W1N 7RJ.
  071 636 7866

Family Planning Sales Ltd   224-225
  28 Kelburne Rd, Cowley, Oxford OX4 3SZ.

Family Tree Magazine   283
  15/16 Highlode Industrial Estate, Stocking
  Fen Rd, Ramsey, Huntingdon, Cambs
  PE17 1RB. 0487 814050

Federation of Family History Societies   283
  c/o Benson Room, Birmingham and Midland
  Institute, Margaret St, Birmingham B3 3BS.

M J Fish & Co Ltd   139, 140
  3 Rivers Way Business Village, Navigation
  Way, Ashton-on-Ribble, Preston PR2 2YP.
  0772 724442

Flying Scholarships for Disabled People   291
  International Air Tattoo, Building 1108, Royal
  Air Force, Fairford, Glos Gl7 4DL.

Foam for Comfort Ltd   178
  401 Otley Old Rd, Cookridge, Leeds
  LS16 7DF. 0532 673770

Fox's Spices Ltd   178
  59 Aston Cantlow Rd, Wilmcote, Stratford-
  upon-Avon CV37 9XN. 0789 266420

Fred Aldous Ltd   284
  P O Box 135, 37 Lever St, Manchester
  M60 1UX. 061 2362477

Freemans plc   179
  139 Clapham Rd, London SW99 0HR.

Frog Frolics   236
  123 Ifield Road, London SW10 9AR.
  071 370 4358/6384

Furniture Recycling Network   146
  c/o SOFA, Pilot House, 41 King's St, Leicester
  LE1 6RN. 0533 545283

Gardena Ltd   287
  0462 686688

Gardeners' Royal Benevolent Society   178
  Bridge House, 139 Kingston Rd, Leatherhead,
  Surrey KT22 7NT.

Gardens for the Disabled Trust   288
  Hayes Farmhouse, Hayes Lane, Peasmarsh,
  East Sussex TN1 6XR. 0424 882345

Gemma   218
  BM Box 5700, London WC1N 3XX.

Gingerbread   218
  35 Wellington Street, London WC2E 7BN.
  071 240 0953

GLAD (Greater London Association for Disabled
People)   276
  336 Brixton Rd, London SW9 7AA.
  071 274 0107

Good Book Guide   281
  91 Great Russell St, London WC1B 3PS.
  071 580 8466

Good Housekeeping Institute   172
  National Magazine House, 72 Broadwick St,
  London W1. 071 439 5000

Griffin Tools   287
  Level St, Brierley Hill, West Midlands,
  DY5 1UA. 0384 77789

John Groom's Association for the Disabled   276
  10 Gloucester Drive, London N4 2LP.
  081 802 7272.

Guild of Disabled Homeworkers   270
  Enterprise Aid Centre, Stag House,
  Woodchester GL5 5EZ. 045383 5623

Handicapped Anglers' Trust   290
  c/o L D Warren, 29 Ironlatch Ave, St Leonards-
  on-Sea, East Sussex TN38 9JE. 0424 427931

Hardy Plant Society Correspondents' Group   286,
288
  c/o Mrs Jane Lucas, 37 Horndean Avenue,
  Wigston Fields, Leicester LE8 1DP.
  0533 881249

Hatchards   115
  187 Piccadilly, London W1V 9DA.
  071 437 3924

Hawkshead Countrywear   179
  Main St, Hawkshead Village, Cumbria
  LA22 0NT. 05394 34000 (Dept 918)

Hawton Ltd   290
  155 Lincoln Avenue, Twickenham Middlesex
  TW2 6NJ. 081 755 1496

Health, Dept of (DoH)   113, 120
  Richmond House, 79 Whitehall, London SW1.
  071 210 3000
  Health Publications Unit   142
  No 2 Site, Heyward Stores, Manchester Rd,
  Heywood OL10 2PZ
Health Education Authority   69
  Hamilton House, Mabledon Place, London
  WC1H 9TX. 071 383 3833
Health Information Network   121
  Algarve House, 1A The Colonnade, High St,
  Maidenhead, Berks SL6 1QL. 0628 778744
Health Information Service   121
  Level 4, Lister Hospital, Coreys Mill Lane,
  Stevenage SG1 4AB. 0438 315414
Health and Safety Executive   260
  Baynards House, 1 Chepstow Place, London
  W2 4TE. 071 221 0870
Healthaction Ltd   155
  P O Box 18, Romsey, Hants SO51 9ZX.
  0794 884556
Healthline (College of Health)   112
  081 983 1133
Healthwise   114, 121, 206, 217
  27 Mortimer St, London W1N 7RU.
  071 636 7866
Help for Health   121
  Wessex Regional Library Unit, Southampton
  General Hospital, Southampton S09 4XY.
  0703 779091
Helping Hand Company (Ledbury) Ltd   161
  Unit 9L, Bromyard Rd Trading Estate,
  Ledbury HR3 1LL. 0531 5678
Herons Bonsai Ltd   288
  Wiremill Lane, Newchapel, near Lingfield,
  Surrey RH7 6HJ. 0342 832657
Highfield Nurseries   287
  Whitminster, Glos GL2 7PL. 0452 740266
HMSO   37
  P O Box 276, London SW8. 071 873 0011
HMV Shop   178
  150 Oxford St, London W1N 0DJ.
  071 631 3423
Hobby Horse Ltd   284
  11 Blue Boar St, Oxford OX1 4EZ.
  0865 247292.
Holiday Care Service   277, 279
  2 Old Bank Chambers, Station Rd, Horley,
  Surrey RH6 9HW. 0293 774535. (Holiday
  helpers: 0293 775137)
Home Improvement Agencies: see Care and
  Repair
Home and Schools Council   236
  81 Rustlings Rd, Sheffield S11 7AB
Home Office   122
  Public Relations Branch, Room 101, 50
  Queen Anne's Gate, London SW1H 9AT.
Home Start Consultancy   143, 235
  2 Salisbury Rd, Leicester LE1 7QR.
  0533 554988
Homecraft Supplies Ltd/Chester-Care   114,
170, 162, 182
  Sidings Rd, Low Moor Estate, Kirkby-in-
  Ashfield, Notts NG17 7JZ. 0623 757955
Homeopathy: see British Homeopathic Assn

Horder Centre   290
  St John's Rd, Crowborough, East Sussex
  TN6 1XP. 0892 665577
Horticultural Therapy Society   288
  Goulds Ground, Vallis Way, Frome, Somerset
  BA11 3DW. 0373 64782
House of Commons   122
  London SW1A 0AA. 071 219 3000 (Public
  Information Office: 071 219 4272)
Housing Debtline   134
  021 359 8501/2/3
HSL High Seat Ltd   163
  Victoria Rd, Dewsbury, WF13 2AB.
  0924 464809
Hugh Steeper Ltd   154
  237/239 Roehampton Lane. London
  SW15 4LB, 081 788 8165

IFL Pen Friend Service   286
  Saltash, Cornwall
IFL Pen Friend Service (UK)   286
  P O Box 117, Leicester LE3 6EE.
In Court Associates   286
  (Ken Nicholls), 26 Laurel Park, St Arvans,
  Chepstow, Gwent NP6 6ED. 02912 71184
Independent Living Fund   132
  PO Box 183, Nottingham, NG8 3RD.
  0602 290423/290427
Index Ltd (Head Office)   178
  100/110 Old Hall St, Liverpool L70 1AB.
Innovations International Ltd   164
  NSP House, 211 Lower Richmond Rd,
  Richmond, Surrey TW9 4LN. 081 878 9111
Inspiration   282
  Unit 7, 7 Haydock St, St Helens, Merseyside
  WA10 1DD. 0744 55543
Institute for Complementary Medicine   72
  21 Portland Place, London W1N 3AF.
  071 636 9543
Institute of Family Therapy   218
  43 New Cavendish St, London W1M 7RG.
  071 935 1651
Institute of Scientific and Technical
Communicators   269
  52 Odencroft Rd, Britwell, Slough, Berkshire
  SL2 2BZ. 0753 691562
Insurance Ombudsman Bureau   139
  31 Southampton Row, London WC1B 5HJ.
  071 242 8613
ISIS Audio Book Tape Library   281
  55 St Thomas' St, Oxford OX1 1JG.
  0865 250333

Jake Mail Order   179
  176 Kennington Park Rd, London SE11 4BT.
  071 735 7577/0665/8296
Janet Coles Beads Ltd   284
  Perdiswell Cottage, Bilford Road, Worcester
  WR3 8QA. 0905 54024
Jewish Marriage Council   218
  23 Ravenhurst Avenue, London NW4 4EL.
  081 203 6311
Jigroll   178
  Freepost, Barton, Cambridge CB3 7BR.
  0223 262592

Microwave Association 166
  8 High St, Hurstpierpoint, West Sussex
  BN6 9TZ. 0273 834 716
Midas Mail Order Ltd 284
  6J Wells Promenade, Ilkley, West Yorkshire
  LS29 9LG
Mills and Boon 282
  Eton House, 18 - 24 Paradise Rd, Richmond,
  Surrey TW9 1SR. 081 948 0444
MIND 89, 111, 218
  22 Harley St, London W1N 2ED.
  071 637 0741
MIS (Mobility Information Service) 186, 187
  Unit 2a, Atcham Estate, Upton Magnor,
  Shrewsbury SY4 4UG. 0743 761889
Monsoon Mail Order 179
  Hammersmith Industrial Est, 74 Winslow Rd,
  London W6 9SF. 081 746 3273
Motability 189
  Gate House, The High, Harlow, Essex
  CM20 1HR. 0279 635666
Mothercare-by-post 236
  0923 210210 or 31616
Mountway Ltd 150
  Dan-y-Bont Mill, Gilwern, Abergavenny,
  Gwent NP7 0DD. 0873 831678
Muriel Braddick Foundation 281
  (Tapes for the Handicapped Association), 14
  Teign Street, Teignmouth, Devon. 0626 6214
Mycoal 155
  Unit 1, Imperial Park, Empress Rd,
  Southampton SO2 0JW. 0703 211068
Myra Coles Shopping List 283
  Tempest Court, Broughton, Skipton, North
  Yorkshire BD23 3AE.

NAIDEX Conventions Ltd 144
  Convex House, 43 Dudley Rd, Tunbridge
  Wells, Kent, TN1 1LE. 0892 544027
Nairn Hydrotherapy Trust 290
  0667 55351
National Ankylosing Spondylitis Society (NASS)
18, 55, 140, 255, 258
  5 Grosvenor Crescent, London SW1X 7EE.
  071 235 9585
National Assn of Carers 217
  29 Chilworth Mews, London W2 3RG.
  071 724 7776
National Assn for the Childless 227
  318 Summer Lane, Birmingham B19 3RL.
  021 3594887
**National Assn of Councils for Voluntary
Service** 272
  P O Box 717, Sheffield S1 1NL. 0742 786636
National Assn of Volunteer Bureaux 272
  St Peter's College, College Rd, Saltley,
  Birmingham B8 3TE. 021 327 0265
National Assn of Women's Clubs 292
  5 Vernon Rise, London WC1X 9EP.
  071 837 1434
National Back Pain Assn (NBPA) 18
  31 - 33 Park Rd, Teddington, Middlesex
  TW11 0AB. 081 977 5474

**National Breakdown's Disabled Drivers'
Scheme** 139
  0532 393939
National Childbirth Trust (NCT) 234, 227, 292
  Alexandra House, Oldham Terrace. London
  W3 6NH. 081 992 8637
National Council for One Parent Families
218, 236
  255 Kentish Town Rd, London NW5 2LX.
  071 267 1361
National Council of Women of Great Britain 292
  36 Danbury St, London N1 8JU. 071 354 2395
National Extension College Trust Ltd 245, 248,
249, 251
  18 Brooklands Ave, Cambridge CB2 2HN.
  0223 316644
National Family Conciliation Council 218
  Shaftesbury Centre, Percy St, Swindon,
  Wiltshire SN2 2AZ. 0793 514055
National Federation of Shopmobility 175
  (Secretary: Liz Reid), 26 Stanley Drive,
  Leicester. 0533 526604
National Federation of Solo Clubs 292
  Room 8, 191 Corporation St, Birmingham
  B4 6RY. 021 236 2879
**National Federation of Spiritual Healers
(NFSH)** 75
  Old Manor Farm Studio, Church St, Sunbury-
  on-Thames, Middlesex TW16 6RG.
  0932 783164
National Federation of Women's Institutes
247, 292
  104 New King's Rd, London SW6 4LY.
  071 371 9300
National Homeworking Unit 270
  3rd Floor, Wolverley House, 18 Digbeth,
  Birmingham. 021 643 6352
**National Institute of Adult Continuing Education
(NIACE)** 247, 280
  19b De Montfort St, Leicester LE1 7GE.
  0533 551451
National Institute of Medical Herbalists 75
  9 Palace Gate, Exeter EX1 1JA. 0392 426022
National Key Scheme: see RADAR   174
National Listening Library 281
  Freepost, 12 Lant St, London SE1 1QH.
  071 407 9417
National Osteoporosis Society 22
  PO Box 10, Radstock, Bath BA3 3YB.
  0761 432472
National Retreat Centre 275
  Liddon House, 24 South Audley St, London
  W1Y 5DL. 071 493 3534
National Trust 146, 178, 276, 286-287
  36 Queen Anne's Gate, London SW1H 9AS.
  071 222 9251
National Union of Students (NUS) 251
  461 Holloway Rd, London N7 6LZ.
  071 272 8900
National Union of Townswomen's Guilds 292
  Chamber of Commerce House, 75 Harborne
  Rd, Edgbaston, Birmingham B15 3DA.
  021 456 3435

National Women's Register 292
9 Bank Plain, Norwich, Norfolk NR2 4SL.
0603 765392

Natural Fibres 155
2 Springfield Lane, Smeeton Westerby,
Leicester LE8 0QW. 053379 2280

Natural History Museum Collection 178
Harrington Dock, Liverpool X, L70 1AX.
051 708 7545

Nature Company 178
Harrington Dock, Liverpool X L70 1AX.
051 708 8202

Nature's Best Health Products 178
Freepost, P O Box 1, Tunbridge Wells
TN2 3EQ. 0892 34143

Neal's Yard DeskTop Publishing Studio 282
14 Neal's Yard, London WC2H 9DP.
071 379 4739

Neatwork 184
The Lee Stables, Coldstream, Berwickshire
TD12 4NN. 0890 3456

Needlecraft Kits 283
P O Box 24, Newtown Abbot, Devon,
TQ12 4UG.

Network for the Handicapped 122, 138
16 Princeton St, London WC1R 4BB.
071 831 8031/7740

New Ways to Work 268
309 Upper St, London N1 2TU. 071 226 4026

Next Directory 179
0345 100500

Nexus 292
Nexus House, 65 High St, Bideford, North
Devon EX39 2AN. 0237 471704/421619

Nightingales Ltd 179
Meadowcroft Mill, off Bury Rd, Rochdale,
Lancs OL11 4AU. 0706 620919

Norland Gazelle Travel Goods Ltd 274
Wallingford Rd, Uxbridge, Middlesex
UB8 2SX. 0895 52555

Nottingham Rehab Ltd 144, 154, 170
17 Ludlow Hill Rd, Melton Rd, West
Bridgford, Nottingham, NG2 6HD.
0602 452000

Observer Helpline 250
Middlesex Polytechnic, Bramley Rd,
Oakwood, London N14 4XS. 081 368 1299

OBUT Boule (UK) 290
Hillside House, Wood Norton, Evesham,
Worcs, WR11 4TE. 0386 860234

Office of Fair Trading 134, 176, 189
Field House, Bream's Buildings, London
EC4A 1PR. 071 242 2858

Open College 248
Freepost TK1006, Brentford, Middlesex
TW8 8BR. 081 847 7788

Open College of the Arts 248
Hound Hill, Worsborough, Barnsley S70 6TU.
0226 730495

Open University 246, 247-248, 251
Walton Hall, Milton Keynes MK7 6AA.
0908 274066. (Adviser on the Education of
Students with Disabilities: 0908 653442)

**Opportunities for People with Disabilities (Head
Office)** 260
1 Princes St, London EC2P 2AH. 071 726 4963

OPUS: see Parentline

Outset (Employment Development Unit) 269
Drake House, 18 Creekside, London SE8 3DZ.
081 692 7141

OwnBase 270
57 Glebe Rd, Egham, Surrey TW20 8BU.

OXFAM Trading 177
Murdock Rd, Bicester, Oxon OX6 7RF.
0869 245011

Pandora Publishing: see Thorsons 236

Panilet Tables 171
Unit 17 Dragon Court, Crofts End Rd, St
George's, Bristol BS5 7XX. 0272 511858

**Parent to Parent Information on Adoption Services
(PPIAS)** 230
Lower Boddington, near Daventry, Northants,
NN11 6YB. 0327 60295

Parentline 234
Rayfa House, 57 Hart Rd, Thundersley, Essex
SS7 3PD. 0268 757077

Parents Anonymous 234
6 Manor Gardens, London N7 6LA.
071 263 8918

Parents with Disabilities 234
c/o Mrs Jo O'Farrell, 6 Forest Rd, Crowthorne,
Berkshire RG11 7EH. 0344 773366

Parents' magazine 235
44 Victory House, Leicester Place, London
WC2H 7BP. 071 437 9011

Park House 276
Sandringham, Kings Lynn, Norfolk PE35 6EH.
0485 43000

Past Times 178
Wootton Business Park, Abingdon, OX13 6LG,
0865 326111

PAT Dogs Scheme, PRO Dogs 101
Rocky Bank, 4 New Rd, Ditton, Maidstone,
Kent ME20 6AD. 0732 848499

Patients' Association 37, 122, 138
18 Victoria Park Square, Bethnal Green,
London E2 9PF. 081 981 5676

Pauline Hephaistos Survey Projects 276
39 Bradley Gdns, West Ealing, London
W13 8HE.

**PCAS (Polytechnics Central Admissions
System** 249
Fulton House, Jessop Ave, Cheltenham
GL50 3SH. 0242 227788

Penny Plain Ltd 179
10 Marlborough Crescent, Newcastle on Tyne
NE1 4EE. 091 232 1124

PHAB 122, 292
12 - 14 London Rd, Croydon, Surrey CR0 2TA.
081 667 9443

Phillips of Axminster 182
Phillips House, West Street, Axminster

Piatkus (Publishers) 270
5 Windmill St, London W1P 1HF. 071 631 0710

Pooh Corner Book Club 236
High St, Hartfield, East Sussex TN7 4AC.
0892 770453

Portia Trust (Future Friends)   205
Workspace, Maryport, Cumbria CA15 8N
Postal Scrabble Club   286
10 Church Lane, Wormley, Herts, EN10 6JT
Practical Parenting   235
IPC Magazines Ltd, Kings Reach Tower,
Stamford St, London SE1 9LS. 071 261 5058
Pre-School Playgroups Association   234
314 Vauxhall Bridge Rd, London SW1V 1AA.
071 828 2417
Prince's Youth Business Trust   270
5 The Pavement, London SW4 0HY.
071 498 3939
Professional Educational Training Aids Ltd   230
127 High St, Hampton Hill, Middlesex
TW12 1NF. 081 941 4456,
Psoriasis Association   22, 193
7 Milton St, Northampton NN2 7JG.
0604 711129

RAC Response: see Royal Automobile Club
RADAR (Royal Assn for Disability and Rehab-
ilitation)   123, 113, 140, 162, 259, 278, 279
25 Mortimer Street, London W1N 8AB.
071 637 5400
RAD-AR Risk Centre (CPM)   49
Dorna House, West End, Woking, Surrey
GU24 9PW.
Raymer Ltd   182
P O Box 16, Henley on Thames, Oxon
RG9 1LL. 0491 578446
Raynaud's and Scleroderma Association   23,
26, 27, 155, 164, 256
112 Crewe Rd, Alsager, Cheshire, ST7 2JA.
0270 872776
Readers' Union Ltd   280
P O Box 6, Brunel House, Newton Abbot,
Devon TQ12 2DW. 0626 69881
Readicut Wool Co Ltd   280, 283
Terry Mills, Ossett, West Yorkshire WF5 9SA.
0924 278027
Red House   236
Cotswold Business Park, Witney, Oxford
OX8 5YF. 0993 771144/774171
Redvale Nurseries   288
St Tudy, Bodmin, Cornwall PL30 3PX.
0208 850378
Rehabilitation Engineering Unit   152
Chailey Heritage, North Chailey, Lewes, East
Sussex BN8 4EF. 082 572 2112
Relate   217, 98, 114, 206, 209, 212, 271
Herbert Gray College, Little Church Street,
Rugby, Warwicks CV21 3AP. 0788 573241
Relax Housewares Ltd   171
Vale Mill, John St, Rochdale OL16 1HR.
0706 353535
Relaxation for Living   107
29 Burwood Park Road, Walton-on-Thames,
Surrey KT12 5LH. 0932 227826
Remploy   253
415 Edgware Rd, London NW2 6LR.
081 452 8020
Richer   179
Royal Mills, Station Road, Steeton, Keighley,
West Yks BD20 6RA

Riding for the Disabled Association   290
Avenue R, National Agricultural Centre,
Kenilworth, Warks CV8 2LY. 0203 696510
Robert Norfolk plc   179
67 Gatwick Rd, Crwaley, West Sussex
RH10 2RD. 0293 553381
Rodda (A E) & Son   178
Scorrier, Redruth, Cornwall TR16 5BU.
0209 820526
Roger Jefcoate: see Electronic Equipment Loan
Service
Rosalie Courage   179
Kit Lane House, Ellisfield, near Basingstoke,
Hampshire. 0255683 386
Rowe, L   286
26 St Andrews Terrace, Roker, Sunderland,
Tyne and Wear SR6 0PB.
Royal Automobile Club (RAC)   139, 186
P O Box 700, Spectrum, Bond St, Bristol
BS99 1RB. 0800 400432
Royal Disability Association   121, 123
Royal National Institute for the Blind   242
224 Great Portland Street, London W14 4XX.
071 388 1266
Royal School of Needlework   284
Mail Order Dept, Little Barrington, Burford,
Oxon OX8 4TE. 0451 4433
Royal Society for the Protection of Birds
(RSPB)   286
The Lodge, Sandy, Beds. 0767 08551
RSA Examinations Board (Publications)   245
Westwood Way, Coventry CN4 8HS.
0203 470033

Safari   286
c/o A Ashby, 33 Mervyn Rd, Ealing, London
W13 9UW.
Samaritans (Central London)   110, *123*, 271
071 734 2800. Also in your local phone book.
Save the Children Fund   177
Trading Department, P O Box 40, Burton-on-
Trent DE14 3LQ. 0326 562511
Scottish Council for Single Parents   218
13 Gayfield Square, Edinburgh EH1 3NX.
031 556 3899
Scottish Education Department   245
Gyleview House, 3 Redheughs Rigg, South
Gyle, Edinburgh EH12 9HH.
Scottish Institute of Adult and Continuing
Education   246
30 Rutland Square, Edinburgh EH1 2BW.
031 229 0331
SCOTVEC (Scottish Vocational Education
Council)   245
Hanover House, 24 Douglas St, Glasgow
G2 7NG. 041 248 7900
Search Press Ltd   280, 281, 284
Wellwood, North Farm Rd, Tunbridge Wells,
Kent TN2 3DR. 0892 510850
Selectus Ltd   154
The Uplands, Biddulph, Stoke-on-Trent
ST8 7RH. 0782 513316
Selfridge Selection   179
Admail 70, Oxford St, London W1E 3YZ.
Freephone 0800 101 101

SHAPE 280
  1 Thorpe Close, London W10 5XL.
  081 960 9245
Sheldon Press 206
  SPCK, Holy Trinity Church, Marylebone
  Road, London NW1 4DU. 071 387 5282
Shopmobility: see National Federation of
  Shopmobility
Skill (National Bureau for Students with
Disabilities) 241, 249
  336 Brixton Rd, London SW9 7AA.
  081 274 0565, 081 737 7166
Small Firms Service 270
  Freephone 0800 222 999
Small Press Group 282
  BM Bozo, London WC1N 3XX. 0234 211606
Snowdon Awards Scheme 251
  c/o Action Research, Vincent House, North
  Parade, Horsham, West Sussex RH12 2DA.
  0403 210406
Snuggler: see Innovations International Ltd
Social Change, Directory of 251
  Radius Works, Back Lane, London NW3 1HL.
  071 435 8171
Social Security Benefits Agency: see Social
Security, Dept of
Social Security, Dept of (DSS) 112, 120, 127
  Freeline 0800 666555. Benefits Enquiry Line:
  0800 882200.
  DSS Leaflets Unit 127
  P O Box 21, Stanmore, Middlesex HA7 1AY
  DSS Mobility Component Unit 187
  102 Norcross, Blackpool FY5 3TA.
  0253 856 123
Society of Indexers 269
  c/o Mrs H C Troughton, 16 Green Rd,
  Birchington, Kent CT7 9JZ. 0843 41115
Solicitors' Family Law Association 218
  P O Box 302, Keston, Kent BR2 6EZ.
  0689 850227
Solo Clubs (National Federation of) 292
  7/8 Ruskin Chambers, 101 Corporation St,
  Birmingham B4 6R4. 021 236 2879
Sparklers Shirts 179
  Eythorne House, Eythorne, near Dover, Kent
  CT15 4BE. 0304 830424
Spencers Trousers 154
  Friendly Works, Sowerby Bridge HX6 2TN.
  0422 833020
SPOD 123, 220, 224-225
  286 Camden Road, London N7 0BJ.
  071 607 8851/2
Sports Council 289
  16 Upper Woburn Place, London WC1H 0QH.
  071 388 1277
St Catherine's House 283
  General Register Office (England and
  Wales), 10 Kingsway, London WC2B 6JP
  General Register Office (Scotland), New
  Register House, West Register St, Edinburgh
  EH1 3YT.
St John's Wools 283, 284
  Parkside Rd, West Bowling, Bradford
  BD5 8DZ. 0274 729031

St Saviour's Nurseries 178
  P O Box 266, Guernsey, Channel Islands.
  O481 65521
Stackpole Trust Support Group 274
  19 Elrington Rd, London E8 3BJ
Stannah Lifts Ltd 162
  Watt Close, East Portway, Andover,
  Hampshire, SP10 3SD. 0264 332244
Stockingfillas Ltd 236
  Tennant House, London Rd, Macclesfield,
  Cheshire SK11 0LW. 0625 511511
Student Loans Company 251
  100 Bothwell St, Glasgow G27 JD
Studio Cards 166, 177
  Birley Bank, Preston PR1 4AE
Suffolk Herbs 287
  Sawyers Farm, Lt. Cornard, Sudbury, Suffolk,
  CO10 0NY. 0787 227247
Suffolk Ornithologists' Group 286
  c/o M Bowling, Sunnyhill, 6 Hardwick Lane,
  Bury St Edmunds, Suffolk
Surgical Advisory Service 63
  108 Whitfield St, London W1P 6BE.
  071 388 1839

Taking a Break 217
  Newcastle upon Tyne X, NE85 2AQ.
Talking Newspaper Association 271
  90 High St, Heathfield, East Sussex TN21 8JD.
  0435 866102
Tamar Neckwear Ltd 155
  21 Tudor Grove, London E9 7QL.
  081 985 4771
Tapes for the Handicapped Association: see
  Muriel Braddick Foundation
Task Force on Concerns of Physically Disabled
Women: see Eurospan
Technical Equipment for Disabled People 146
  John Wright, National Organiser, 'Hazeldene',
  Ightham, Sevenoaks, Kent TN15 9AD.
  0732 883818
Thorsons Publishers Ltd 206
  Denington Estate, Wellingborough, Northants
  NN8 2RQ. 0933 440033
Thousand and One Lamps Ltd 149
  4 Barmeston Rd, London SE6 2UX.
  081 698 7238
Together 179
  Rainbow Home Shopping Ltd, The Galleries,
  Preston, Lancs PR1 4WN. 0772 202707
Thrasher, G A and I P 288
  Honiton, Devon EX14 8SX. 0404 42617
Three Jay & Co 154
  0992 442974
Trading by Post Ltd 179
  Freepost, Waverley Mills, Langholm,
  Dumfriesshire DG13 0BR. 03873 80092
Traidcraft plc 177
  Kingsway, Gateshead, Tyne and Wear
  NE11 0NE. 091 491 0591
Transport, Dept of, (Door-to-Door Guide) 278
  Freepost, Victoria Rd, South Ruislip, Middlesex
  HA4 0NZ. 081 841 3425

INDEX

Notes

1   *Appendix 2* lists organisations and businesses mentioned in the book, together with their addresses and relevant page references. These are not duplicated in this index.

2   Individual rheumatic disorders, eg ankylosing spondylitis, rheumatoid arthritis: only selected page numbers appear here, since these disorders form the subject matter of the whole book. The entries for 'arthritis', 'rheumatic disorders', 'doctors', 'disability', are similarly intentionally selective.

3   Alphabetical arrangement is word-by-word. Prepositions have been ignored in determining order.